MRI of Musculoskeletal Masses: A Practical Text and Atlas

MRI of Musculoskeletal Masses: A Practical Text and Atlas

Alan Laorr, M.D.
Musculoskeletal Radiologist
Suburban Radiologic Consultants
Minneapolis, Minnesota

Clyde A. Helms, M.D.
Professor of Radiology
Duke University Medical Center
Durham, North Carolina

IGAKU-SHOIN NEW YORK • TOKYO

Published and distributed by

IGAKU-SHOIN Medical Publishers, Inc.
One Madison Avenue, New York, New York 10010

IGAKU-SHOIN Ltd.,
5–24–3 Hongo, Bunkyo-ku, Tokyo 113–91

Library of Congress Cataloging-in-Publication Data

Laorr, Alan.
MRI of musculoskeletal masses : a practical text and atlas / Alan Laorr, Clyde A. Helms.
p. cm.
Includes bibliographical references and index.
1. Musculoskeletal system—Tumors—Magnetic resonance imaging. 2. Musculoskeletal system—Cysts—Magnetic resonance imaging. 3. Musculoskeletal system—Tumors—Magnetic resonance imaging—Atlases. 4. Muculoskeletal system—Cysts—Magnetic resonance imaging—Atlases. I. Helms, Clyde A. II. Title.
[DNLM: 1. Bone and Bones—radiography. 2. Bones and Bones—radiography—atlases. 3. Magnetic Resonance Imaging—methods. 4. Magnetic Resonance Imaging—methods—atlases. WE 141L298m 1996]
RC280.M83L35 1996
616.99'2707548—dc20
DNLM/DLC
for Library of Congress 96-24302
CIP

ISBN: 0-89640-320-3 (New York)
ISBN: 4-260-14320-4 (Tokyo)

Printed and bound in the U.S.A.
10 9 8 7 6 5 4 3 2 1

PREFACE

This text/atlas discusses and illustrates a variety of musculoskeletal masses and their appearance with MR imaging. In many cases, the MRI features are characteristic. The entities included are equally divided between tumors and lesions which can present clinically or on MR exams as masses. In this regard, the book is intended to fill a void among the many excellent currently available texts on musculoskeletal MRI and bone tumors. It is not meant to be a complete textbook, and many rare lesions have purposely been excluded. We have tried to limit the topics to those lesions which might fall within the realm of a busy private practice or outpatient academic setting. Many of the masses are commonly or fairly commonly encountered in a high-volume practice. Some uncommon lesions have also been included, usually as a result of unique or interesting MRI features or due to recent emphasis in the literature. A concise and uniform format was chosen in order to facilitate use as a quick reference or as an easily readable text. Each entity is described with respect to its definition, clinical features, location, implications, MRI appearance, and differential diagnosis. References for additional reading are also provided for each topic. We hope that this book will be useful to both the novice and experienced musculoskeletal MR reader, as well as to clinicians involved in the diagnosis and treatment of musculoskeletal disorders.

Alan Laorr, M.D.
Clyde A. Helms, M.D.

Acknowledgments

I would like to express my appreciation and indebtedness to Harry K. Genant, M.D. and my former colleagues at the University of California, San Francisco. Many thanks are owed to James O. Johnston, M.D. for his contributions as well as his tumor conferences, which were a joy to attend. I would also like to acknowledge my current associates within Suburban Radiologic Consultants, Ltd., with whom it is a privilege to work. Finally, this book could not have been completed without the understanding and support of my wife Jill, who also directly contributed by transcribing the entire text and providing extensive editorial assistance.

AL

To Jill, my wife and best friend
and
To Anna and Eric, who make our lives complete

AL

FOREWORD

Only a decade ago the diagnostic tools available to a physician concerned with a musculoskeletal mass were, typically, a history, a careful physical examination, and a radiograph, followed by surgical exploration, and then a tissue diagnosis by a pathologist. With the recent development of magnetic resonance (MR) imaging technology, it is now possible to visualize the anatomy of a bone or soft tissue mass with such clarity that invasive biopsy is, in a great many cases, no longer necessary. Often, solely on the basis of MR imaging, a definitive diagnosis of a mass can be made and, if malignant, the surgeon can plan an effective limb sparing procedure.

The authors of this text offer lucid discussion of musculoskeletal conditions both from a clinical and an MR radiological perspective. Of particular value is the differential diagnostic approach, providing the clinician with guidance for the diagnostic work-up of a wide array of neoplastic and pseudo-tumorous conditions. This practical and comprehensive book deserves a place on the shelf of all those concerned with the differential diagnosis of musculoskeletal masses, including the diagnostic radiologist, orthopaedic surgeon, pathologist, rheumatologist, and general physician.

James O. Johnston, M.D.
Professor of Clinical Orthopaedics
and Clinical Radiology
University of California, San Francisco

Contents

SECTION I

SOFT TISSUE

1 Fat-Containing Tumors

Lipoma

Definition. Lipomas are composed of lobular collections of adipose tissue. They contain multiple fibrous septa and are surrounded by a thin fibrous capsule.

Clinical Features. Lipomas are among the most common and widely distributed soft tissue tumors. Most commonly, lipomas occur in the extremities of adult women, presenting as slow growing, asymptomatic, soft, mobile subcutaneous masses. They are uncommon in children and may rarely be congenital or familial.

Location. Lipomas may arise from fatty tissue in any part of the body. They are most often subcutaneous and only infrequently found in the deeper soft tissues. When deep, they are categorized as intermuscular, intramuscular, parosteal, or intraosseous.

Implications. Lipomas are benign lesions which are cured with surgical excision. Incomplete excision is likely to result in recurrence.

MRI Findings. Lipomas typically appear as masses with smooth, lobulated margins and internal septations. They demonstrate signal intensity which parallels subcutaneous fat on all pulse sequences. These masses demonstrate homogeneous high signal intensity on T1-weighted sequences, becoming intermediate in intensity with T2-weighting.

Differential Diagnosis. If the above MR criteria are met, the diagnosis of lipoma can be made. The most critical differentiation to make is between a lipoma and liposarcoma. Unlike lipomas, liposarcomas have a wide range of signal intensity patterns because of their histologic composition and varying degrees of tumor necrosis and vascularity. Many liposarcomas have a long T1, which results in much lower signal intensity than normal fat on T1-weighted images; these lesions are easily distinguished from lipomas. However, a well-differentiated liposarcoma may be composed predominantly of lipomatous tissue. In general, a fatty mass with internal septations which demonstrates homogenous signal intensity that parallels subcutaneous fat on all pulse sequences can be presumed to represent a benign lipoma. Any inhomogeneity or other aberration from this pattern should raise the possibility of an atypical lipoma or well-differentiated liposarcoma. At the very least, such a lesion should be followed very closely clinically.

References

Madewell J, Sweet D. Tumors and tumor-like lesions in or about joints. In: *Resnick: Bone and Joint Imaging.* Philadelphia, PA, W.B. Saunders Company; 1989; p 1182.

Laorr A, Greenspan A. Hand lipomas: Detection and characterization by magnetic resonance imaging. *Can Assoc Radiol J* 44:14–18, 1993.

Murphy W, Hurst G, Duerk J, et al. Atypical appearance of lipomatous tumors on MR images: High signal intensity with fat-suppression STIR sequences. *JMRI* 1:477–480, 1991.

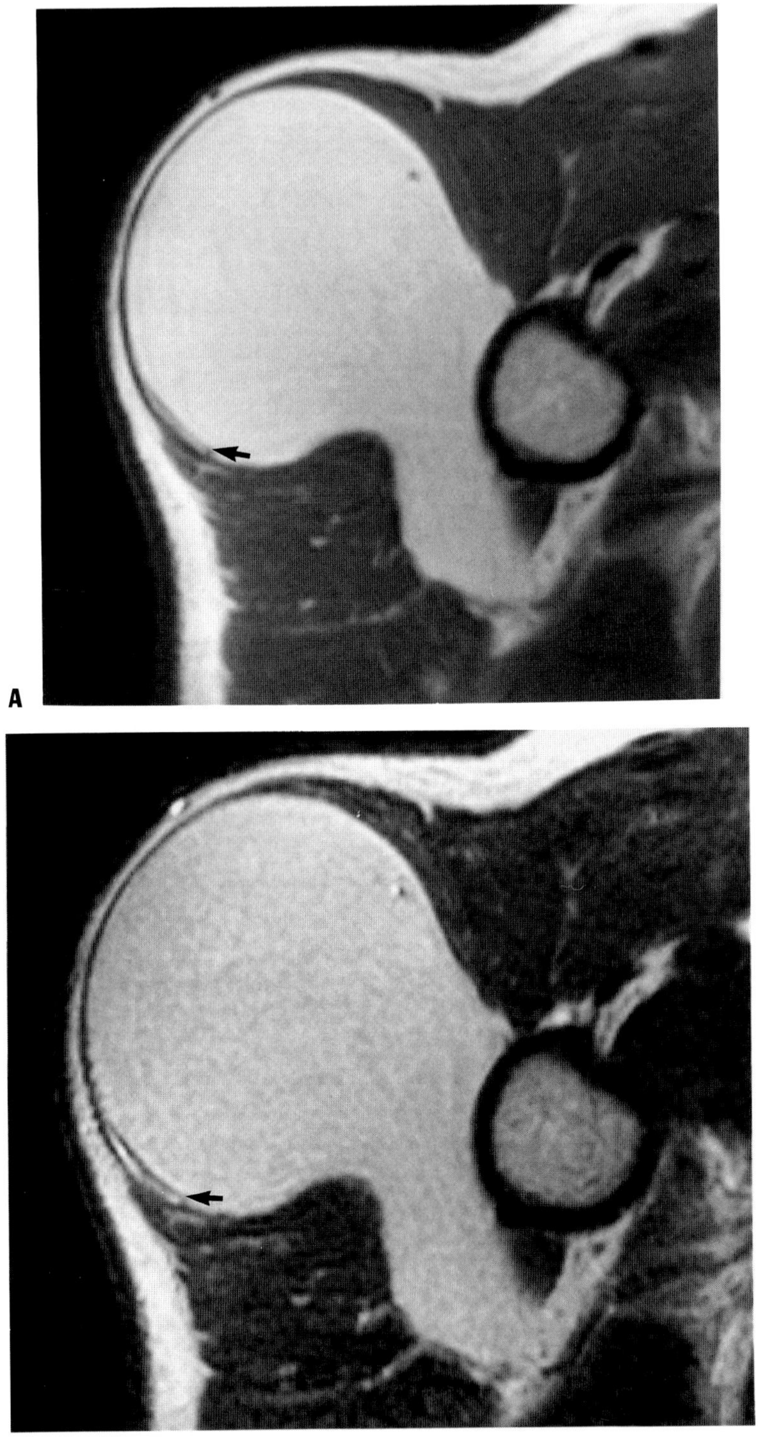

FIGURE 1.1 A 73-year-old male with a palpable right shoulder mass. MRI findings are diagnostic of a lipoma. Axial (A) T1-weighted (600/16) and (B) T2-weighted (2500/70) images reveal a lobulated mass with homogeneous signal intensity paralleling that of the adjacent subcutaneous fat. An internal septation is present (arrows) as well as a thin peripheral rim of low signal representing a fibrous capsule.

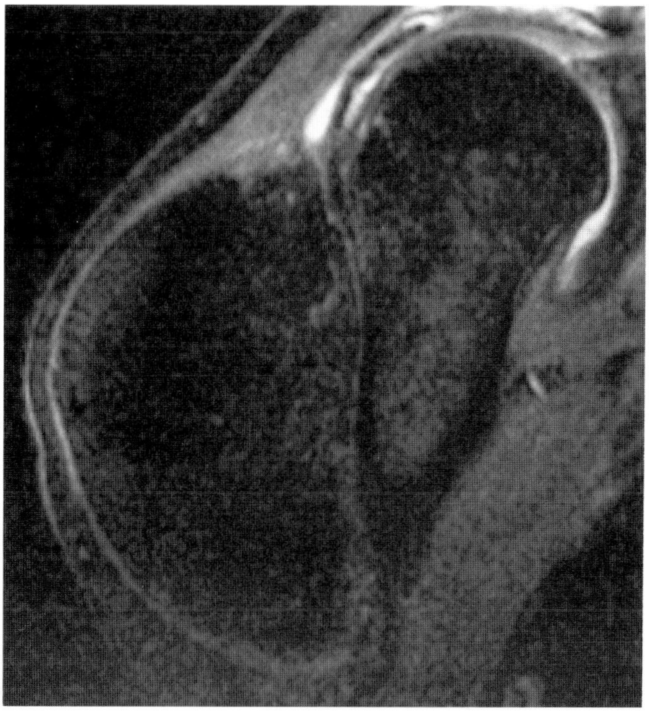
C

Figure 1.1 (continued) (C) Coronal FMPIR image (3000/28, TI-150) demonstrates uniform fat-suppression of the lipoma which remains isointense to the adjacent subcutaneous fat.

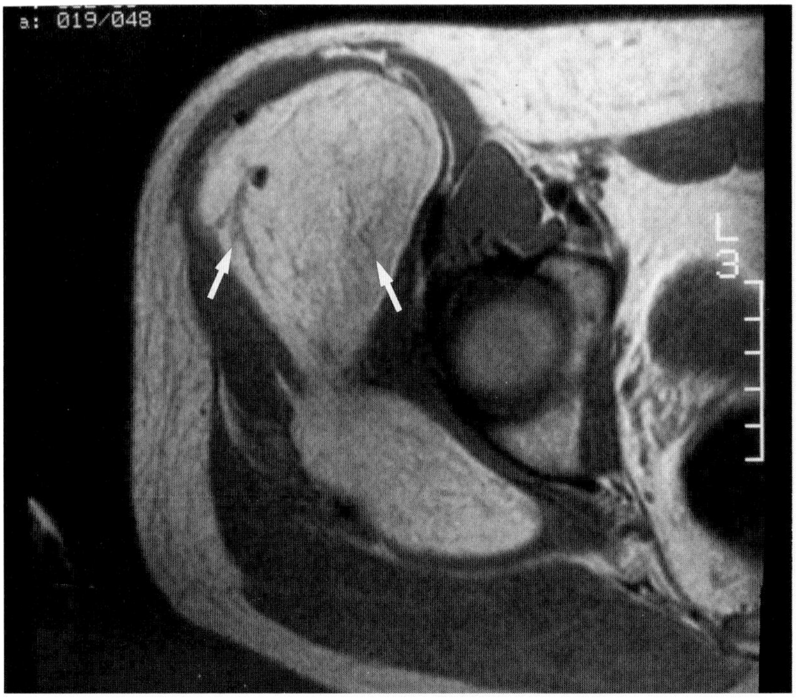

A

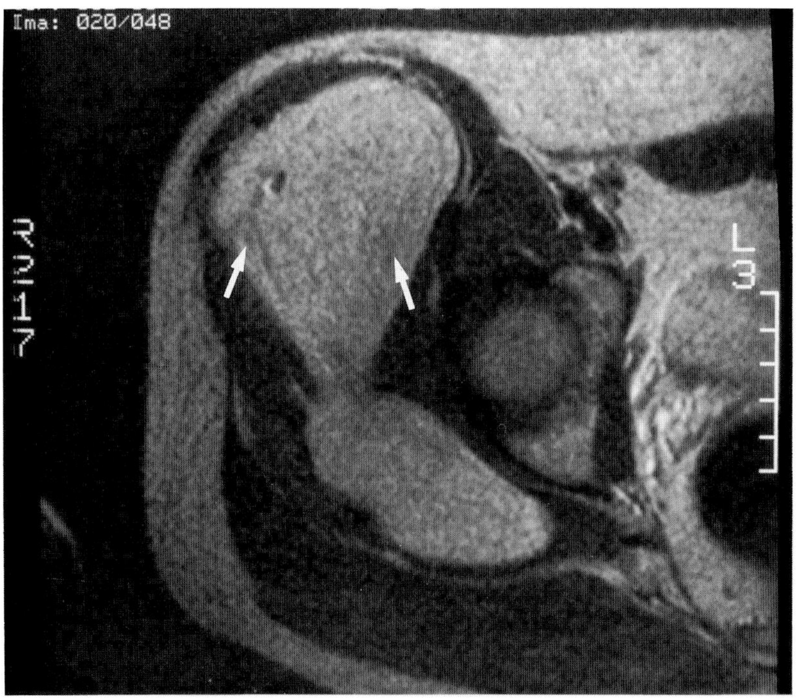

B

FIGURE 1.2 Large lipoma involving the musculature about the right hip. Axial (A) proton density (2000/20) and (B) T2-weighted (2000/60) images reveal a mass with signal which is isointense to that of the adjacent fat. Note the low signal internal fibrous septations (arrows).

Atypical Lipoma

Definition. Atypical lipomas are soft tissue tumors which differ from simple lipomas in that they are composed of mature adipose cells interspersed with areas containing a variable mixture of multinucleated giant cells, collagen bundles, and adipocytes with large, hyperchromic nuclei. Although these histopathologic features resemble those of liposarcoma, atypical lipomas exhibit benign clinical behavior. Atypical lipomas lie between simple lipomas and well-differentiated liposarcomas within the spectrum of lipomatous neoplasms. These lesions have also been termed spindle cell lipomas and pleomorphic lipomas.

Clinical Features. Adults are typically affected. These lesions usually present as large, nontender, slowly-growing masses. Subcutaneous lesions may be soft and mobile. Deep lesions may be difficult to evaluate clinically.

Location. Atypical lipomas may arise from fatty tissue in any part of the body. They may be subcutaneous or deep (intramuscular).

Implications. These lesions exhibit benign clinical behavior, but may recur locally following surgical excision. Unlike liposarcomas, these lesions are not associated with distant metastasis. Sarcomatous dedifferentiation has been described.

MRI Findings. Atypical lipomas contain a large amount of mature fatty tissue which appears isointense to subcutaneous fat on all pulse sequences. Within some fatty areas, a thin wispy strand-like network of nonlipomatous tissue is seen. This network demonstrates hypointense signal on all pulse sequences and most likely represents fibrocytic, collagenous areas of the tumor. Confluent nonlipomatous areas of high-signal intensity on T2-weighted sequences may be seen, which may represent pleomorphic adipose cells and giant cells.

Differential Diagnosis. These lesions can be distinguished from simple lipomas, which typically appear as homogenous masses, with the exception of internal septations. The signal within simple lipomas should parallel the signal of subcutaneous fat on all pulse sequences. Liposarcomas have a wide range of appearances on MRI based upon their fatty content. Most liposarcomas contain no identifiable fatty tissue on imaging studies. More well-differentiated liposarcomas contain fatty tissue which is readily seen on MRI. It is probably not possible to distinguish between atypical lipomas and more well-differentiated liposarcomas by MR imaging. Both atypical lipoma and well-differentiated liposarcoma should be included in the differential diagnosis of a lipomatous lesion that fails to meet the criteria for a simple lipoma.

Reference

Bush C, Spanier S, Gillespy T. Imaging of atypical lipomas of the extremities: Report of three cases. *Skeletal Radiol* 17:472–475, 1988.

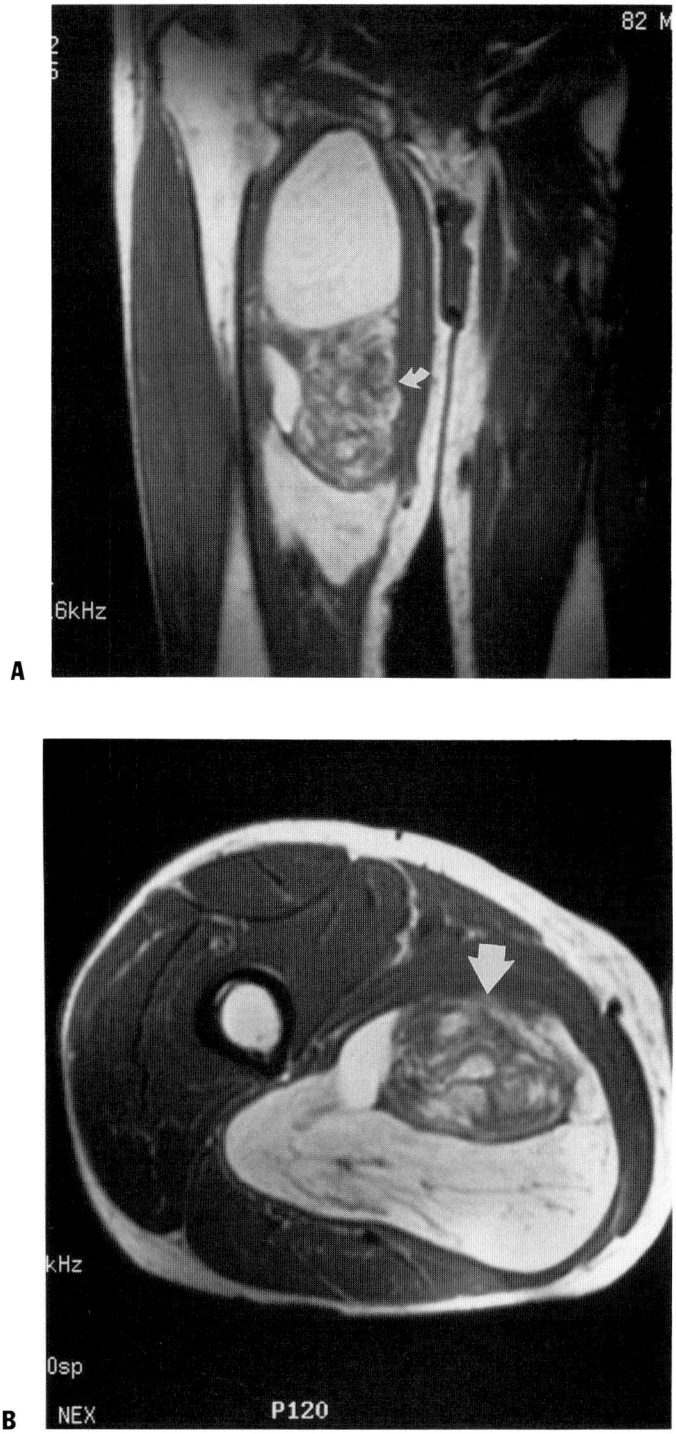

Figure 1.3 An 82-year-old male with a large right thigh mass. T1-weighted (A) coronal (666/10) and (B) axial (516/11) images reveal a fat-containing mass with a prominent area of heterogeneous signal intensity (arrows).

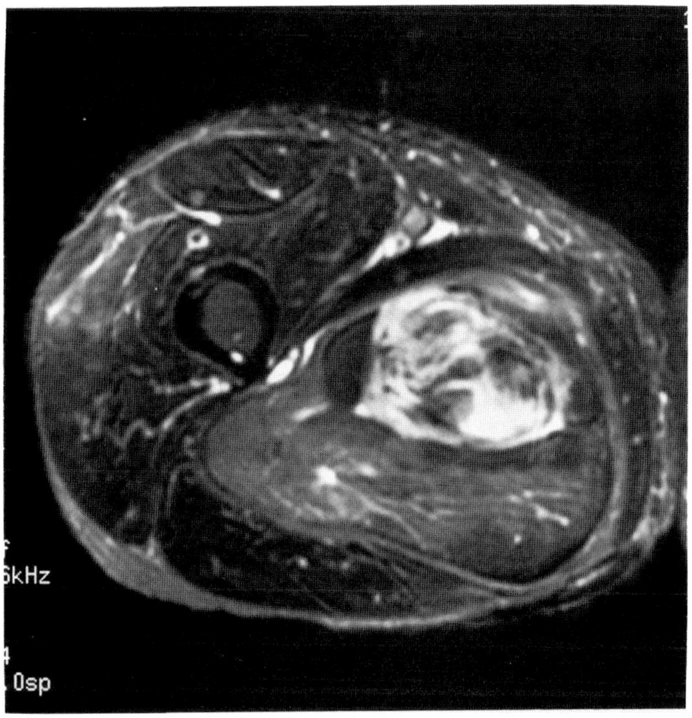

C

FIGURE 1.3 (continued) This area becomes very bright on a (C) FSE T2-weighted fat suppression sequence (3100/102). Based upon the MRI features, this lesion could represent an atypical lipoma or well-differentiated liposarcoma. The mass continues to be stable on periodic follow-up examination and has been given the presumptive clinical diagnosis of an atypical lipoma.

Parosteal Lipoma

Definition. Parosteal lipomas are lipomas which are contiguous with the underlying periosteum. They are otherwise similar to subcutaneous lipomas. The etiology is unknown. Occasionally, these lesions are associated with reactive changes in the adjacent bone including hyperostosis, osseous bowing, and cortical erosion.

Clinical Features. These lesions are rare, representing only 0.3% of all lipomas. Over half of affected patients are between the ages of 40 and 70 years old. Patients typically present with a nontender, immobile mass that has been present and slowly growing for an average of 8 to 10 years. Size is variable, however, the lesions are often large by the time of presentation. Due to the overlying musculature, the consistency of the mass is often difficult to evaluate clinically. Symptoms of nerve compression may be present.

Location. Parosteal lipomas arise almost exclusively as solitary lesions adjacent to the long bones of the upper and lower extremities, especially the proximal radius and femur. However, lesions have been reported at numerous locations throughout the appendicular and axial skeleton.

Implications. At surgery, these lesions are often firmly attached to the periosteum, especially when associated osseous changes are present. Occasionally, the lesion is loosely adherent or nonadherent to the underlying bone. These lesions are benign and there has not been a reported case of a parosteal liposarcoma. MRI has proven useful for surgical planning.

MRI Findings. MRI reveals a fatty mass that is intimately associated with the underlying bone. Characteristically, the mass has smooth, lobulated margins and contains internal septa. The mass demonstrates uniformly high signal intensity on T1-weighted images and intermediate signal intensity with T2-weighting. The signal intensity of the mass parallels subcutaneous fat on all pulse sequences. When reactive osseous changes are present, the newly formed bone must be contiguous with the underlying bone for the diagnosis to be confirmed. The amount of cortical hyperostosis may range from a small area of cortical thickening to exuberant bony excrescences. The associated hyperostosis demonstrates markedly hypointense signal on all pulse sequences, paralleling that of cortical bone.

Differential Diagnosis. The MRI findings are diagnostic. Although a well-differentiated parosteal liposarcoma is a theoretical differential diagnostic possibility, no such lesion has been reported.

References

Murphey M, Johnson D, Bhati P, et al. Parosteal lipoma: MR imaging characteristics. *AJR* 162:105–110, 1994.

Laorr A, Greenspan A. Parosteal lipoma with hyperostosis: Report of two pathologically proven cases evaluated by magnetic resonance imaging. *Can Assoc Radiol J* 44:285–290. 1993.

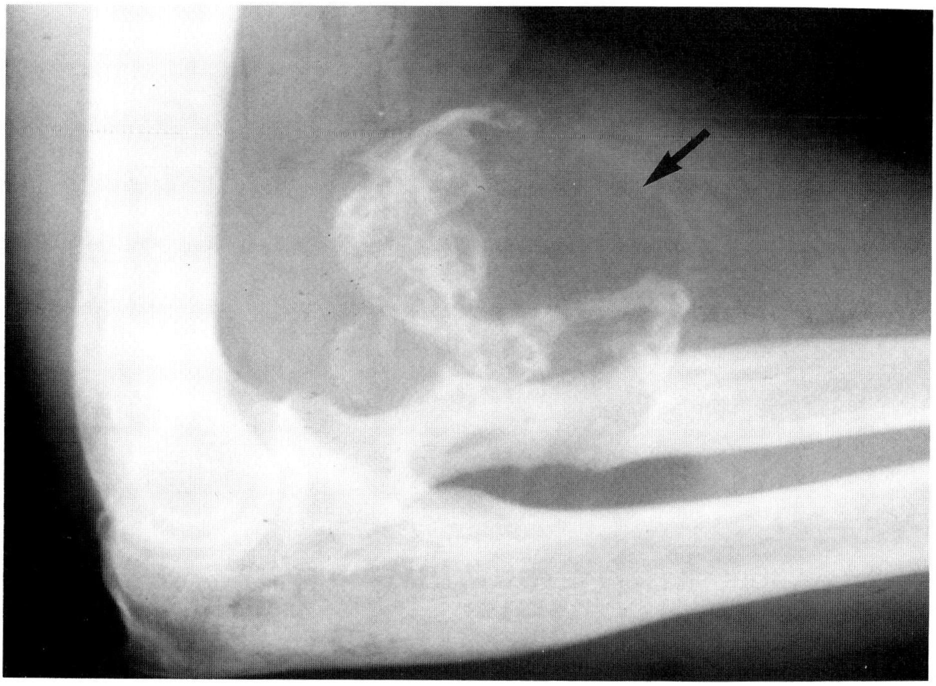

A

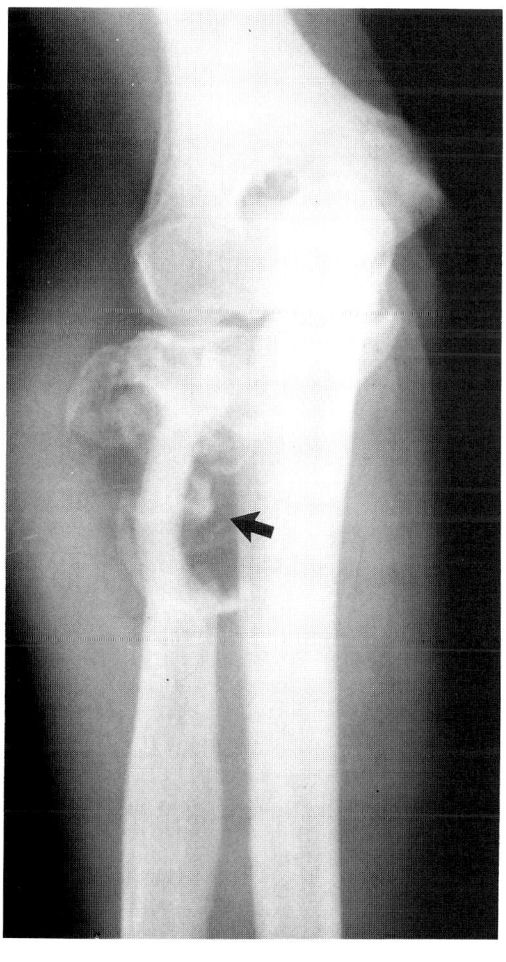

B

Figure 1.4 An 80-year-old man who presented with a slow-growing mass in the antecubital region. (A), (B) A low density soft tissue mass (arrows) is seen adjacent to the proximal radius with prominent associated osseous excrescences and cortical erosion.

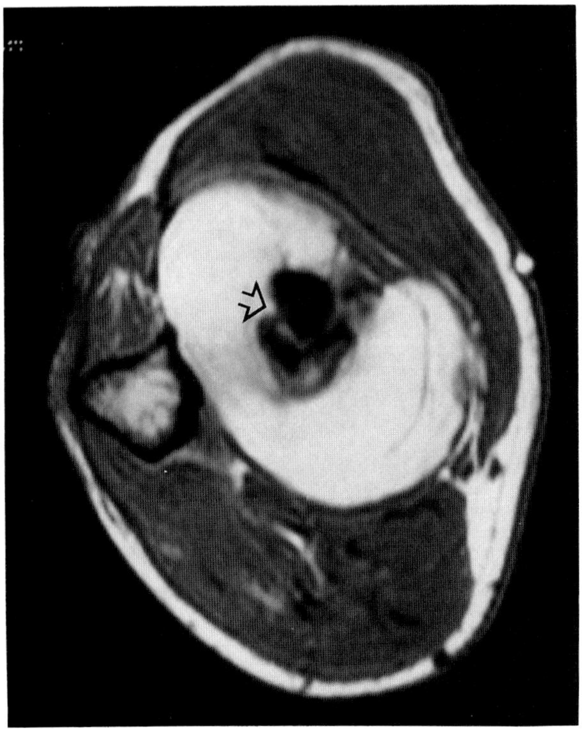

C

D

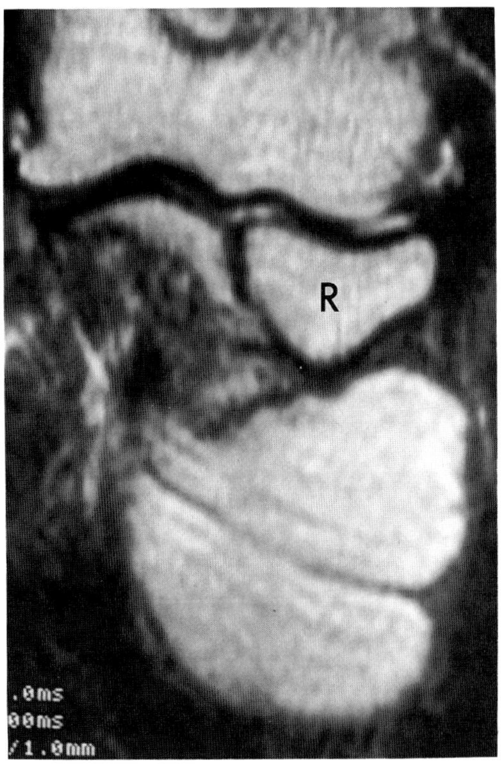

FIGURE 1.4 (continued) (C) Axial T1-weighted (817/20) and (D) coronal T2-weighted (2000/80) images reveal a fatty mass surrounding the proximal radius (R) consistent with a parosteal lipoma. Note the areas of signal void (open arrow) from the associated hyperostosis. (Reprinted from *CARJ* 1993;44:285–290, by permission of the publisher).

Liposarcoma

Definition. Liposarcomas are malignant mesenchymal neoplasms which have a variable fatty component. These lesions arise de novo, rather than from pre-existing lipomas. Histologically, they are categorized as well-differentiated, myxoid, round cell, and pleomorphic. The myxoid variety is most common, accounting for approximately half of all cases. Well-differentiated liposarcomas contain abundant fatty tissue. The remaining subtypes of liposarcoma may contain little or no fatty elements on imaging studies.

Clinical Features. Liposarcoma is the second most common malignant soft tissue neoplasm, behind only malignant fibrous histiocytoma. It is seen most frequently between the ages of 40 and 60 years, but all ages may be affected. This lesion is extremely rare in childhood. There is a slight male predominance. Typically, liposarcoma presents as a firm palpable mass. Symptoms depend on the size of the mass, location, and involvement of neurovascular structures.

Location. The most common musculoskeletal locations are the gluteal region and lower extremity, particularly around the quadriceps muscle and the popliteal fossa.

Implications. Distant metastasis may be present at the time of diagnosis. These lesions may recur following surgery. Well-differentiated liposarcomas are associated with an excellent prognosis. The round cell and pleomorphic subtypes have the poorest prognosis.

MRI Findings. Liposarcomas have a wide range of signal intensity patterns due to their histologic composition and varying degrees of tumor necrosis and vascularity. Well-differentiated liposarcomas contain a large amount of fat, which appears as hyperintense on T1-weighted images and of intermediate intensity on T2-weighted sequences. This signal parallels the adjacent subcutaneous fat on all pulse sequences. In addition to the fatty tissue, there are typically some areas of low signal intensity with T1-weighting, which become hyperintense with T2-weighting. The remaining subtypes of liposarcoma may contain little or no fat identifiable on MRI. These lesions appear hypointense on T1-weighted images and hyperintense with T2-weighting. Central necrosis (i.e., fluid) and hemorrhage may be seen. The lesion may contain calcification, which appears as hypointense foci on all pulse sequences. This hypointense signal may become more prominent on gradient echo images due to magnetic susceptibility.

Differential Diagnosis. Well-differentiated liposarcomas may resemble simple lipomas on MRI. A lipoma appears as an encapsulated mass with signal that parallels subcutaneous fat on all pulse sequences. The signal intensity is typically homogeneous, with the exception of thin internal fibrous septa. A well-differentiated liposarcoma is probably not distinguishable from an atypical lipoma on MRI. While the identification of fatty signal intensity suggests the diagnosis of liposarcoma or lipoma, fat has been reported in a variety of other soft tissue sarcomas as well. A soft tissue hemangioma may contain a large amount of fatty tissue, but is usually distinguishable based upon the identification of vascular channels. Most liposarcomas demonstrate nonspecific signal characteristics (low on T1-weighted images, high on T2-weighted images) and cannot be differentiated from other soft tissue sarcomas. Numerous benign soft tissue lesions may also have a similar appearance.

References

Kransdorf M, Jelinek J, Moser R, et al. Soft-tissue masses: Diagnosis using MR imaging. *AJR* 153:541–547, 1989.

Sundaram M, McGuire M, Herbold D. Magnetic resonance imaging of soft tissue masses: An evaluation of fifty-three histologically proven tumors. *Magn Reson Imaging* 6:237–248, 1988.

Resnick D. *Bone and Joint Imaging.* Philadelphia, PA: W.B. Saunders Company; 1989; pp 1188, 1263.

Bush C, Spanier S, Gillespy T. Imaging of atypical lipomas of the extremities: Report of three cases. *Skeletal Radiol* 17:472–475, 1988.

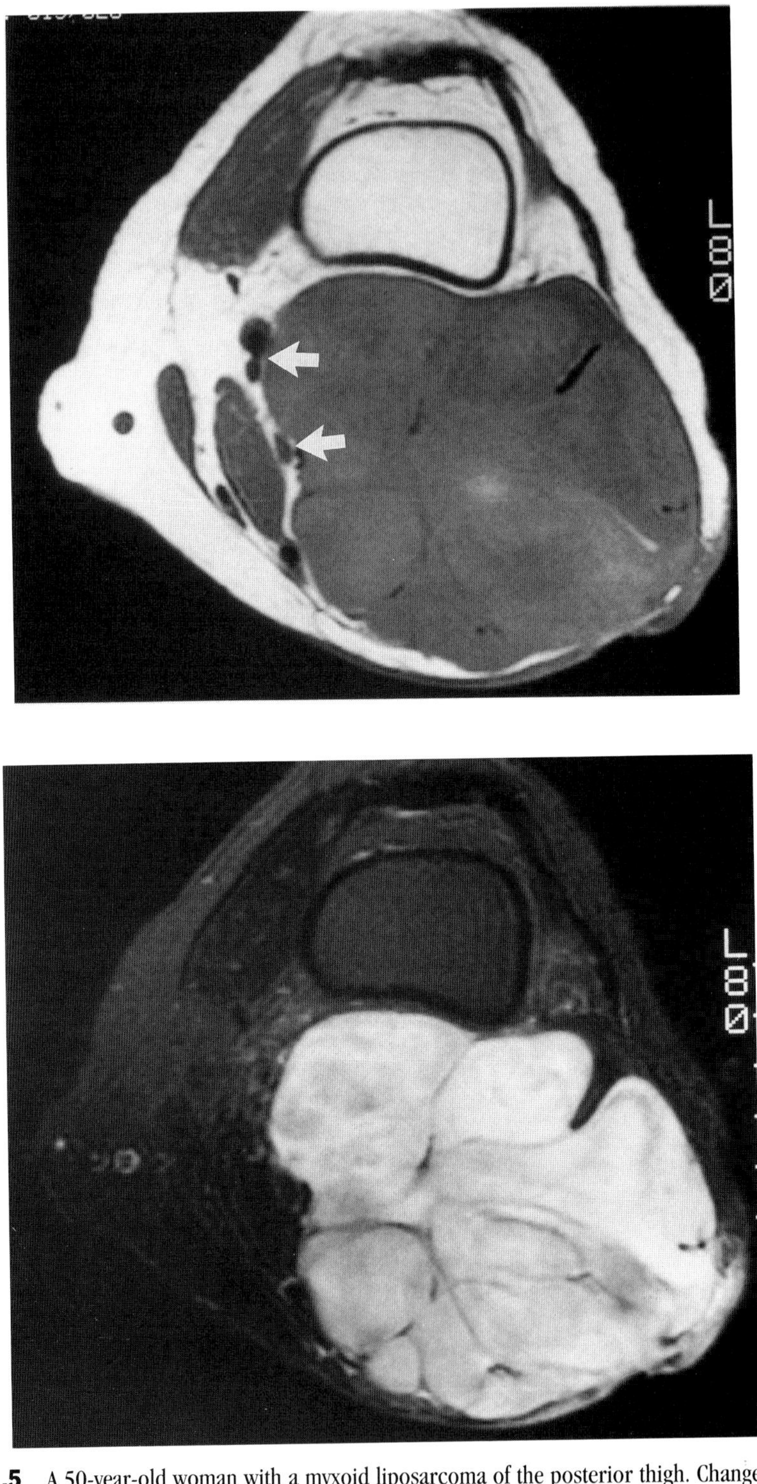

A

B

Figure 1.5 A 50-year-old woman with a myxoid liposarcoma of the posterior thigh. Changes in the adjacent subcutaneous tissue likely reflect recent biopsy. (A) Axial T1-weighted image (666/19) reveals an intermediate signal intensity mass causing medial displacement of the neurovascular structures (arrows). Note the absence of fatty signal intensity within the mass. (B) Axial FSE T2-weighted fat suppression image (3000/85) reveals heterogeneous hyperintense signal. The MR appearance of this mass is nonspecific.

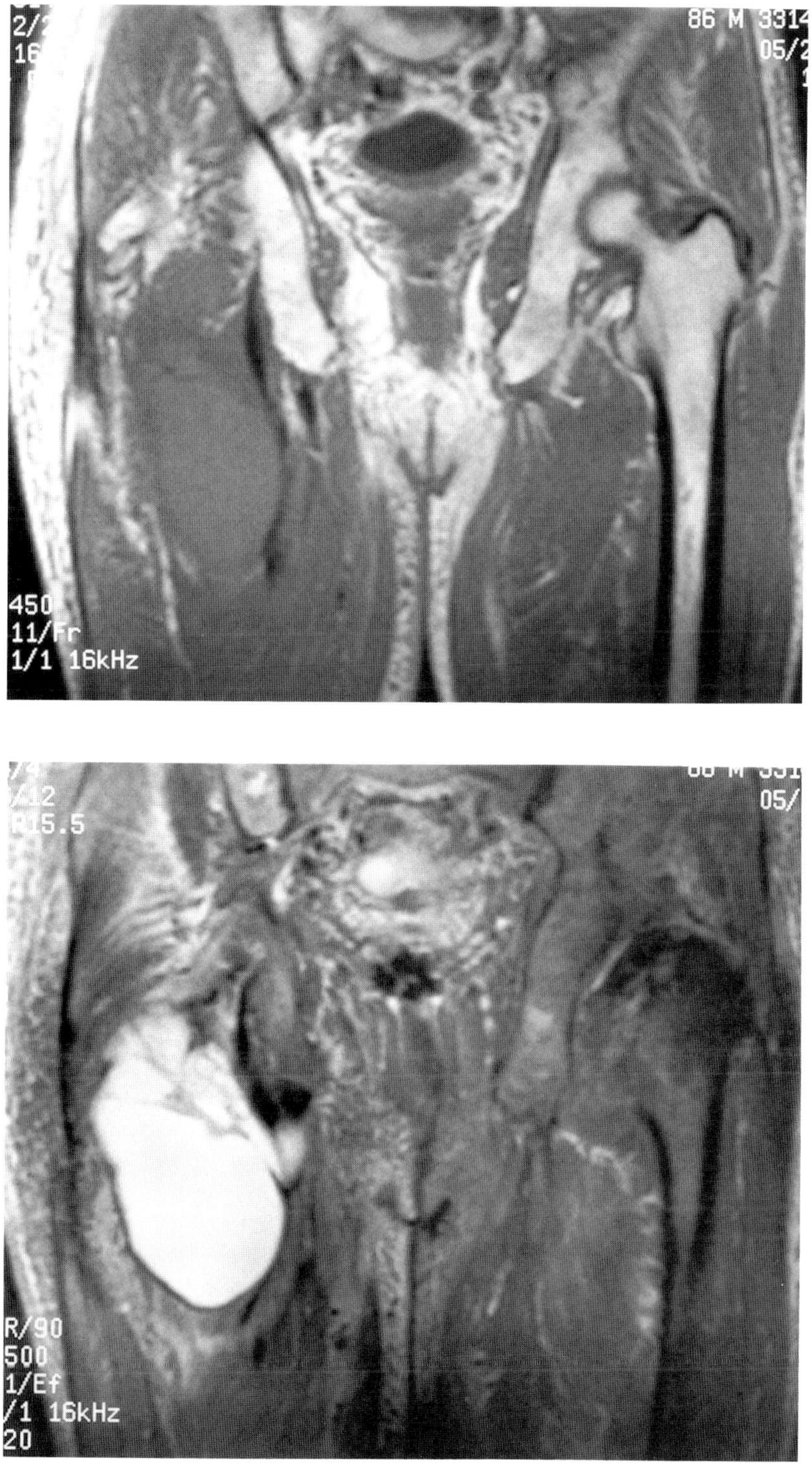

A

B

FIGURE 1.6 An 86-year-old male with a myxoid liposarcoma of the right gluteal region. Coronal (A) T1-weighted (450/11) and (B) FMPIR (3500/51, TI-120) images demonstrate a multilobulated mass of fairly uniform signal intensity. Note the absence of identifiable fatty tissue with T1-weighting and the marked hyperintensity on the FMPIR image. This appearance is common for myxoid liposarcoma, although the MR features are nonspecific and may be seen with numerous other entities.

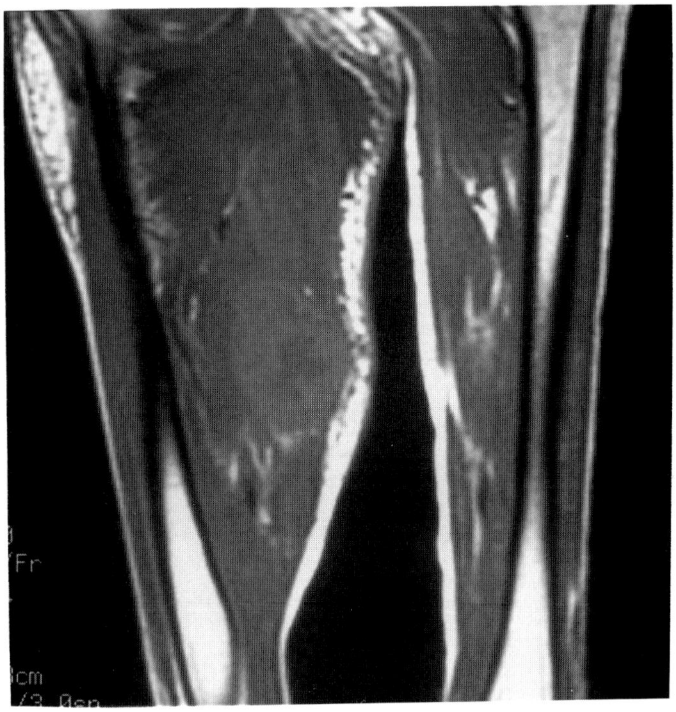

A

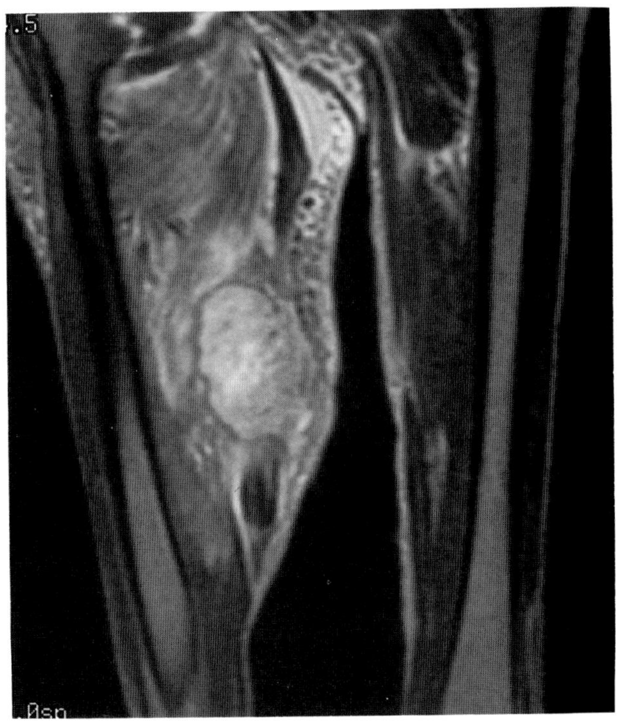

B

FIGURE 1.7 A 62-year-old male presented with a three-week history of right thigh pain, swelling, and tenderness. An abscess was suspected clinically. (A) Coronal T1-weighted (800/15) image demonstrates an intermediate signal intensity mass containing a central area of lower signal. Marked surrounding soft tissue swelling is present. (B) Coronal T2-weighted (2000/80) image reveals a hyperintense lesion with a central area of very bright signal corresponding to necrosis. The lesion is predominantly solid, making an abscess unlikely. Note the prominent increased signal within the adductor muscles consistent with edema. Microscopic extension of tumor throughout this area cannot be excluded. Pathologic examination revealed a high-grade liposarcoma.

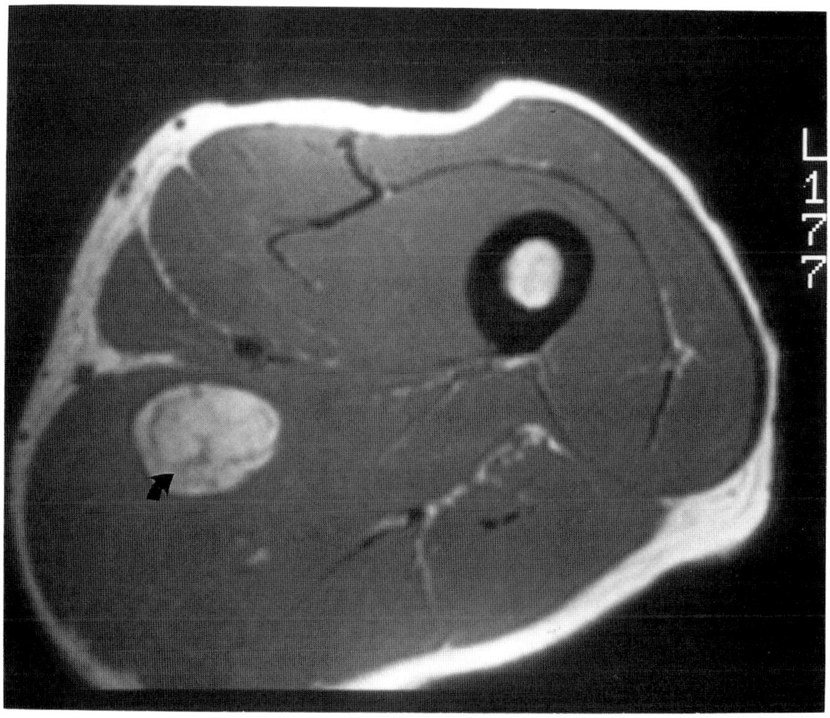

A

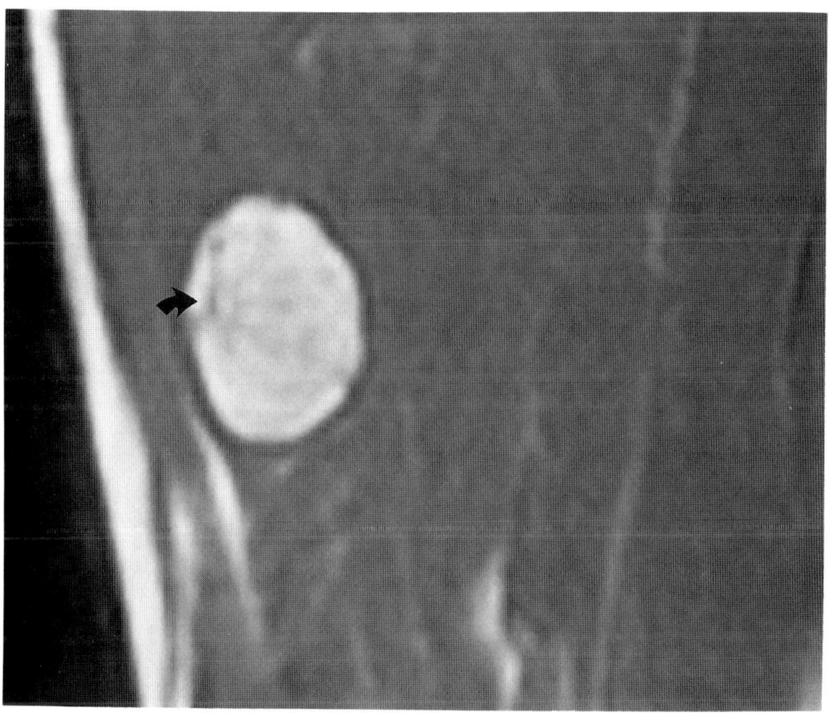

B

FIGURE 1.8 A 36-year-old male with a three-month history of an enlarging thigh mass. (A) Axial and (B) coronal T1-weighted images (600/10) reveal a well-marginated fat-containing mass in the adductor magnus muscle. Very slight internal inhomogeneity is noted (arrows).

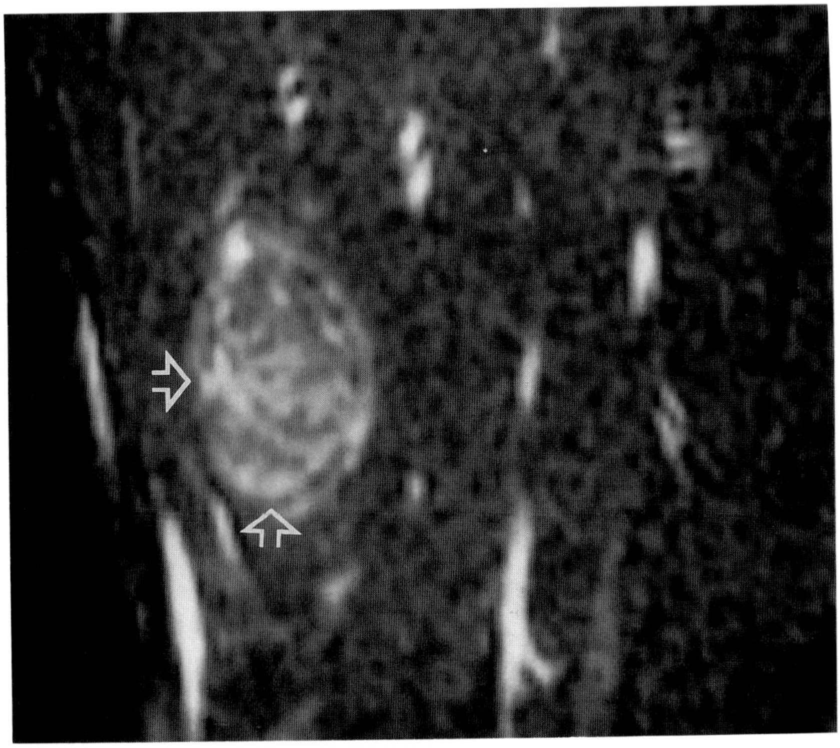

C

FIGURE 1.8 (continued) (C) Coronal FMPIR image (3100/51, TI-150) reveals some areas of bright signal within the lesion (open arrows). Based upon the MR findings and the patient's age, this lesion was felt to most likely represent an atypical lipoma. Liposarcoma was also mentioned as a possibility in light of the heterogeneous signal. Pathologic examination revealed liposarcoma.

2 Fibrous Lesions

Malignant Fibrous Histiocytoma of Soft Tissue

Definition. Malignant fibrous histiocytoma (MFH) is a soft tissue sarcoma consisting of fibroblastic and histiocytic proliferation. There are varying amounts of collagen and myxoid tissue within the stroma. These tumors demonstrate invasion of the surrounding tissue histologically and commonly contain areas of hemorrhage and necrosis. Occasionally, foci of metaplastic ossification/calcification are present.

Clinical Features. MFH is the most common soft tissue sarcoma in adults, usually occurring between 40 and 70 years of age with a male predominance. It generally presents as a painless soft tissue mass, which has enlarged over several months duration.

Location. The most common locations of MFH, in decreasing frequency, are the lower extremity (50%), upper extremity, and retroperitoneum. Extremity lesions typically involve the deep fascia or muscle.

Implications. The overall prognosis of soft tissue MFH is unfavorable. Larger and more deeply positioned lesions are associated with a poorer prognosis. Most cases are treated with preoperative chemotherapy followed by wide en bloc resection. Local recurrence and metastasis are common.

MRI Findings. MFH of soft tissue typically appears as a partially or poorly defined, multilobular mass. The signal intensity is generally isointense or slightly hyperintense to muscle on T1-weighted images. Typically, heterogeneous hyperintense signal is seen on T2-weighted sequences and there may be large focal areas of very bright signal intensity corresponding to hemorrhage, necrosis, or myxoid tissue, which are common in MFH. Variably-sized low-signal internal septations are seen on T2-weighted sequences. Areas of low signal intensity, which represent areas of collagen and hypocellularity, may be present on T2-weighted images. Foci of ossification/calcification may also be seen which appear as hypointense signal on all pulse sequences. Fluid-fluid levels may be present. There is a propensity for cortical involvement.

Differential Diagnosis. The vast majority of these lesions exhibit nonspecific signal characteristics, i.e., hypointense signal with T1-weighting and heterogeneous hyperintense signal with T2-weighting. This appearance can be seen with any of the soft tissue sarcomas. A similar appearance may also be seen with numerous benign soft tissue lesions, which may appear poorly defined on MRI. Bone involvement is more typical of MFH than other soft tissue sarcomas.

References

Miller T, Hermann G, Abdelwahab I, et al. MRI of malignant fibrous histiocytoma of soft tissue: Analysis of 13 cases with pathologic correlation. *Skeletal Radiol* 23:271–275, 1994.

Murphey M, Gross T, Rosenthal H. Musculoskeletal malignant fibrous histiocytoma: Radiologic-pathologic correlation. *RadioGraphics* 14:807–826, 1994.

Kransdorf M, Jelinek J, Moser R, et al. Soft-tissue masses: Diagnosis using MR imaging. *AJR* 153:541–547. 1989.

Sundaram M, McGuire M, Herbold D. Magnetic resonance imaging of soft tissue masses: An evaluation of fifty-three histologically proven tumors. *Magn Reson Imaging* 6:237–248, 1988.

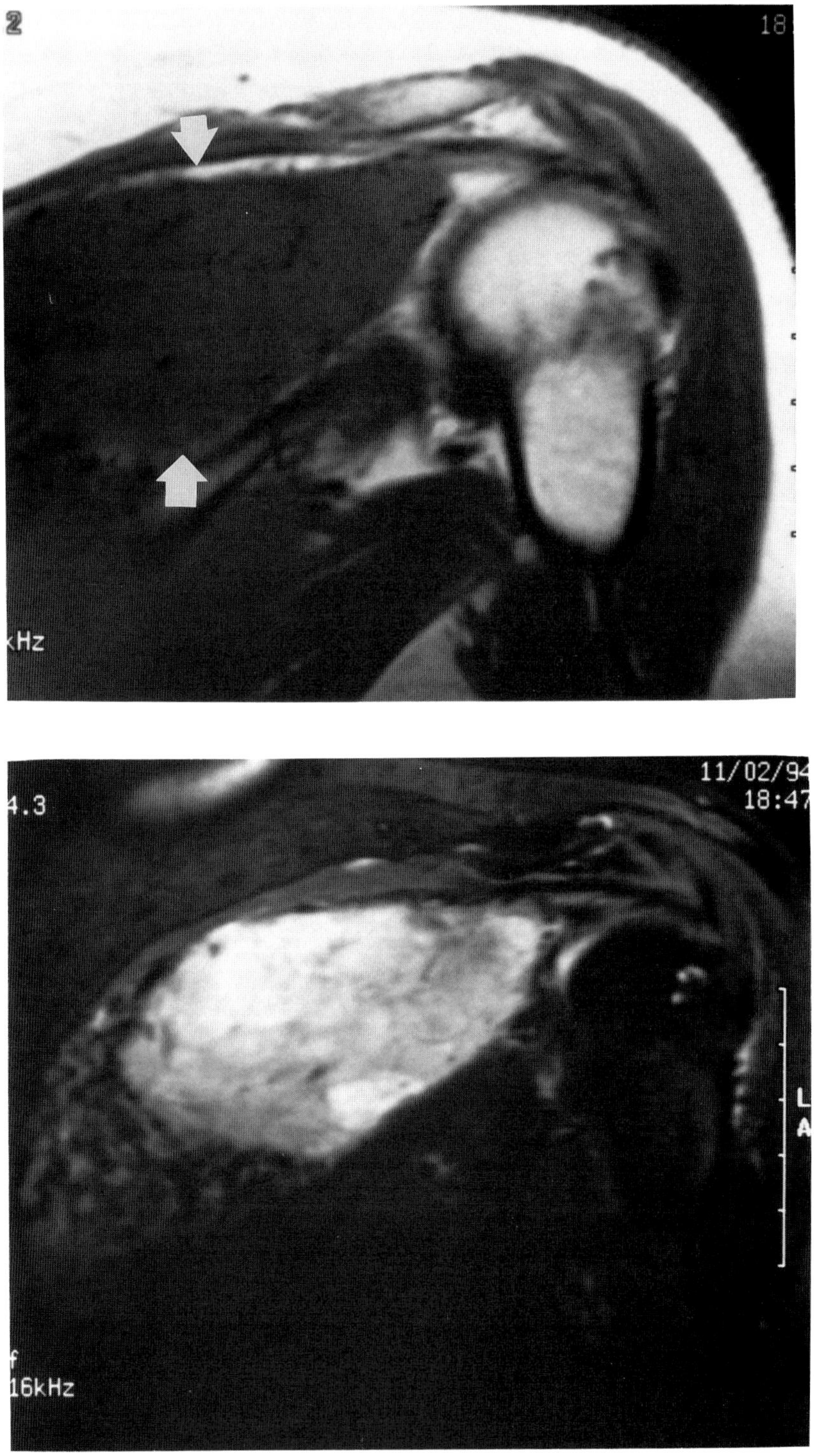

FIGURE 2.1 A 43-year-old woman presented with symptoms of possible rotator cuff tear. Biopsy revealed malignant fibrous histiocytoma. (A) Coronal T1-weighted image (516/15) demonstrates a large mass (arrows) involving the infraspinatus muscle. The mass is isointense with muscle. (B) Coronal FSE T2-weighted fat suppression image (4050/63) demonstrates heterogeneous, predominantly high signal intensity within the mass.

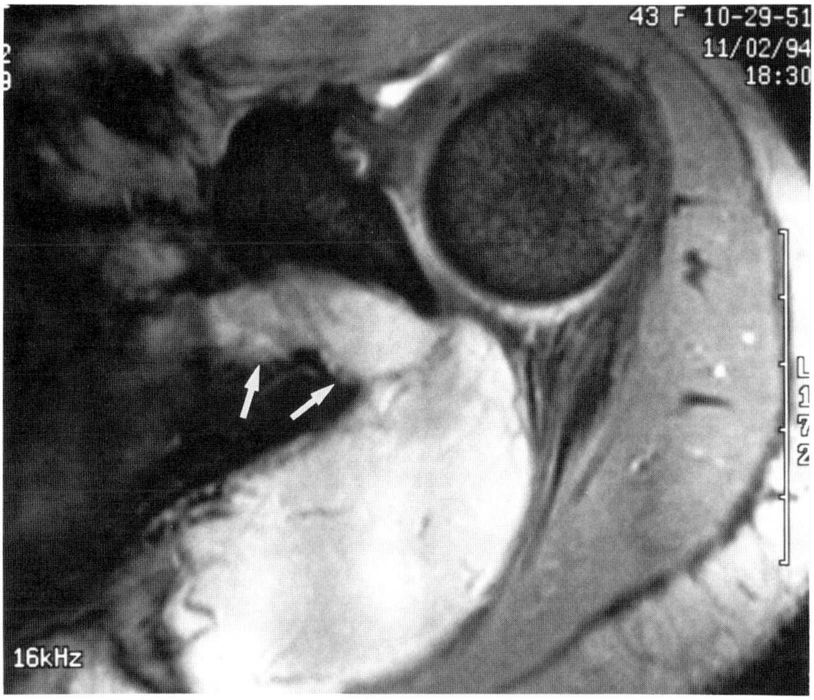

C

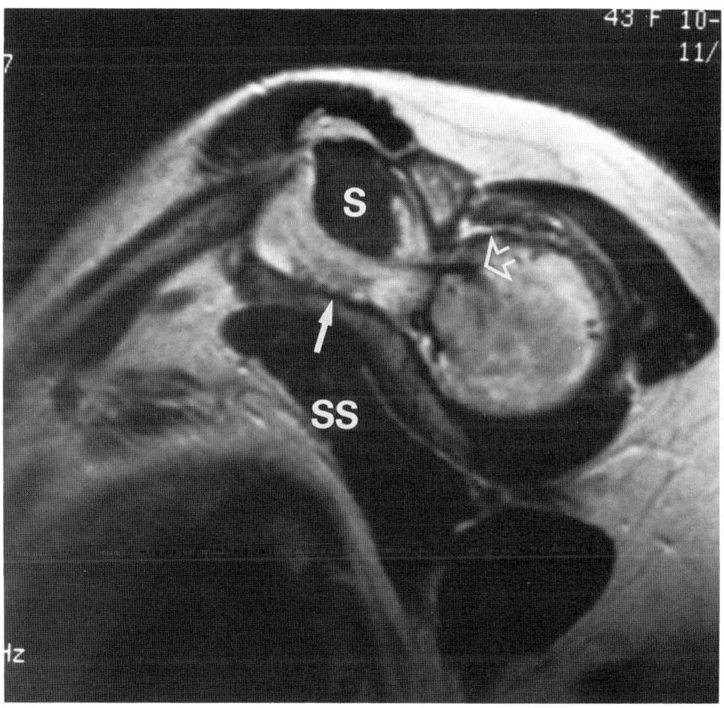

D

Figure 2.1 (continued) (C) Axial GRE (500/20, 20 degrees) and (D) sagittal FSE T2-weighted (4883/95) images reveal extension of the mass through the spinoglenoid and suprascapular notches (thin arrows) with mass effect on the supraspinatus muscle (S). Note the area of low signal (open arrow), which may be due to collagen or hypocellularity. Subscapularis muscle (SS).

Fibrosarcoma of Soft Tissue

Definition. Fibrosarcoma of soft tissue is a malignant neoplasm consisting of fibroblastic proliferation. Histologically, these lesions demonstrate invasion of the surrounding tissue and there are commonly areas of hemorrhage and necrosis.

Clinical Features. Fibrosarcoma of soft tissue may be seen at any age. There is a male predominance. Symptoms depend on size, location, and neurovascular involvement.

Location. These tumors occur most commonly in the extremities, especially the thigh and around the knee.

Implications. The prognosis depends on the histologic grade, size, and location of the mass. Local recurrence and metastasis are common.

MRI Findings. Fibrosarcoma of soft tissue typically appears as a partially or poorly defined mass with nonspecific signal characteristics. The signal intensity is generally hypointense (approximately isointense to muscle) on T1-weighted images and hyperintense on T2-weighted sequences. There is variable heterogeneity on T2-weighted images depending on the amount of hemorrhage and necrosis present as well as the cellularity and fibrous content. Areas of low signal intensity on T2-weighted sequences, which correspond to areas of collagen and hypocellularity, may be present.

Differential Diagnosis. Most of these lesions demonstrate nonspecific signal characteristics with an appearance that may be seen with any of the soft tissue sarcomas. If fibrosarcoma is considered as a diagnostic possibility, it would be prudent to also include the more common soft tissue sarcomas such as malignant fibrous histiocytoma, liposarcoma, and rhabdomyosarcoma. Numerous benign soft tissue lesions could also have a similar appearance.

Reference

Kransdorf M, Jelinek J, Moser R, et al. Soft-tissue masses: Diagnosis using MR imaging. *AJR* 153:541–547, 1989.

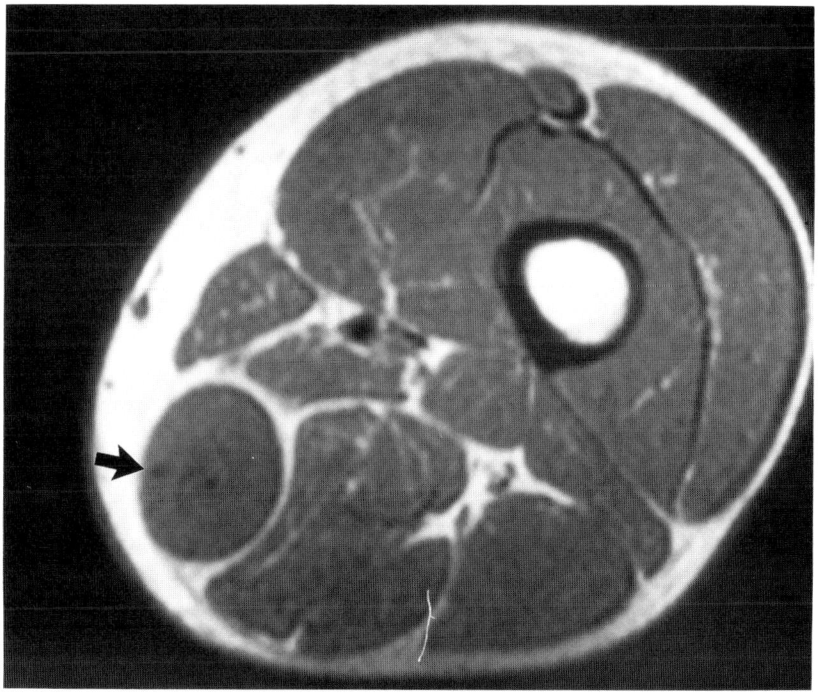

A

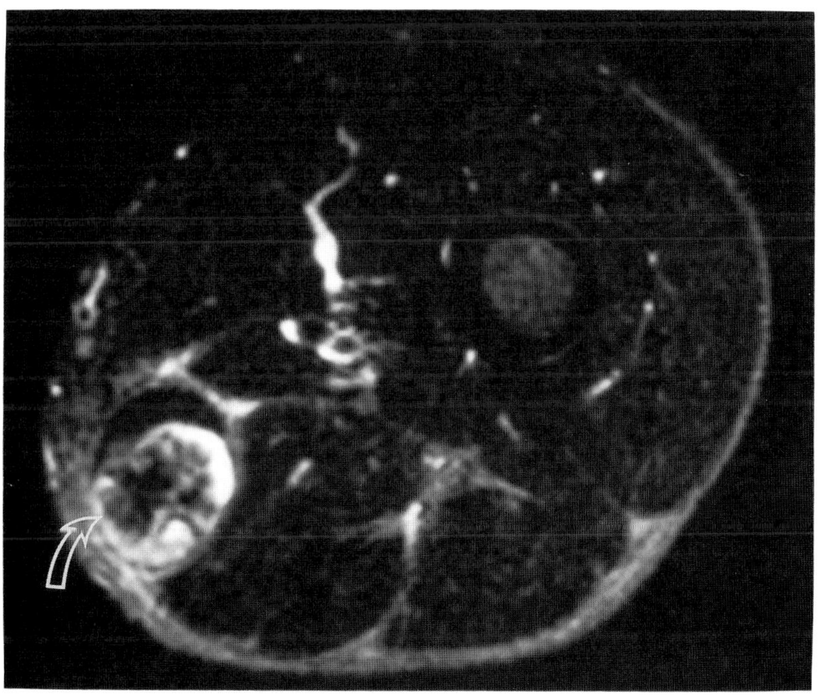

B

FIGURE 2.2 A 46-year-old male with fibrosarcoma of the gracilis muscle. (A) Axial T1-weighted image demonstrates a well-marginated mass which is isointense with adjacent muscle. (B) Axial FSE T2-weighted fat suppression image reveals heterogeneous signal intensity. Hypointense areas (arrows) likely correspond to collagen or hypocellularity.

Fibromatosis (Soft Tissue Desmoid Tumor)

Definition. The fibromatoses consist of a group of benign soft tissue tumors characterized by fibrous tissue proliferation. They have been classified into superficial (fascial) and deep (musculoaponeurotic) groups. An example of a superficial fibromatosis is plantar fibromatosis, which has been described in more detail because of its unique features (*see* Index). Histologically, these lesions are identical to desmoplastic fibroma of bone (intraosseous desmoid) and consist of fibroblasts within a matrix containing variable amounts of collagen. In addition, there may be areas of myxoid change, hemorrhage, inflammation, and vascularity. These lesions exhibit infiltrative growth and microscopic invasion into adjacent soft tissues. They have also been referred to by the name aggressive fibromatosis.

Clinical Features. The fibromatoses are uncommon tumors typically occurring between puberty and 40 years of age. Patients usually present with a painless palpable mass lesion.

Location. Superficial fibromatoses arise from fascia or an aponeurosis. Deep fibromatoses can occur in any musculoskeletal location, but may also involve the abdominal wall or be intra-abdominal.

Implications. Fibromatoses are locally aggressive lesions which do not metastasize. The infiltrative growth pattern is responsible for the high rate of local recurrence, which has been reported in up to 50% of patients. The margins of surgical resection should be wide, in hopes of preventing local recurrence.

MRI Findings. The fibromatoses typically appear as round or oval masses which are usually well-marginated on MRI, despite the infiltrative nature on pathologic examination. The signal characteristics are highly variable and dependent on the histologic composition of a particular lesion. The signal intensity is usually heterogeneous. On T1-weighted images, the lesions are usually isointense or minimally hyperintense in relation to muscle. However, they may appear hyperintense on T1-weighted images if there is abundant myxoid material. On T2-weighted sequences, the majority of lesions will exhibit a predominant signal intensity that is between that of muscle and fat or approximately isointense to fat. Lesions (or areas within the lesions) which are very hypocellular or contain abundant collagen will appear hypointense on T2-weighted sequences. Conversely, hypercellular lesions or areas with relatively little collagen will exhibit high signal intensity with T2-weighting.

Differential Diagnosis. The MRI findings of fibromatosis are variable and nonspecific. Some lesions are relatively hypocellular and contain large amounts of dense collagen. These lesions will appear hypointense on T2-weighted sequences, which should suggest fibromatosis as a possible diagnosis, although other fibrous soft tissue tumors and giant cell tumor of tendon sheath can have this appearance. Other lesions will exhibit high signal with T2-weighting and can therefore not be distinguished from the majority of soft tissue neoplasms.

References

Kransdorf M, Jelinek J, Moser R, et al. Magnetic resonance appearance of fibromatosis. A report of 14 cases and review of the literature. *Skeletal Radiol* 19:495–499, 1990.

Quinn S, Erickson S, Dee P, et al. MR imaging in fibromatosis: Results in 26 patients with pathologic correlation. *AJR* 156:539–542, 1991.

Feld R, Burk D, McCue P, et al. MRI of aggressive fibromatosis: Frequent appearance of high signal intensity on T2-weighted images. *Magn Reson Imaging* 8:583–588, 1990.

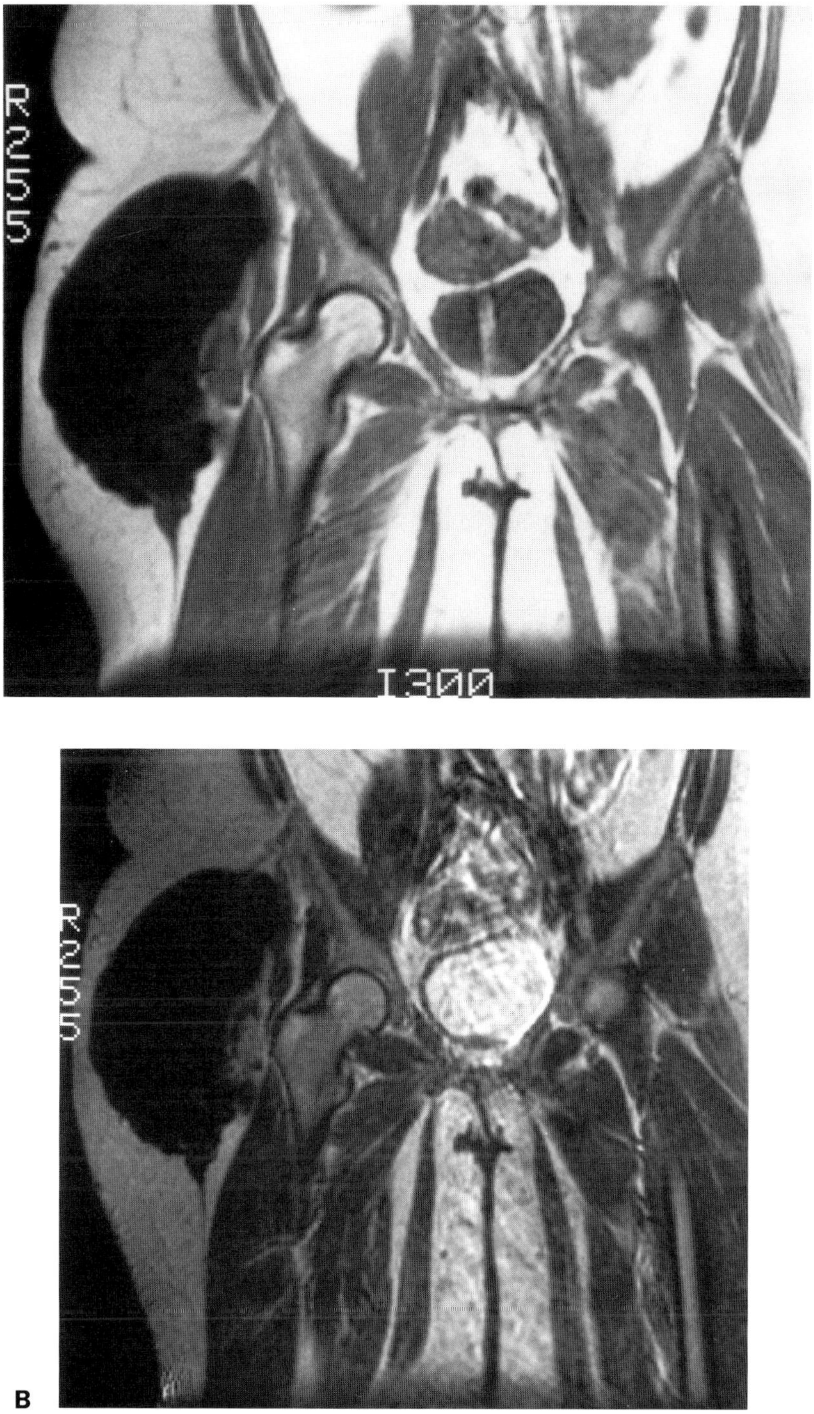

A

B

FIGURE 2.3 A 29-year-old woman with a large right hip region mass. Coronal (A) T1-weighted (800/20) and (B) T2-weighted (2100/80) scans reveal a large, slightly lobulated mass with homogeneous hypointense signal. The marked low signal with T2-weighting suggests the presence of fibrous tissue. This lesion proved to be a desmoid tumor.

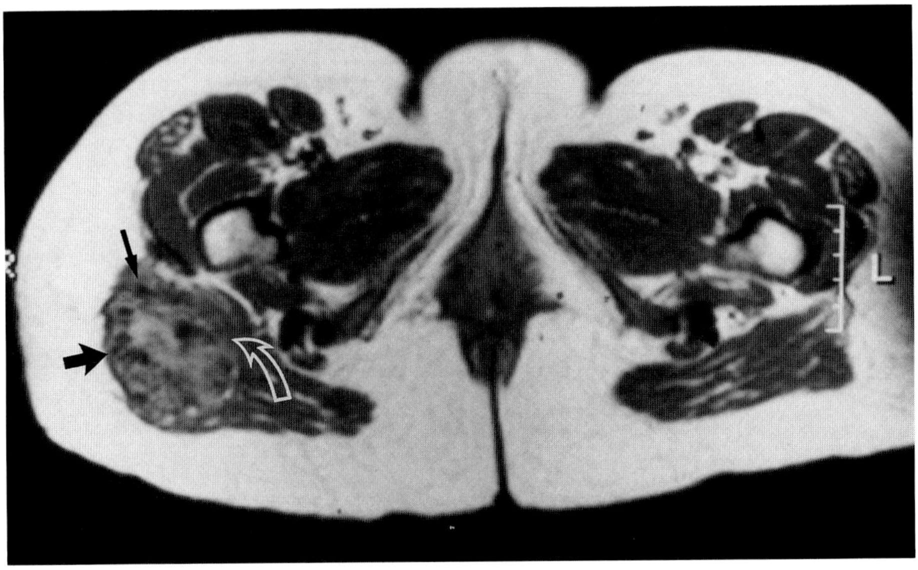

A

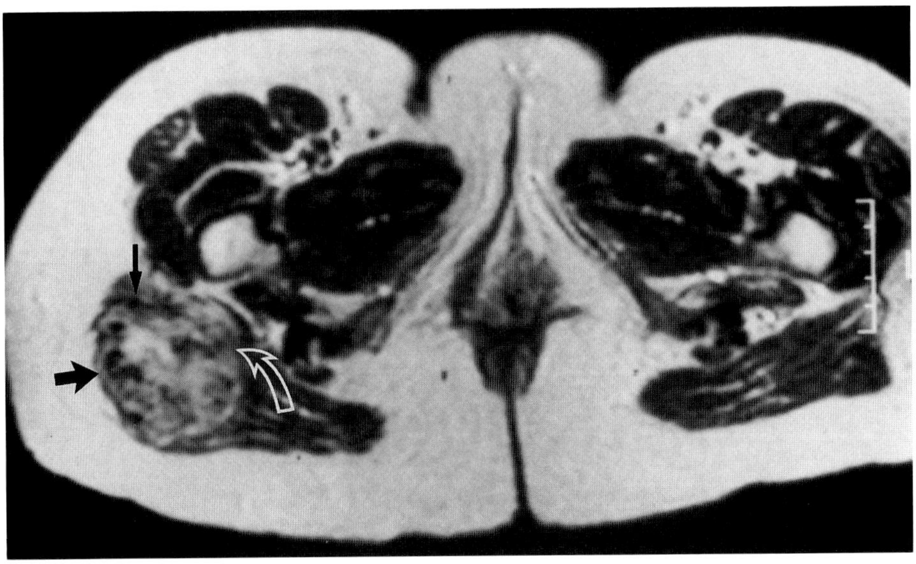

B

FIGURE 2.4 A 45-year-old woman with a desmoid tumor of the right gluteal region. (A) T1-weighted (700/40) and (B) T2-weighted (2200/30) axial scans demonstrate a heterogeneous mass involving the right gluteus maximus muscle. The relatively bright areas with T1-weighting likely correspond to myxoid material. The areas of very low signal on both images (arrows) likely represent collagenous or hypocellular foci.

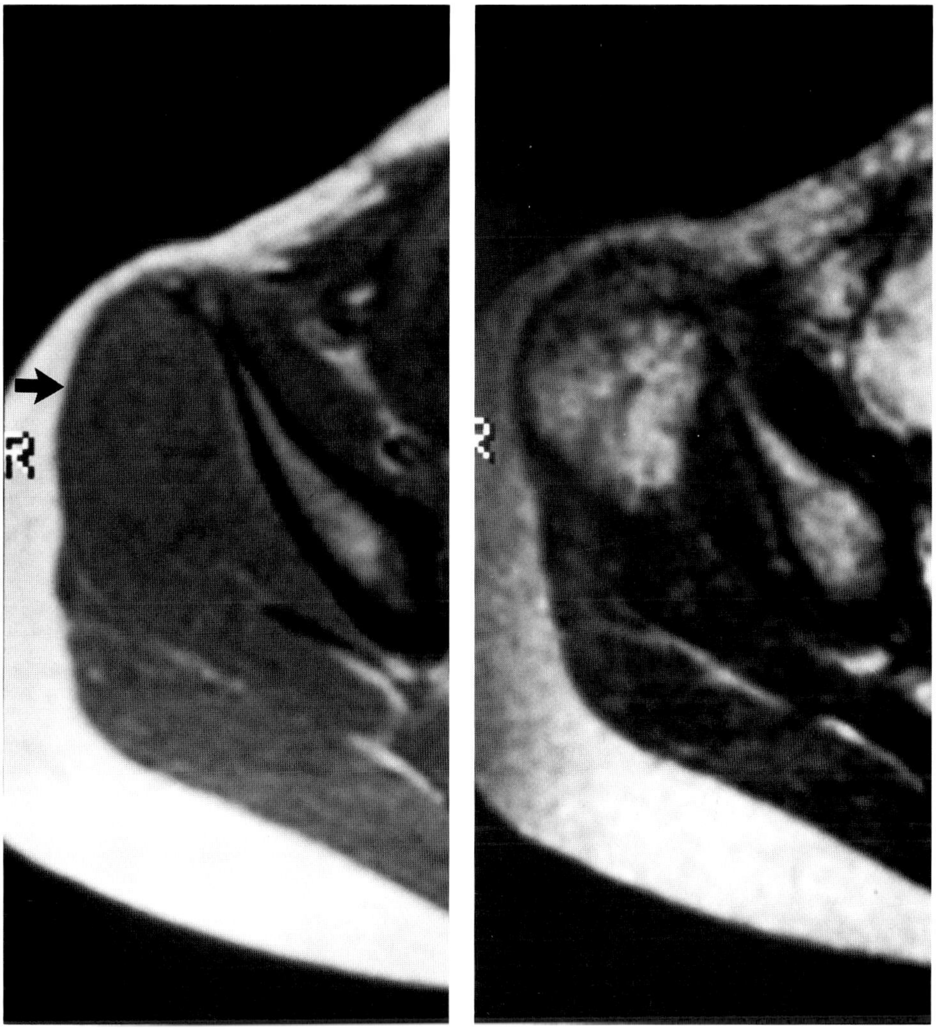

A **B**

FIGURE 2.5 Soft tissue desmoid tumor involving the right gluteal muscles in a 26-year-old woman with Gardner's syndrome. Nonspecific MRI appearance. (A) Axial T1-weighted (400/15) scan reveals a mass (arrow) which is isointense with adjacent muscle. (B) Axial T2-weighted (2000/80) image demonstrates predominantly hyperintense signal within the mass. This MRI appearance is nonspecific, although the hypointense foci with T2-weighting may very well represent foci of fibrous tissue.

Plantar Fibromatosis

Definition. Plantar fibromatosis refers to a specific lesion within the group of fibromatoses and is described here separately (*see* Index for fibromatosis discussion) due to its special implications to musculoskeletal imaging. It is a benign, locally aggressive neoplasm of the subcutaneous tissues of the foot which is intimately associated with the plantar aponeurosis. The lesion contains a large amount of collagen and is characterized by a focal proliferation of fibroblasts.

Clinical Features. Plantar fibromatosis tends to remain asymptomatic for long periods of time and manifests as single or multiple firm, fixed subcutaneous nodules located on the plantar aspect of the foot. Symptoms may result from mass effect or from local invasion of adjacent neurovascular structures or muscles. These lesions may be seen in childhood or adulthood.

Location. Plantar fibromatosis is located in the subcutaneous tissues of the plantar aspect of the foot and is intimately associated with the aponeurosis. Most lesions are located immediately superficial to the aponeurosis, but lesions may also be centered on the aponeurosis or deep to the aponeurosis. Most cases involve the medial aspect of the middle or distal aponeurosis. Multiple or bilateral lesions may be present.

Implications. Treatment of plantar fibromatosis depends on patient symptomatology and the extent of the lesion. Mildly symptomatic lesions may be treated with orthotics. Painful or deeply infiltrating lesions are treated as low-grade malignancies with wide surgical excision and possibly radiation therapy or chemotherapy. Experienced surgeons can usually make this diagnosis based upon the clinical findings, but the number of lesions and full extent of involvement may not be clinically evident. MRI has proven useful for preoperative evaluation because incomplete excision of this lesion may result in a very aggressive recurrence.

MRI Findings. This condition appears as a mass associated with the plantar aponeurosis possessing a well-circumscribed lower margin and an infiltrative upper margin that occasionally grows into the deep plantar soft tissues. Most lesions demonstrate heterogeneous hypointense signal on T1-weighted and T2-weighted sequences. The lesions are generally isointense or minimally hyperintense when compared with adjacent muscle. The lesions generally appear hyperintense on STIR images. Most lesions show heterogeneous, marked enhancement following gadolinium administration, however, mild or absent enhancement may be present. These lesions are of variable size with larger lesions tending to be more heterogeneous.

Differential Diagnosis. The unique signal characteristics and location of plantar fibromatosis allow a confident diagnosis in the majority of cases. Other entities in this region which demonstrate hypointense signal on both T1-weighted and T2-weighted sequences include callus and scarring. However, callus is typically located beneath the metatarsal heads and distal to the aponeurosis and appears contiguous with a thickened skin margin. Scarring can be differentiated by the absence of a discrete mass, the presence of associated skin thickening, and a history of previous surgery or trauma in the involved area. Both callus and scarring can show enhancement following gadolinium administration.

References

Morrison W, Schweitzer M, Wapner K, et al. Plantar fibromatosis: A benign aggressive neoplasm with a characteristic appearance on MR images. *Radiology* 193:841–845, 1994.

Kransdorf M, Jelinek J, Moser R, et al. Magnetic resonance appearance of fibromatosis. A report of 14 cases and review of the literature. *Skeletal Radiol* 19:495–499, 1990.

Quinn S, Erickson S, Dee P, et al. MR imaging in fibromatosis: Results in 26 patients with pathologic correlation. *AJR* 156:539–542, 1991.

Feld R, Burk D, McCue P, et al. MRI of aggressive fibromatosis: Frequent appearance of high signal intensity on T2-weighted images. *Magn Reson Imaging* 8:583–588, 1990.

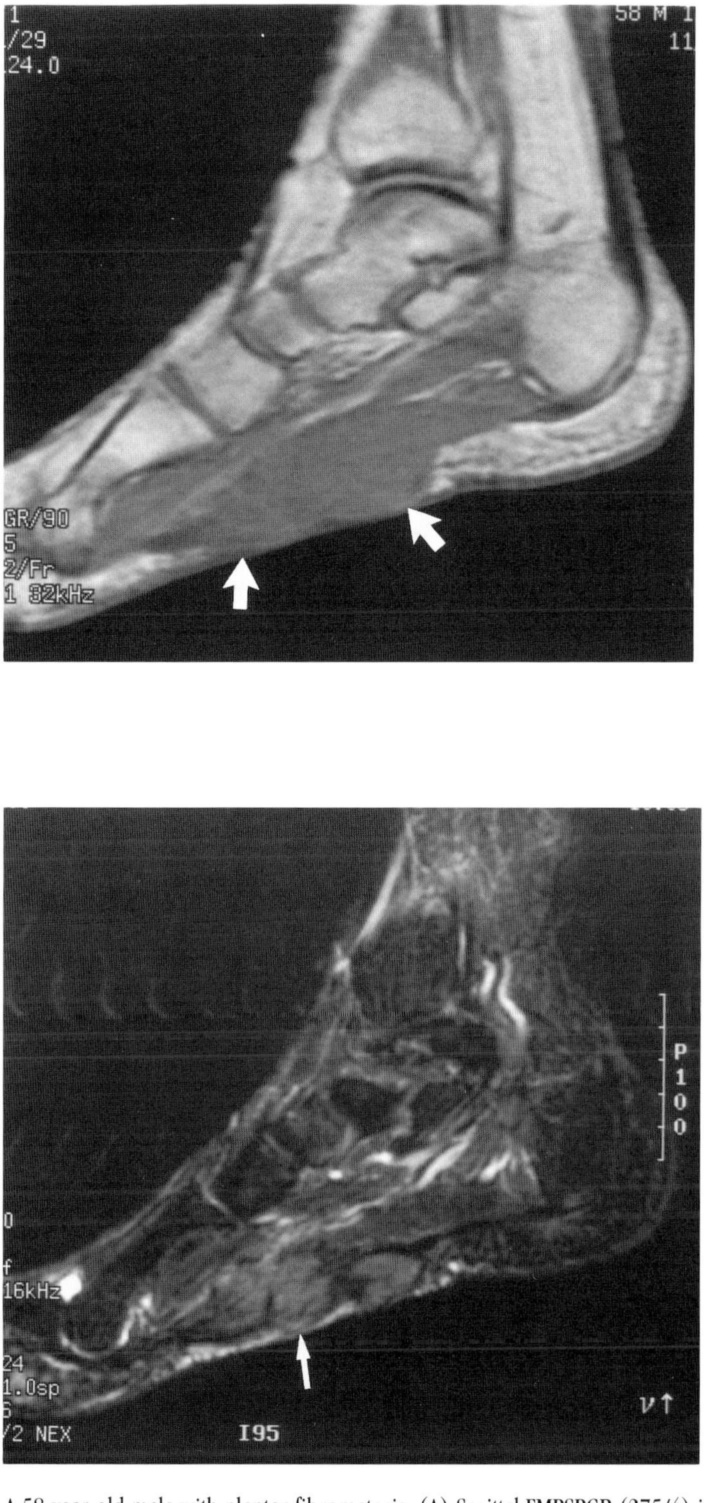

A

B

FIGURE 2.6 A 58-year-old male with plantar fibromatosis. (A) Sagittal FMPSPGR (275/4) image demonstrates a mass (arrows) within the plantar subcutaneous tissues which is associated with the middle and distal portions of the plantar aponeurosis. The signal intensity is approximately isointense to muscle. (B) Sagittal FMPIR image (4233/68) reveals that the signal (thin arrow) is slightly hyperintense to muscle, but much lower than that typically seen with most soft tissue masses.

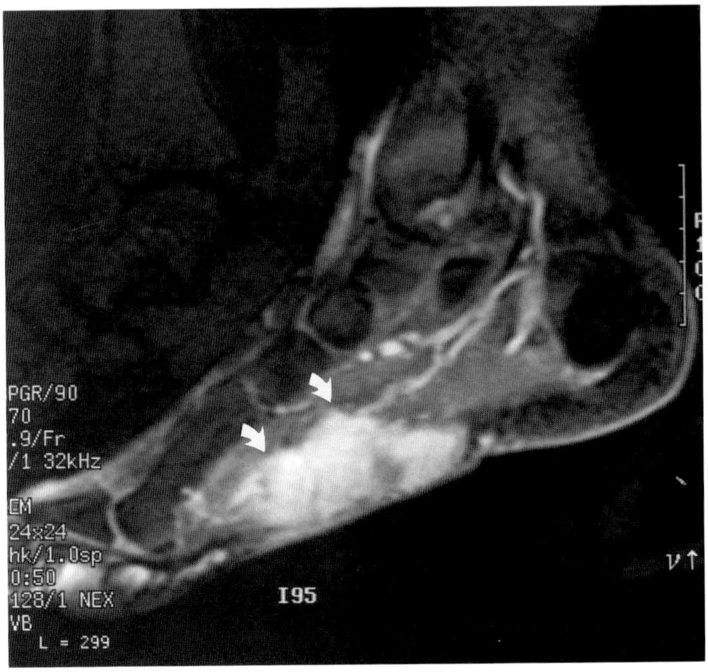

C

FIGURE 2.6 (continued) (C) Sagittal FMPSPGR fat suppression (170/3) image following gadolinium administration shows marked enhancement of the lesion which extends deep (curved arrows) to the aponeurosis. (Courtesy of Mark Schweitzer, MD).

Elastofibroma

Definition. Elastofibroma is a slow-growing, fibroblastic pseudotumor composed histologically of elastic fibers, collagen, and mature adipose tissue. It is not a true neoplasm, but rather is thought to arise from periosteal fibroblasts with deranged elastogenesis as a result of repetitive trauma or mechanical stress, such as friction between the tip of the scapula and the chest wall.

Clinical Features. The majority of elastofibromas are asymptomatic and clinically occult. At autopsy, these lesions are not uncommon and have been reported to occur in 24% of women and 11% of men greater than 55 years of age. Most elastofibromas occur in elderly patients (average age 70), although these lesions have been reported to occur in young patients including children. The lesions are usually small (3 cm or less) but may be as large as 20 cm in size. The most common presenting symptom is stiffness, which is present in about 25% of patients. Pain is present in about 10% of patients and there may be a painful clicking sensation associated with movement as the scapula rubs across the lesion. Large lesions may present as soft tissue masses. These lesions may remain stable in size or may grow slowly over a period of many years.

Location. The classic location of elastofibroma is between the inferior scapular tip and the chest wall. This site is involved in 99% of reported cases and bilateral lesions are present in 10–66%. The tumor is located deep to the serratus anterior, rhomboid major, and latissimus dorsi muscles. The subscapularis muscle is typically either displaced or infiltrated by the lesion. Synchronous lesions in the infraolecranon region are present in 16% of patients. Additional less common sites include the thoracic wall, ischial tuberosity, greater trochanter, deltoid, axilla, hand, foot, and thigh.

Implications. Indications for surgery include symptomatology, large lesions (some recommend surgery for lesions greater than 5 cm), and cosmetic concerns. Complete surgical resection is curative. Local recurrence following surgery is uncommon (about 7%) and related to incomplete excision. Biopsy should not be performed solely for diagnostic reasons. Familiarity with the imaging and clinical features of elastofibroma should allow the correct radiologic diagnosis and prevent unnecessary or radical surgery.

MRI Findings. On both T1- and T2-weighted images, elastofibromas typically exhibit hypointense signal (isointense to muscle), corresponding to the predominant dense fibrous tissue content. Within the mass, there are interspersed linear and curvilinear areas of higher signal intensity (isointense to fat), reflecting the mature adipose tissue component. The mass generally has a lenticular, ovoid, or flat shape with the long axis in the craniocaudal dimension. The mass is typically fairly well-defined without surrounding edema.

Differential Diagnosis. The MR signal characteristics of elastofibroma are not typical for the majority of musculoskeletal masses. Other lesions which may exhibit decreased signal intensity on T2-weighted sequences included desmoplastic fibroma and malignant fibrous histiocytoma, as well as lesions containing calcium or hemosiderin. Masses which contain bright signal with T1-weighting include hematoma and hemorrhagic lesions (due to methemoglobin), as well as fat-containing lesions such as lipoma, liposarcoma, and hemangioma. Nevertheless, the classic location and unusual signal characteristics of elastofibroma should allow the presumptive diagnosis to be made.

References

Kransdorf M, Meis J, Montgomery E. Elastofibroma: MR and CT appearance with radiologic-pathologic correlation. *AJR* 159:575–579, 1992.

Massengill A, Sundaram M, Kathol M, et al. Elastofibroma dorsi: A radiologic diagnosis. *Skeletal Radiol* 22:121–123, 1993.

Pechman D, Kenan S, Abdelwahab I, et al. Case report 839. *Skeletal Radiol* 23:459–461, 1994.

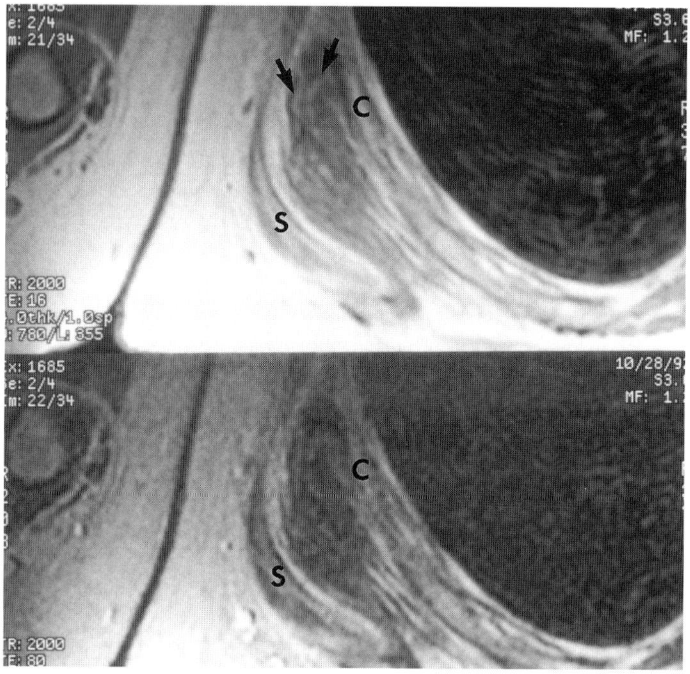

FIGURE 2.7 A 72-year-old woman with right-sided elastofibroma. Axial dual-echo T2-weighted images (2000/16,80) reveal a lenticular-shaped mass. The predominant signal intensity is isointense to adjacent muscle due to the dense fibrous content. In addition, there are some linear areas of higher signal intensity (arrows) corresponding to fatty tissue. Note the classic location between the inferior scapula (S) and chest wall (C).

Scar Tissue/Fibrosis

Definition. Scar tissue consists of variable amounts of fibrous and granulation tissue, depending on the age and maturity of the lesion. Scar tissue develops following surgery or other types of tissue injury. An interesting type of scar tissue is hypertrophic scar, which is defined as an enlarged or elevated scar which is confined to the original tissue injury site. Histologically, hypertrophic scar exhibits increased cellularity and vascularity, inflammation, hemorrhage, and abundant collagen. Hypertrophic scar, similar to keloid scar, is characterized by excessive collagen production due to an abnormality of the tissue repair process.

Clinical Features. Scar/fibrotic tissue is commonly seen on MR examinations following surgery. It may also occur following other types of soft tissue injury such as trauma and burns. A hypertrophic scar may rarely occur in the deep soft tissues following previous tumor resection and present as an enlarging mass which is suspicious for recurrent neoplasm.

Location. Scar/fibrosis may occur in any soft tissue location. Hypertrophic scars most commonly occur in the skin, but may occur deep within the soft tissues.

Implications. Scar tissue may mimic a neoplastic process on MRI. A hypertrophic scar may simulate recurrent tumor on MRI as well as on physical examination.

MRI Findings. Scar/fibrotic tissue may appear as a focal ill-defined or well-defined mass on MRI. The signal is hypointense on T1-weighted images. The signal intensity on T2-weighted sequences varies with the histologic composition. Mature scar tissue/fibrosis tends to appear hypointense with T2-weighting due to the presence of abundant collagen. Immature scar contains granulation tissue, which tends to appear hyperintense on T2-weighted sequences and enhance following gadolinium administration. Hypertrophic scar may appear bright on T2-weighted sequences due to hypercellularity, inflammation, and hemorrhage.

Differential Diagnosis. The MR appearances of scar tissue are variable and nonspecific. A lesion found in an area of previous surgery or trauma which exhibits low signal with T2-weighting can generally be presumed to represent scar/fibrosis, although this appearance could be seen with various lesions including fibrous tumors. A lesion exhibiting increased signal with T2-weighting in an area of previous tumor resection is always concerning for recurrent neoplasm, but could also represent fibrogranulation tissue or hypertrophic scar. Comparison with the initial postoperative MR examination should enable differentiation of fibrogranulation tissue from recurrent tumor. In rare instances of hypertrophic scar formation, biopsy is the only reliable means of excluding recurrent neoplasm. The preservation of normal muscle architecture and parenchymal pattern has been described as a helpful sign in distinguishing areas of increased signal on T2-weighted images due to scar and other postsurgical and radiation change from recurrent tumor. This so-called "texture sign" should be evaluated on T1-weighted images orthogonal to the muscle long axis.

References

O'Connell J, English J, Beauchamp C, et al. Intramuscular hypertrophic scar: An unusual complication following soft tissue sarcoma resection. *Skeletal Radiol* 24:305–307, 1995.

Biondetti P, Erhman R. Soft-tissue sarcomas: Use of textural patterns in skeletal muscle as a diagnostic feature in postoperative MR imaging. *Radiology* 183:845–848, 1992.

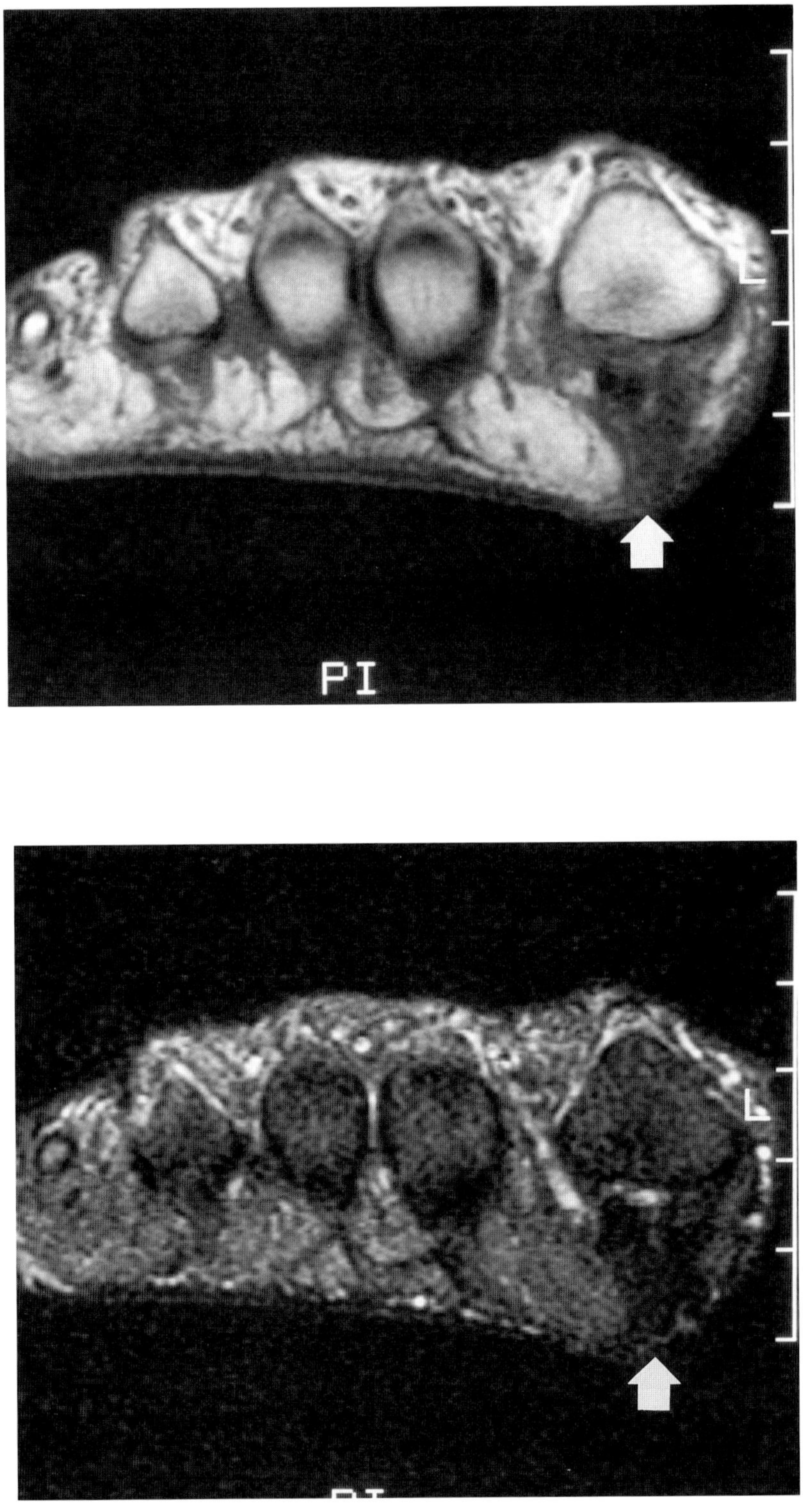

A

B

FIGURE 2.8 Fibrosis within the plantar soft tissues adjacent to the first metatarsal head in a 48-year-old woman who presented with a palpable mass. Axial (A) T1-weighted (633/19) and (B) FSE T2-weighted fat suppression (3500/100) images reveal a plantar soft tissue lesion (arrows). On both sequences, the lesion exhibits low signal intensity, which is typical of fibrosis.

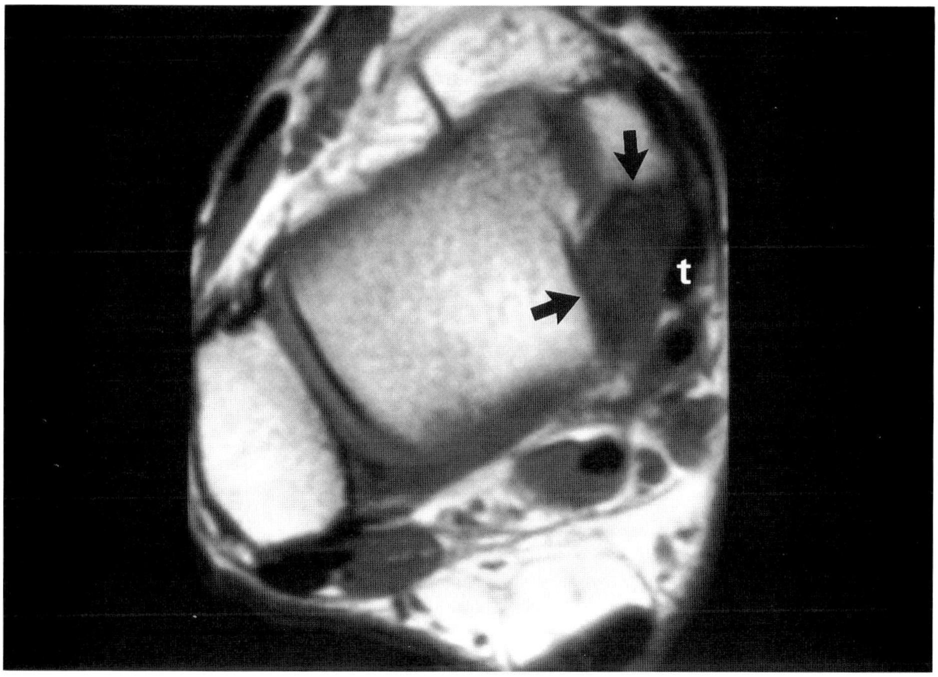

A

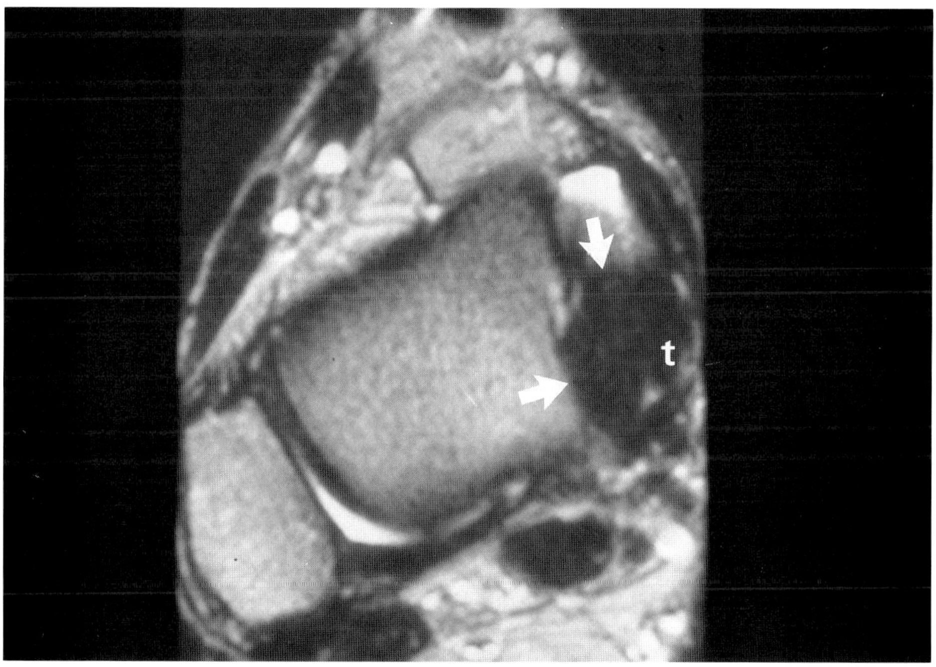

B

FIGURE 2.9 A 38-year-old male who had sustained a medial malleolar fracture six months previously presented with persistent medial ankle pain. Axial (A) T1-weighted and (B) FSE T2-weighted images reveal a focal lesion of low signal intensity (arrows) within the tibiotalar portion of the tarsal tunnel, immediately deep to the tibialis posterior tendon (t). The appearance is consistent with fibrosis/scar tissue related to the previous injury.

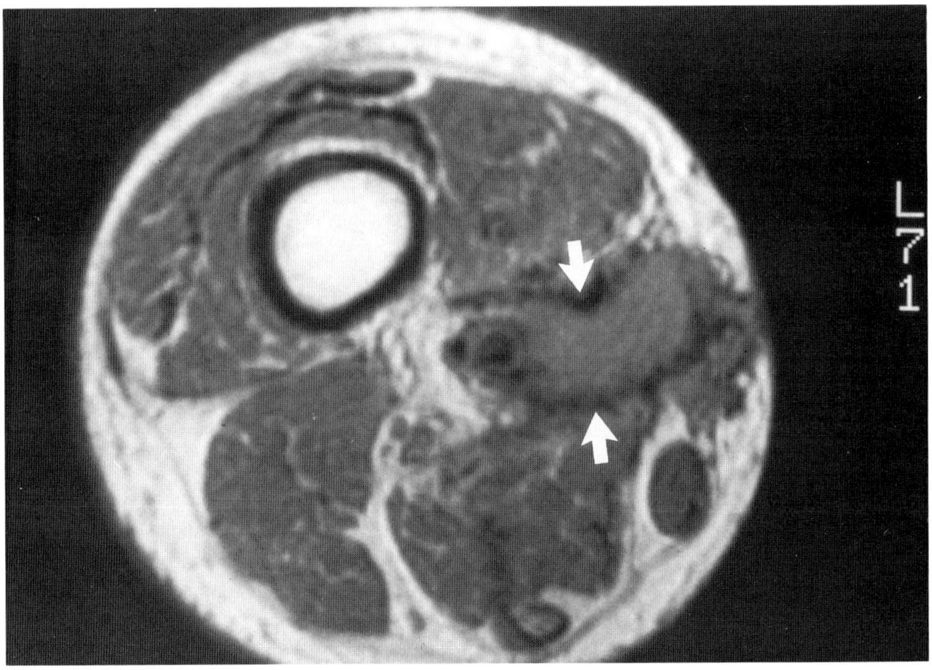

A

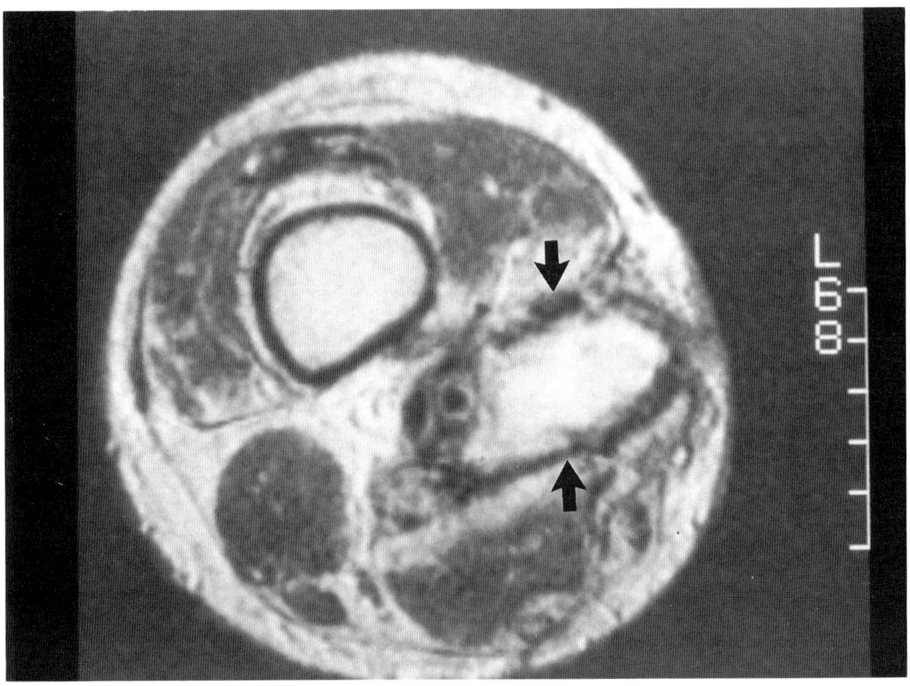

B

FIGURE 2.10 Hypertrophic scar in a patient with prior liposarcoma resection. This lesion presented as a palpable mass which was worrisome for tumor recurrence. (A) T1-weighted and (B) T2-weighted axial scans demonstrate a fairly well-marginated mass adjacent to the neurovascular structures of the left thigh. In light of the hyperintense signal with T2-weighting, recurrent neoplasm cannot be excluded. The peripheral rim of low signal (arrows) likely corresponds to mature scar tissue/fibrosis.

Morton Neuroma

Definition. Morton (interdigital) neuroma is a benign non-neoplastic lesion consisting of perineural fibrosis of a plantar digital nerve with associated vascular and perivascular proliferation. This lesion probably results from compression of the interdigital nerve against the intermetatarsal ligament and may be exacerbated by a fluid-filled intermetatarsal bursa. The most likely cause is wearing ill-fitting shoes (especially high-heels), which place increased force on the metatarsal heads.

Clinical Features. This condition typically affects middle-aged and older patients and presents with pain and/or numbness in the intermetatarsal head region. Pain often radiates into the toes. Symptoms are aggravated by walking and are relieved by rest. Frequently, there is a palpable lesion in the involved interspace and symptoms may be reproduced by compression of this area. The association with high-heeled shoes presumably accounts for the marked female predominance (female:male 7.5–18:1).

Location. These lesions occur between the metatarsal heads, most commonly in the 3–4 interspace, followed by the 2–3 interspace and less commonly the 1–2 web space. The majority of the lesion generally extends just distal to the transverse intermetatarsal ligament, but a smaller portion may extend along the plantar digital nerve proximally.

Implications. Therapeutic alternatives for Morton neuroma include change in footwear, steroid injection, radiofrequency therapy, transverse metatarsal ligament release, neurolysis, and surgical excision. Causes of persistent pain following surgical resection include formation of a recurrent amputation stump neuroma, incomplete excision, and the presence of a second lesion in a different interdigital space.

MRI Findings. The diagnosis of Morton neuroma can usually be made clinically. However, if the clinical findings are atypical or imaging is requested, MR is the imaging modality of choice for diagnosis and localization. The lesions are typically 7 mm or less in size. On T1-weighted images, they exhibit isointense to slightly hyperintense signal in relation to muscle. On T2-weighted sequences, the lesions appear slightly hypointense or isointense to fat and tend to be poorly visualized. The relatively low signal on T2-weighted images likely reflects the dense fibrocollagenous content. The lesions demonstrate moderate to marked enhancement following gadolinium administration and contrast-enhanced T1-weighted fat-suppressed imaging has been advocated as the technique which best depicts these lesions. On T2-weighted sequences, foci of high signal intensity may be seen proximal to the lesion, presumably representing fluid-filled intermetatarsal bursae. Larger lesions can result in mild splaying of the adjacent metatarsal heads.

Differential Diagnosis. In the majority of cases, the typical location and clinical history should enable a presumptive diagnosis of Morton neuroma. The signal characteristics are also unusual in that most soft tissue masses exhibit signal which is hyperintense to fat on T2-weighted sequences. A flexor tendon tear with adjacent inflammatory reaction can resemble a Morton neuroma on MRI, but clinical history should permit differentiation.

References

Erickson S, Canale P, Carrera G, et al. Interdigital (Morton) neuroma: High-resolution MR imaging with a solenoid coil. *Radiology* 181:833–836, 1991.

Terk M, Kwong P, Suthar M, et al. Morton Neuroma: Evaluation with MR imaging performed with contrast enhancement and fat suppression. *Radiology* 189:239–241, 1993.

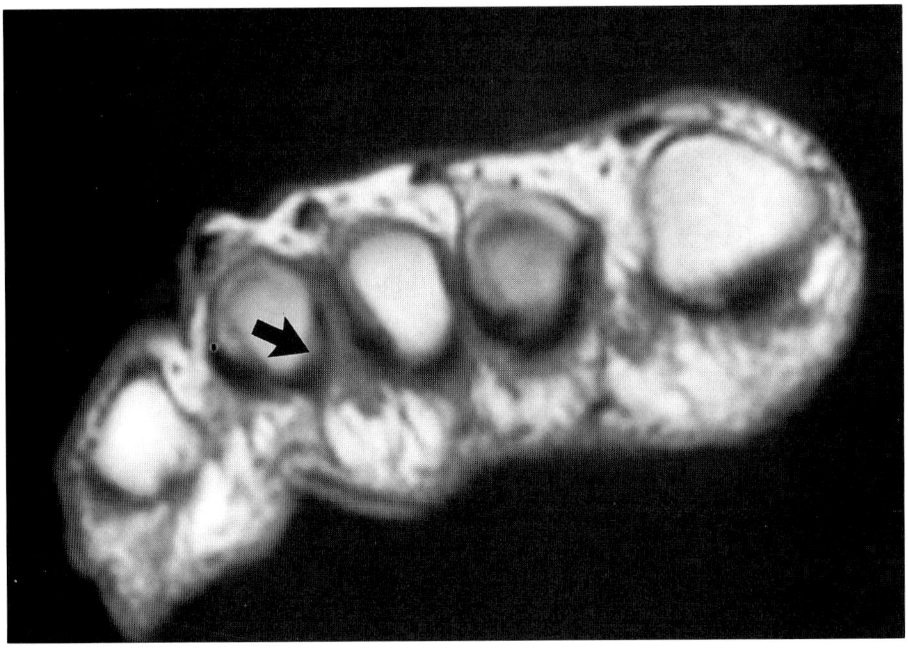

A

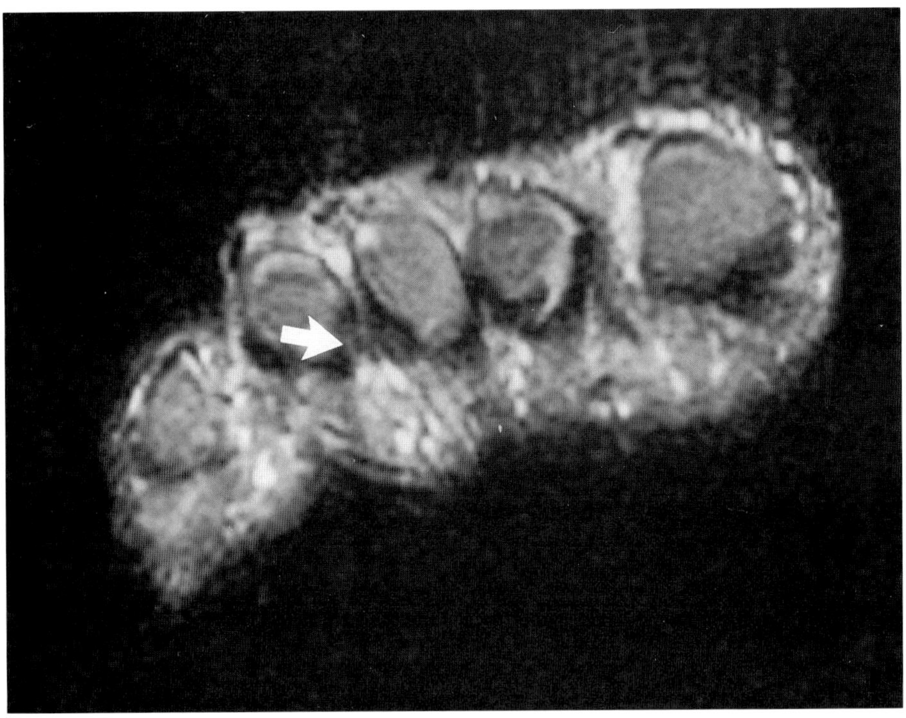

B

FIGURE 2.11 Morton neuroma in a 46-year-old woman. (A) Coronal T1-weighted image (693/16) reveals a small mass (arrow) between the 3rd and 4th metatarsal heads. The signal is approximately isointense to muscle. The lesion is not as well-visualized on the (B) Coronal FSE T2-weighted fat suppression image (3733/84) and exhibits low signal intensity (white arrow).

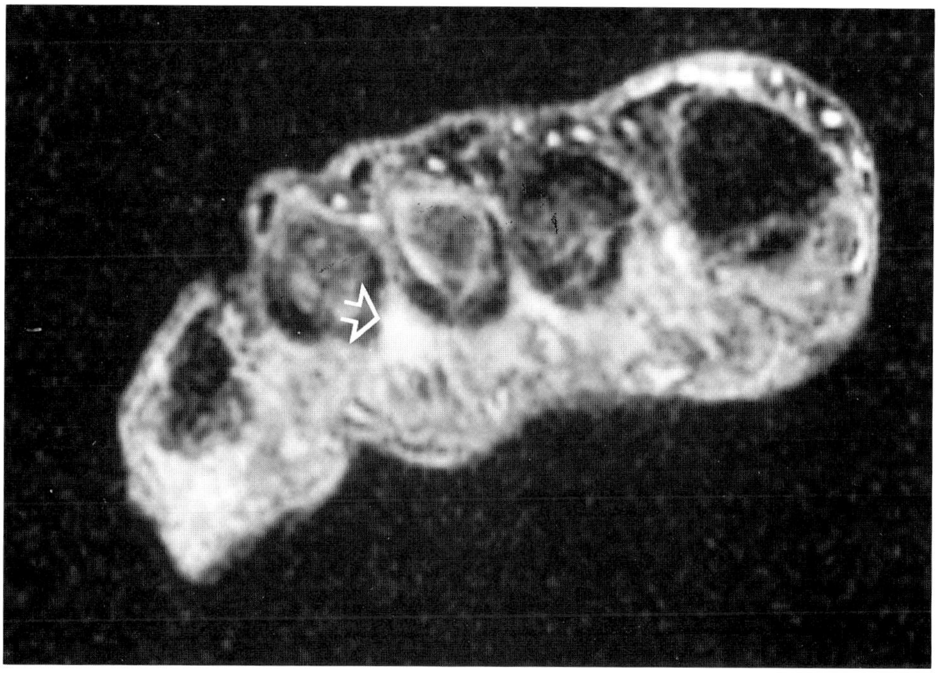

C

FIGURE 2.11 (continued) (C) Coronal T1-weighted fat suppression (533/20) image following gadolinium administration best depicts the lesion which exhibits prominent enhancement (open arrow). (Courtesy of Mark Schweitzer, MD)

3 Cystic Masses

Ganglion Cyst

Definition. Ganglion cysts are tumor-like lesions filled with viscous, gelatinous material. They do not have a synovial lining. These lesions rarely communicate with the synovium of a joint or tendon sheath.

Clinical Features. Ganglion cysts are the most common mass of the hand and wrist. They usually affect young adults between 25 and 45 years of age. These cysts may be incidental, but frequently present as palpable masses. Depending on the size and location, they may be associated with pain, tenderness, functional impairment, or symptoms of nerve compression. For example, a ganglion cyst arising from the proximal tibiofibular joint may present with a common peroneal nerve palsy.

Location. Ganglion cysts are usually attached to a tendon sheath, particularly in the hand, wrist, and foot. They may also arise from tendons or within muscles.

Implications. Asymptomatic lesions do not require therapy, but they may be removed for cosmetic reasons. Lesions associated with nerve compression (i.e., tarsal tunnel syndrome, carpal tunnel syndrome, peroneal neuropathy) should be surgically excised. Demonstration of fluid extensions from a ganglion cyst to the joint capsule could represent capsular components of the cyst. Incomplete resection of such capsular components may lead to recurrence.

MRI Findings. Ganglion cysts typically appear as well-marginated masses demonstrating homogeneous hypointense signal on T1-weighted images and bright signal intensity with T2-weighting. These lesions may be hypointense or isointense to adjacent muscle on T1-weighted images depending on the proteinaceous content. Ganglion cysts may be multiloculated or septated. They may or may not have a definable connection to a joint.

Differential Diagnosis. The fluid content of these lesions accounts for marked hyperintense homogeneous signal on T2-weighted sequences, which is not seen with most neoplastic processes. Around the knee, these lesions can be distinguished from a meniscal cyst by the absence of a meniscal tear extending into the lesion.

References

Burk D, Dalinka M, Kanal E, et al. Meniscal and ganglion cysts of the knee: MR Evaluation. *AJR* 150:331–336, 1988.

Bianchi S, Abdelwahab I, Kenan S, et al. Intramuscular ganglia arising from the superior tibiofibular joint: CT and MR evaluation. *Skeletal Radiol* 24:253–256, 1995.

Resnick D. *Bone and Joint Imaging*. Philadelphia, PA: W.B. Saunders Company; 1989, pp 1187, 1266.

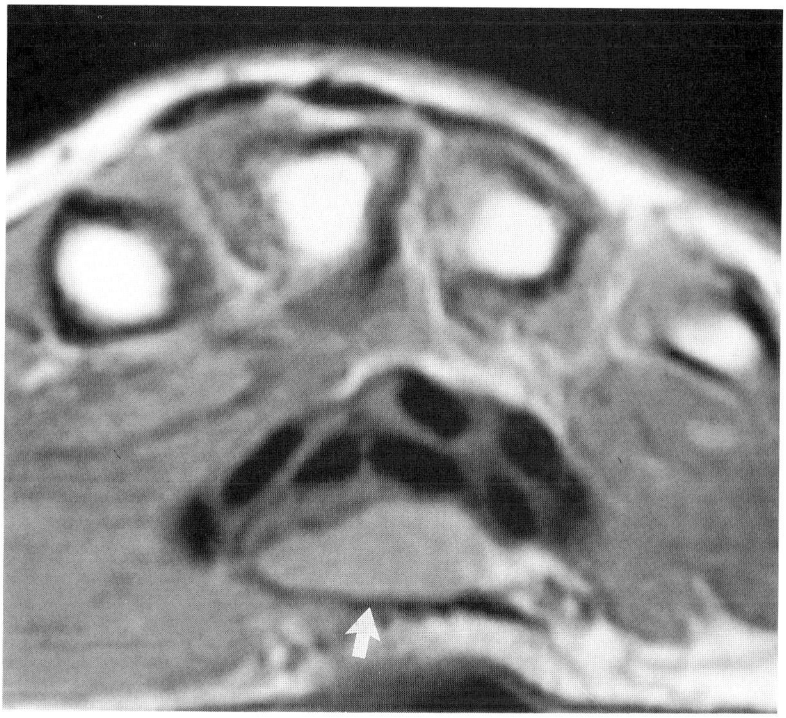

A

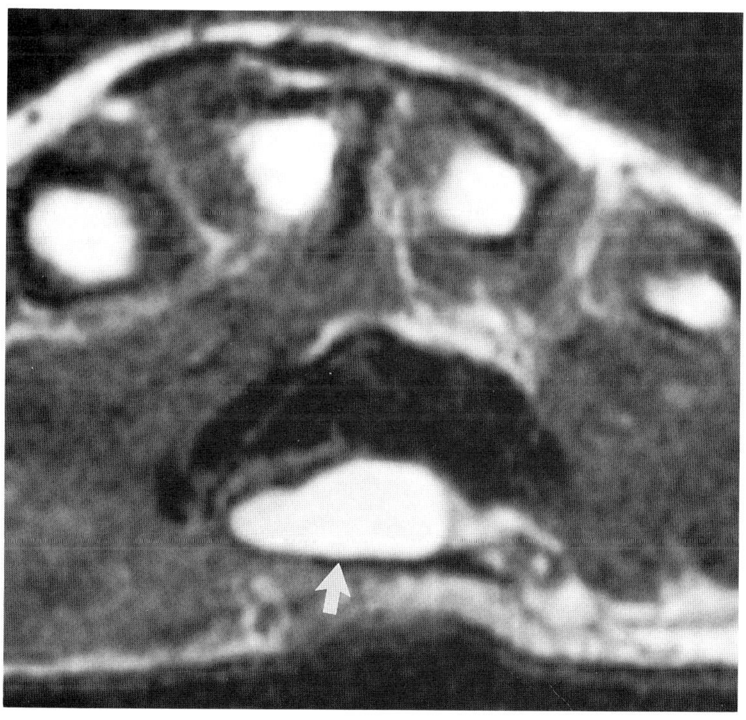

B

FIGURE 3.1 A 37-year-old woman with a palpable mass of the proximal hand. (A) Proton density (1700/30) and (B) T2-weighted (1700/80) axial images reveal a well-marginated mass (arrows) volar to the flexor tendons of the proximal hand. The appearance is consistent with a ganglion cyst, which was confirmed surgically.

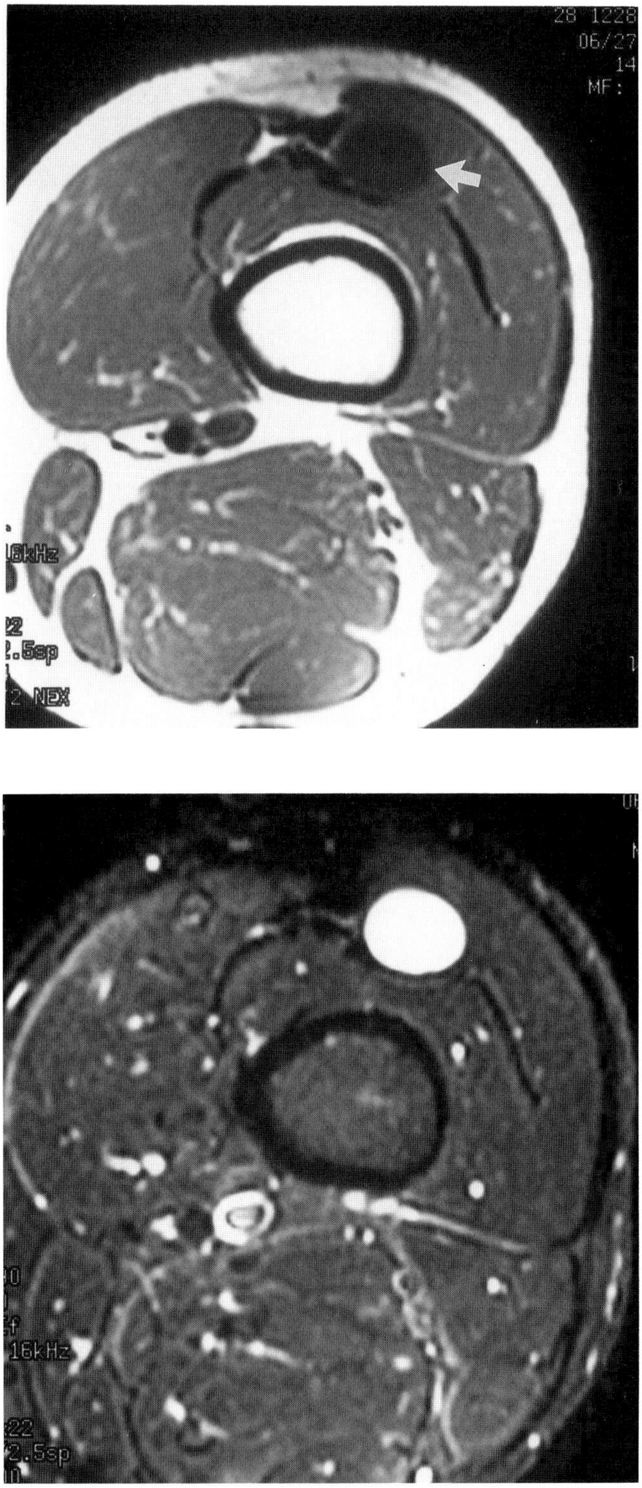

A

B

FIGURE 3.2 A 28-year-old male presented with a palpable mass above the knee anteriorly. (A) Axial T1-weighted image (600/11) demonstrates a well-marginated, homogeneously hypointense mass (arrow) within the distal rectus femoris muscle. (B) Axial FMPIR scan (5000/51, TI-140) demonstrates marked hyperintense and homogeneous signal suggesting a cystic lesion. Surgical resection confirmed the presence of an intramuscular ganglion cyst.

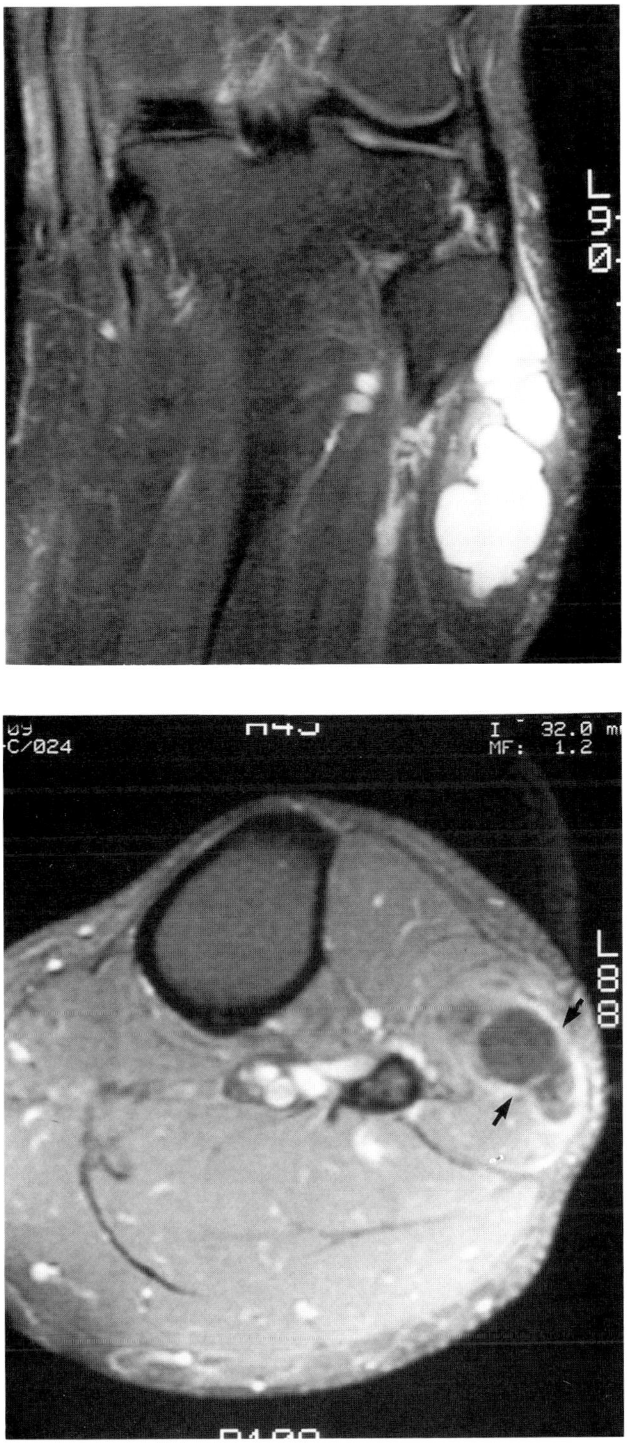

A

B

FIGURE 3.3 A 46-year-old male with a ganglion cyst adjacent to the proximal tibiofibular joint. (A) Coronal FSE T2-weighted fat suppression image (4300/51) reveals a multilobulated, septated lesion with homogeneously bright signal intensity. This appearance is typical of a ganglion cyst. Although not routinely recommended, intravenous gadolinium can be useful in differentiating a fluid-filled lesion from a solid mass since the former will not exhibit central enhancement. (B) Contrast-enhanced axial T1-weighted image with fat suppression (559/12) reveals only peripheral rim enhancement (arrows) of this cystic lesion.

Synovial Cyst

Definition. Synovial cysts are fluid-containing lesions consisting of a continuation or herniation of the synovial membrane through the joint capsule. Unlike ganglion cysts, they contain a true synovial lining. Chronic joint effusions and capsular distension related to inflammation may contribute to the development of these lesions. Rheumatoid arthritis is a well-recognized etiology of synovial cysts. They can also occur in association with trauma, osteoarthritis, neuropathic joint disease, surgery, and various chronic inflammatory conditions.

Clinical Features. Synovial cysts are commonly asymptomatic and noted incidentally on MR examinations. However, they may present as palpable masses or cause pain. Larger lesions may result in limited range of motion or compression of neurovascular structures. They may rupture, hemorrhage, dissect, or become infected.

Location. Synovial cysts are typically periarticular in location, but they may dissect away from the joint. The most common synovial cyst is a popliteal cyst, which arises from the gastrocnemiosemimembranosus bursa. After the knee, the most frequent sites include the shoulder, elbow, ankle, and hip.

Implications. Asymptomatic lesions do not require therapy. Nonoperative treatment is generally adequate in managing symptomatic cysts. Therapy should be directed at the underlying disease process (such as rheumatoid arthritis), if identified. Some authors have advocated repeated joint aspiration and intra-articular corticosteroid injection. Surgical treatment can also be used and typically consists of excision with or without capsular repair.

MRI Findings. Synovial cysts typically appear as well-marginated masses demonstrating homogeneous hypointense signal on T1-weighted images and uniform bright signal intensity with T2-weighting. There may be heterogeneous signal in the presence of internal debris, hemorrhage, or infection. In addition, synovial cysts may contain loose bodies. They can be multilobulated or septated and may have a definable connection to the adjacent joint.

Differential Diagnosis. These lesions typically exhibit markedly hyperintense homogeneous signal on T2-weighted sequences, which is not seen with most neoplastic processes. Synovial cysts have identical signal characteristics to ganglion cysts, but may have a definable connection to a joint. The differential diagnosis depends primarily on the specific site and joint involved. Around the knee, a synovial cyst can be distinguished from a meniscal cyst by the absence of a meniscal tear extending into the lesion.

References

Cosgarea A, Weng M, McIntyre J, et al. Giant synovial cyst of the shoulder presenting as a chest wall mass. *Am J of Orthoped* 24:432–434, 1995.

Allan R, Keen R, Hine A. Case Report 855. *Skeletal Radiol* 23:462–464, 1994.

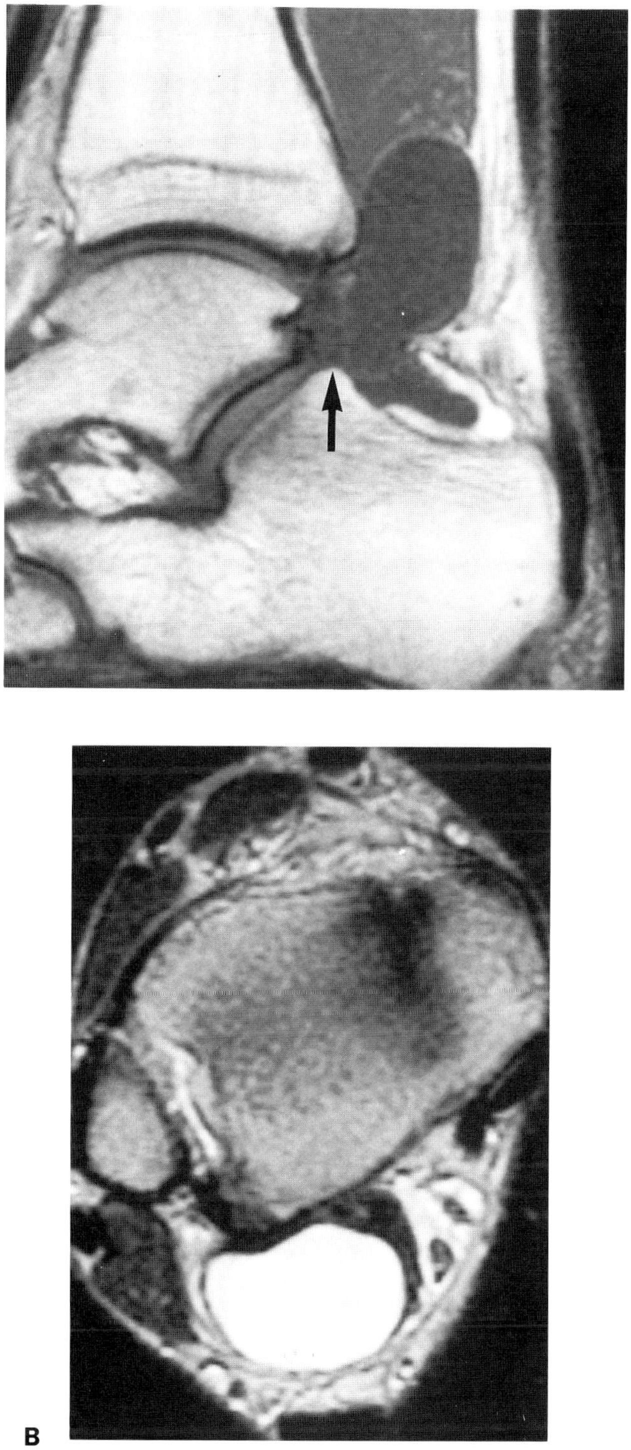

A

B

FIGURE 3.4 A 30-year-old male with a history of several prior ankle sprain injuries presents with a painful, palpable mass of 10 days duration. (A) Sagittal T1-weighted image (500/20) demonstrates a lobulated lesion with homogeneously low signal arising from the posterior ankle joint space (arrow). (B) Axial T2-weighted image (2000/70) demonstrates homogeneously bright signal within the lesion. The MR appearance is consistent with a synovial cyst.

Meniscal Cyst

Definition. Meniscal cysts are associated with an underlying horizontal or complex meniscal tear. The cysts form as synovial fluid is forced out through the meniscal tear and accumulates at the meniscocapsular margin. Most meniscal cysts contain a gelatinous substance with a high proteinaceous content. Some authors use the term intrameniscal cyst to refer to the cystic component within the meniscus and refer to the portion extruded outside the meniscus as a parameniscal component. We prefer to use the term meniscal cyst to refer to both the intrameniscal and extrameniscal components.

Clinical Features. Meniscal cysts are seen in approximately 1% of meniscectomies. Lateral meniscal cysts typically present with swelling and tenderness near the lateral joint line. A tense, hard lump may be palpated. Pain is typically dull and worsened with exercise. Medial meniscal cysts are more likely to be asymptomatic and large. Meniscal cysts have a male predominance and a peak incidence in the third to fourth decades of life. Large posterior medial meniscal cysts may be mistaken clinically for popliteal cysts.

Location. Lateral cysts are three to four times more common than medial cysts. The cysts are often multiple. Medial meniscal cysts are found posteriorly. A weak zone immediately posterior to the medial collateral ligament allows synovial fluid to penetrate the capsule and expand in an unrestricted fashion to form clinically apparent cysts. Progressive posterior dissection may occur secondary to repeated knee flexion and the cyst may be located away from the joint line, connected to the meniscus by a long, thin stalk. Lateral meniscal cysts are usually contained by the joint capsule and fill a potential space adjacent to the midportion of the lateral meniscus between the fibular collateral ligament and the iliotibial band.

Implications. Meniscal cysts are always associated with an underlying meniscal tear. However, the tear can be an intrasubstance tear and not extend to an articular surface. If this is the case, the meniscal tear and cyst could be overlooked at arthroscopy if the surgeon is not informed preoperatively. Successful treatment requires meniscal surgery. Recurrence of the cyst following resection is common unless the meniscal tear is treated.

MRI Findings. Meniscal cysts appear as well-marginated masses which may be multiloculated. Signal intensity is nearly always homogeneous, demonstrating hypointense signal on T1-weighted images and bright signal intensity with T2-weighting. On T1-weighted images, the signal may be hypointense or isointense to adjacent muscle depending on the proteinaceous content. Septation is common.

Differential Diagnosis. Meniscal cysts can be differentiated from other isolated fluid collections about the knee by the identification of a meniscal tear extending into the lesion.

References

Burk D, Dalinka M, Kanal E, et al. Meniscal and ganglion cysts of the knee: MR evaluation. *AJR* 150:331–336, 1988.

Munk P, Helms C. *MRI of the Knee.* Gaithersburg, MD: Aspen Publishers; 1992, pp. 72–73.

Mink J, Reicher M, Crues J. *Magnetic Resonance Imaging of the Knee.* New York, NY: Raven Press; 1987; pp 77–79.

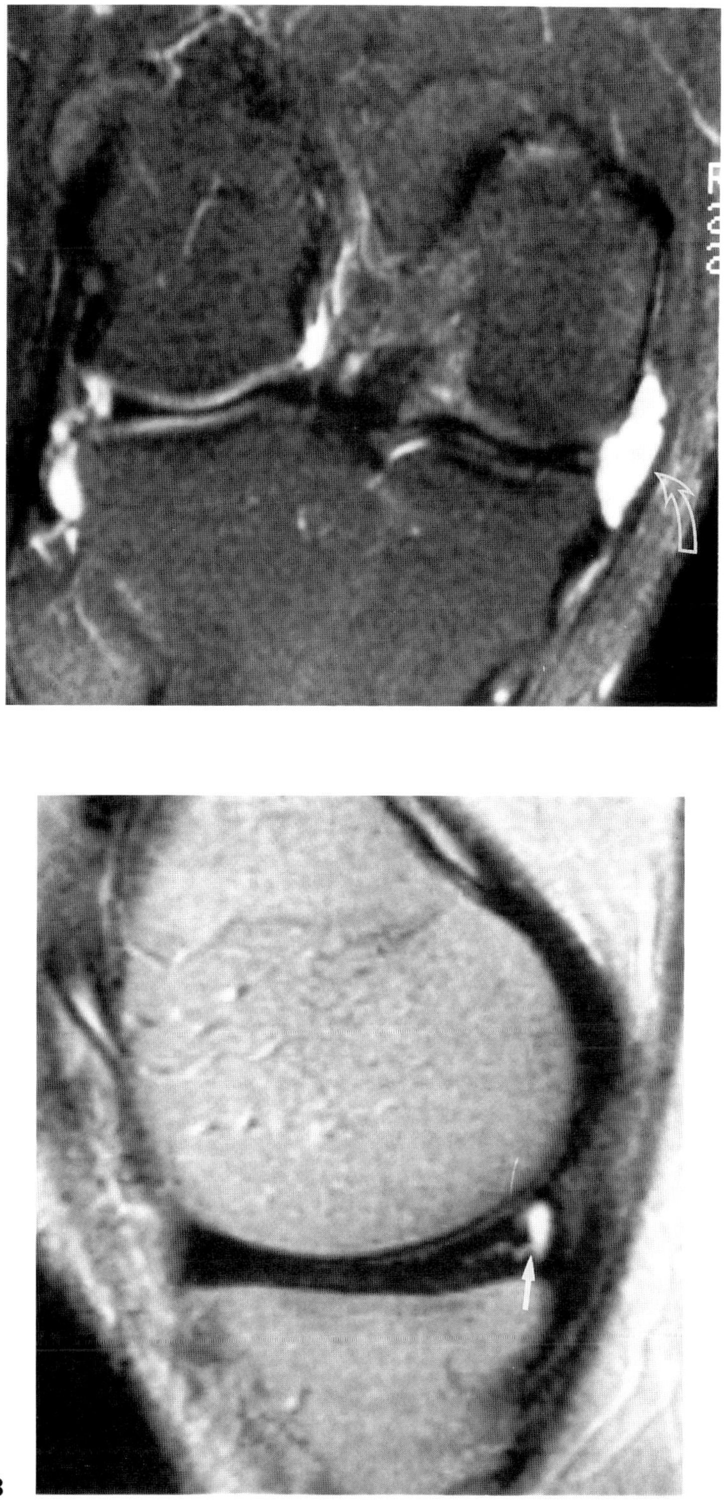

A

B

FIGURE 3.5 A 40-year-old male with medial knee pain. (A) Coronal FSE T2-weighted fat suppression image (4150/54) demonstrates a lobulated cystic mass (open arrow) adjacent to a horizontal tear in the posterior horn of the medial meniscus. (B) Sagittal FSE T2-weighted image (3900/120) confirms communication of the cyst with the meniscal tear (arrow). Findings are diagnostic of a meniscal cyst.

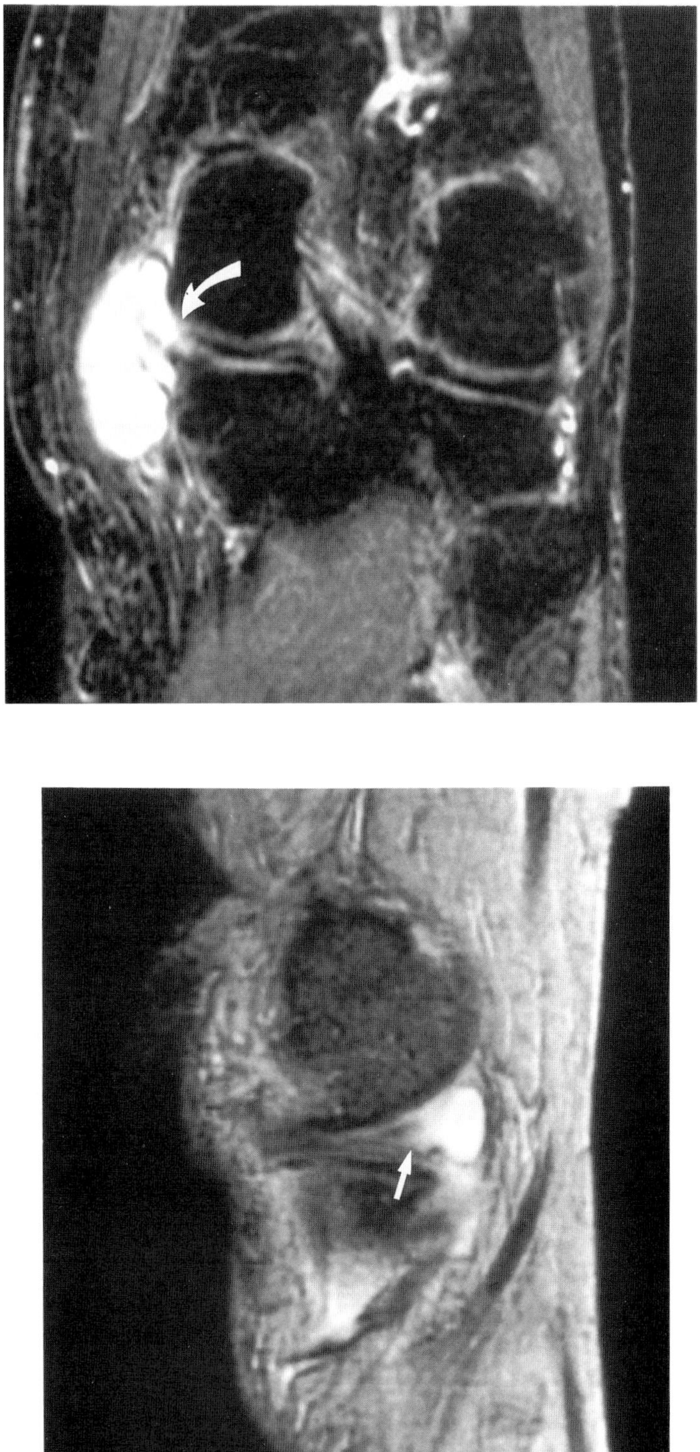

A

B

FIGURE 3.6 An 83-year-old female with medial knee pain. (A) Coronal IR (1500/35, TI-160) and (B) sagittal MPGR (600/20, 30 degrees) images reveal a prominent medial meniscal cyst associated with a tear in the posterior horn. The key to differentiating this entity from other cystic masses is identifying communication of the cyst with a meniscal tear (arrows).

Glenoid Labral Cyst

Definition. This entity consists of a ganglion cyst adjacent to the glenoid labrum associated with an underlying labral tear. Histologically, this cystic lesion contains proteinaceous or mucinous material. The exact pathogenesis of a labral cyst is not known. However, it is postulated that a labral cyst develops when glenohumeral joint fluid is extruded through a labral or capsular tear into the adjacent tissues. This is analogous to the mechanism thought to be responsible for the development of meniscal cysts and some labral cysts of the hip. A communication between the glenohumeral joint and labral cyst can be confirmed at arthroscopy. A labral cyst may cause a pressure erosion in the adjacent bone.

Clinical Features. Labral cysts are seen in approximately 4% of shoulder MR examinations. There is a male predominance. Teens and adults of all ages may be affected. There is often evidence of glenohumeral joint instability on physical examination. Less commonly, there is infraspinatus muscle weakness and atrophy (with or without involvement of the supraspinatus) due to suprascapular nerve compression by the cyst.

Location. Labral cysts are most commonly located posterosuperior to the glenoid. This can be explained by the fact that the posterosuperior capsule above the posterior band of the inferior glenohumeral ligament is a relatively weak area compared to the thicker anterior capsule. The cysts commonly extend into the spinoglenoid notch, suprascapular notch, or both.

Implications. Since labral cysts occur in the presence of a labral tear, they are commonly associated with shoulder instability. Patients who have subluxation (as opposed to dislocation) may present with nonspecific, generalized shoulder pain making the clinical diagnosis of instability difficult. In addition, the clinical diagnosis of instability may require specific testing which is not routinely performed in patients presenting with shoulder pain. Therefore, identification of a labral cyst on MRI may be the initial indicator of shoulder instability. Labral cysts can cause a compression neuropathy of the suprascapular nerve resulting in rotator cuff muscle weakness and atrophy. Cysts in the suprascapular notch may compress the proximal suprascapular nerve resulting in pain and denervation of the supraspinatus and infraspinatus muscles. Cysts in the spinoglenoid notch can compress the distal suprascapular nerve, producing pain and denervation of the infraspinatus muscle only. Resection or percutaneous aspiration of a labral cyst without repair of the associated labral tear commonly results in cyst recurrence. Therefore, surgeons must use an intra-articular surgical approach (not an extra-articular approach) in order to successfully treat this lesion. On MR examination, the underlying labral tear may be subtle and identification of a cystic mass adjacent to the glenoid should prompt a careful evaluation of the labrocapsular structures. MRI may occasionally fail to reveal the associated labral tear because it may heal with fibrosis. MRI is the method of choice in diagnosing labral cysts, which may not be seen during routine arthroscopy.

MRI Findings. On MRI, these cystic masses are seen in the paralabral soft tissues and are almost always in contact with or connected to an underlying labral tear. Occasionally, the underlying labral tear is not identified due to fibrosis. The cysts may be round, oval, or multiloculated and typically range between 3 mm and 4 cm in size. The cysts demonstrate homogeneous hypointense signal on T1-weighted images and uniform bright signal intensity on T2-weighted sequences. The signal intensity should be similar or identical to that of the adjacent joint fluid. On occasion, the cyst causes a pressure erosion in the adjacent bony glenoid. In these cases, the cyst appears partially located within the bone.

Differential Diagnosis. Normal blood vessels in the spinoglenoid notch should not be confused for a labral cyst. These vessels are normally small and can be traced on sequential images. A dilated vein or varix in the spinoglenoid notch may be more difficult to distinguish. It typically has a tubular configuration compared with the multilobulated or septated appearance of most labral cysts. If differentiation is not possible, a flow-sensitive sequence (such as MR venography) or intravenous gadolinium could be used to make this distinction. Anterior labral cysts may be confused with fluid in the subscapularis or subcoracoid bursa. In most cases, labral cysts can be differentiated by their multilobulated or septated appearance and contiguity with a labral tear. Bursal fluid is typically not septated and should be identifiable by its normal anatomic location.

References

Tirman P, Feller J, Janzen D, et al. Association of glenoid labral cysts with labral tear and glenohumeral instability: Radiologic findings and clinical significance. *Radiology* 190:653–658, 1994.

Fritz R, Helms C, Steinbach L, et al. Suprascapular nerve entrapment: Evaluation with MR Imaging. *Radiology* 182:437–444, 1992.

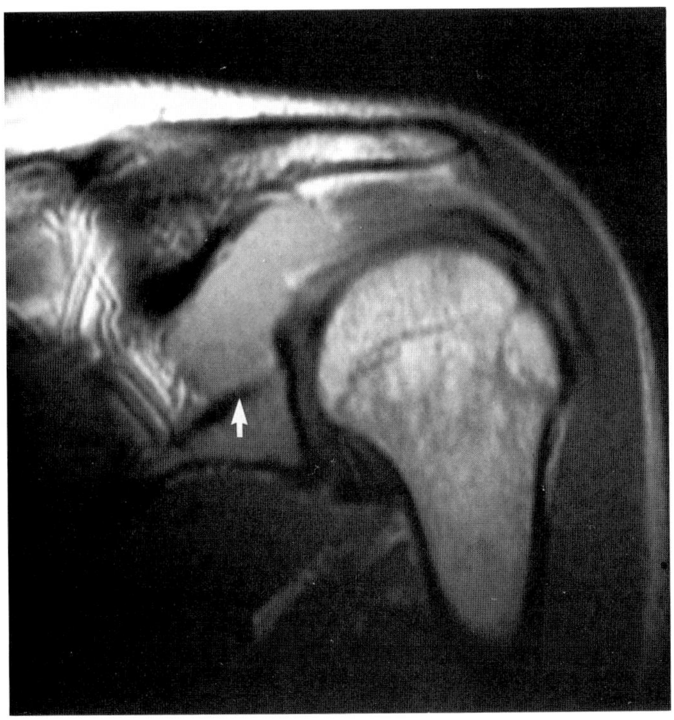

A

FIGURE 3.7 A 36-year-old male with a labral cyst in the spinoglenoid notch. (A) Proton density (2000/20) and (B) T2-weighted (2000/70) coronal images reveal an elongated, well-marginated mass with small lobulations in the region of the spinoglenoid notch (arrows). The lesion exhibits fluid-like signal characteristics. (C) Sagittal T2-weighted image (2000/70) demonstrates slight posterior displacement of the infraspinatus muscle (I) by the cyst (curved arrow). There is increased signal and mild atrophy of the infraspinatus muscle consistent with compression of the distal suprascapular nerve. Note the normal appearance of the supraspinatus muscle (S). Suprascapular nerve entrapment from a cyst in the suprascapular notch would affect both supraspinatus and infraspinatus muscles. Subscapularis (SS), Teres minor (T).

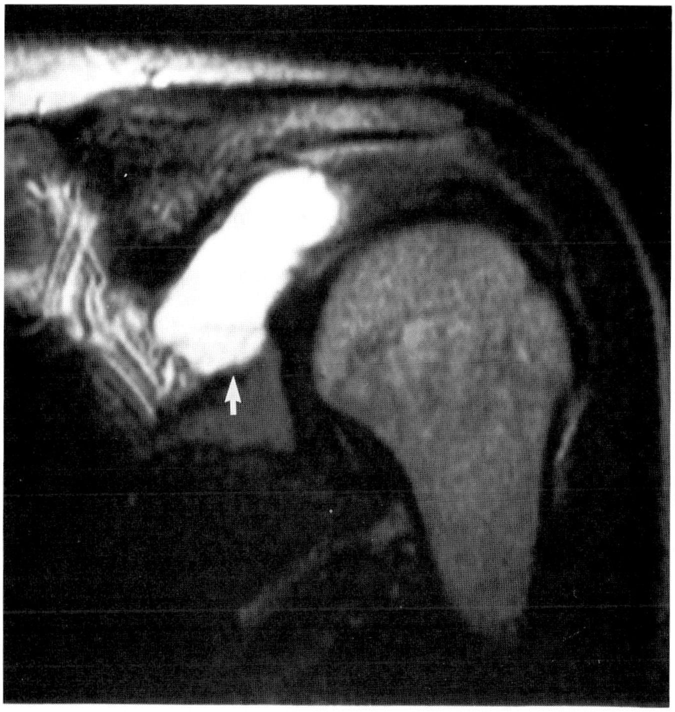

B

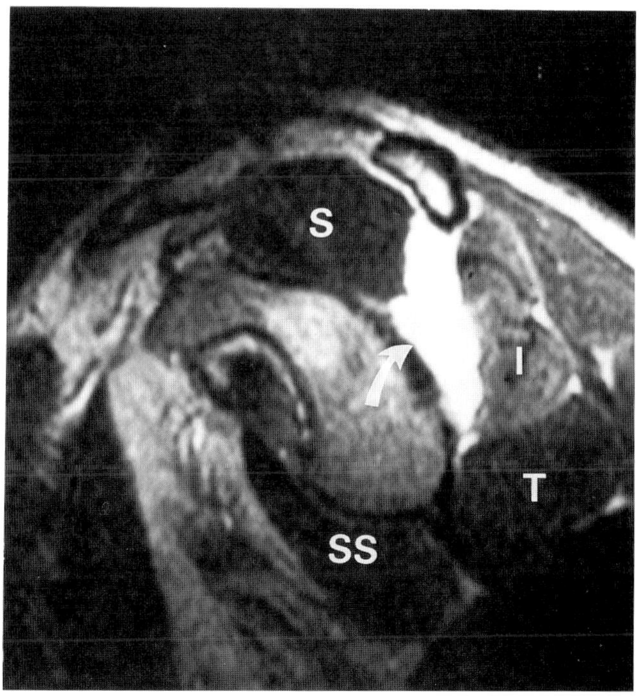

C

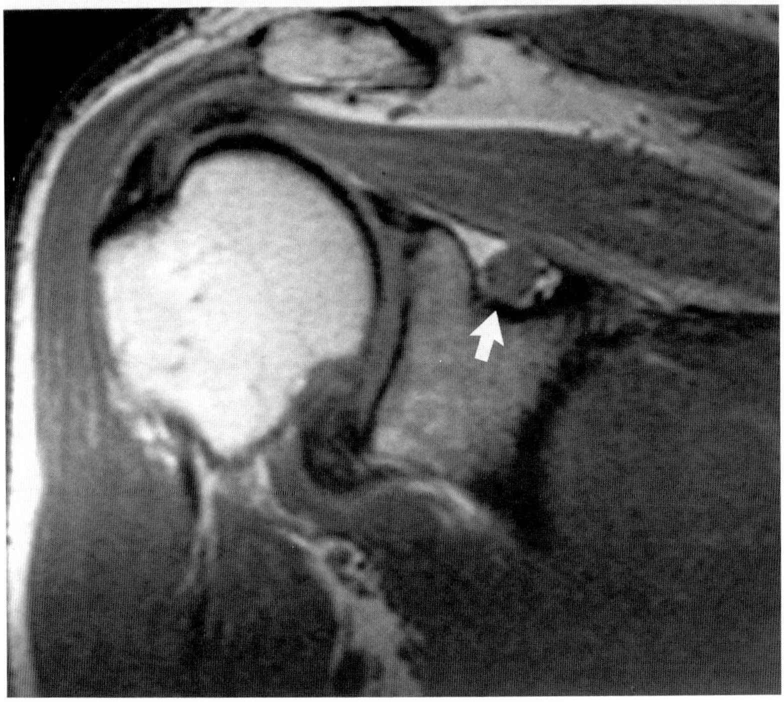

A

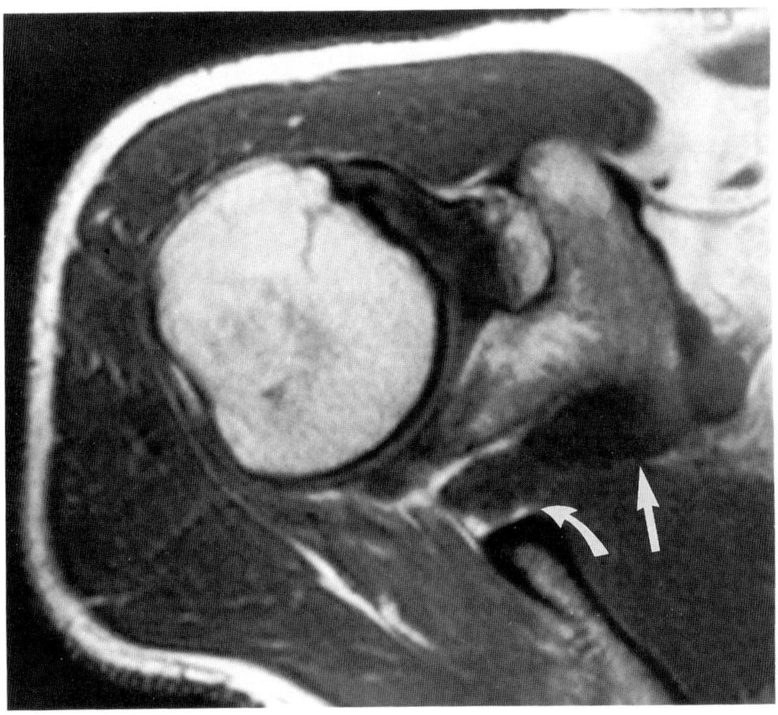

B

FIGURE 3.8 A 46-year-old male with extension of a labral cyst into the suprascapular notch. (A) Coronal proton density image (1850/20) reveals a well-marginated lesion within the suprascapular notch (arrow). (B) T1-weighted (700/20) and (C) T2-weighted (1850/80) axial images reveal a tubular cystic lesion extending across the spinoglenoid (curved arrows) and suprascapular (long arrows) notches.

c

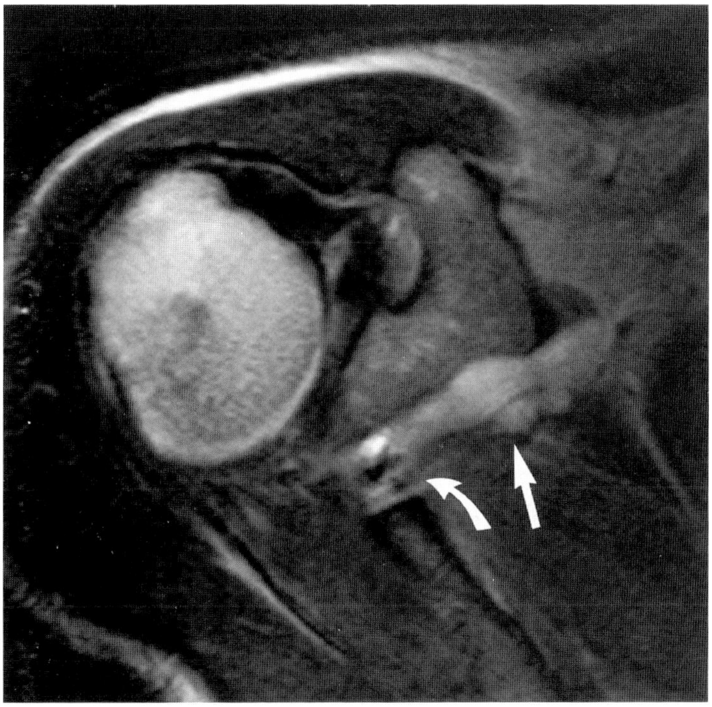

Labral Cyst of the Hip

Definition. Labral cysts of the hip are juxta-acetabular lesions which contain mucoid material and synovial elements. They may be ganglion or synovial cysts. Ganglia are lined by flat, spindle-shaped cells, whereas synovial cysts are lined by synovium. Labral cysts of the hip may arise via several pathogenic pathways. Many of these cysts are associated with a labral tear. A para-acetabular cyst may then form when synovial fluid and/or synovial tissue is forced through the labral tear as a result of elevated intra-articular pressure. This is analogous to the mechanism thought to be responsible for the development of meniscal cysts and glenoid labral cysts. Labral tears may result from acute trauma or from chronic mechanical stresses. Labral cysts are more likely to occur in an unstable hip joint. Acetabular dysplasia and osteoarthritis are associated with labral cyst development. Acetabular dysplasia may lead to mechanical deformation and tear of the labrum. Osteoarthritis is commonly associated with superolateral migration of the femoral head which may cause excessive pressure on the labrum. Additional postulated mechanisms include: (1) an intraosseous acetabular ganglion cyst could erode through the lateral bony margin into the adjacent soft tissues, (2) increased muscle contraction forces may result in juxta-acetabular cyst formation due to degenerative changes at a tendon insertion site, (3) primary degeneration may result in cyst formation in the periosteum, joint capsule, or labrum or possibly in a bursa or tendon sheath, and (4) the labrum itself may undergo ganglionic transformation.

Clinical Features. Para-acetabular cysts have been reported to be present on up to 8% of hip MR examinations. Adults of all ages may be affected. Most patients have a history of remote trauma or acetabular dysplasia. Patients typically complain of intermittent hip discomfort and pain. The hip pain may be localized or radiating, which may simulate sciatica. Physical examination reveals pain upon hip flexion and internal rotation. Labral tears may be associated with instability or clicking.

Location. These juxta-acetabular lesions occur unilaterally, more frequently on the right. They are most commonly located posterosuperior to the acetabulum, presumably because the posterosuperior labrum is most vulnerable to mechanical stress.

Implications. Labral cysts are a fairly frequent cause of hip pain. Identification of a paralabral cyst should provoke a careful evaluation for labral pathology. If untreated, labral cysts tend to enlarge over time. Nonweight-bearing often provides relief of symptomatology, but surgery is the most definitive therapy. For those cysts associated with a labral tear, resection of the cyst should also be accompanied by repair (suturing or partial resection) of the torn labrum. Surgery typically results in immediate relief of symptoms. In those cases associated with severe acetabular dysplasia or osteoarthritis, total hip arthroplasty is often performed.

MRI Findings. Labral cysts of the hip appear as well-marginated round, oval, or multiloculated masses which are in contact with a portion of the acetabular labrum. Most often, they are associated with a tear of the adjacent labrum and a direct connection with the tear may be visualized. The cysts, which are typically between 3 mm and 3 cm in size, exhibit low to intermediate signal intensity on T1-weighted images and bright signal intensity on T2-weighted sequences. The cysts may appear hyperintense to adjacent synovial fluid on T1-weighted sequences due to a high proteinaceous content. The signal intensity may appear homogeneous or may be heterogeneous if internal debris is present. The cysts may cause erosion in the adjacent bony acetabulum.

Differential Diagnosis. Labral cysts can be distinguished from bursal fluid in most cases because of their intimate association with the labrum and the presence of associated labral pathology. The fluid content of these lesions accounts for the marked hyperintensity on T2-weighted sequences, which is not seen with most neoplastic processes.

References

Schnarkowski P, Steinbach L, Tirman P, et al. Labral cysts of the hip: MR features and clinical significance. (In Press).

Haller J, Resnick D, Greenway G, et al. Juxtaacetabular ganglionic (or synovial) cysts: CT and MR features. *JCAT* 13:976–983, 1989.

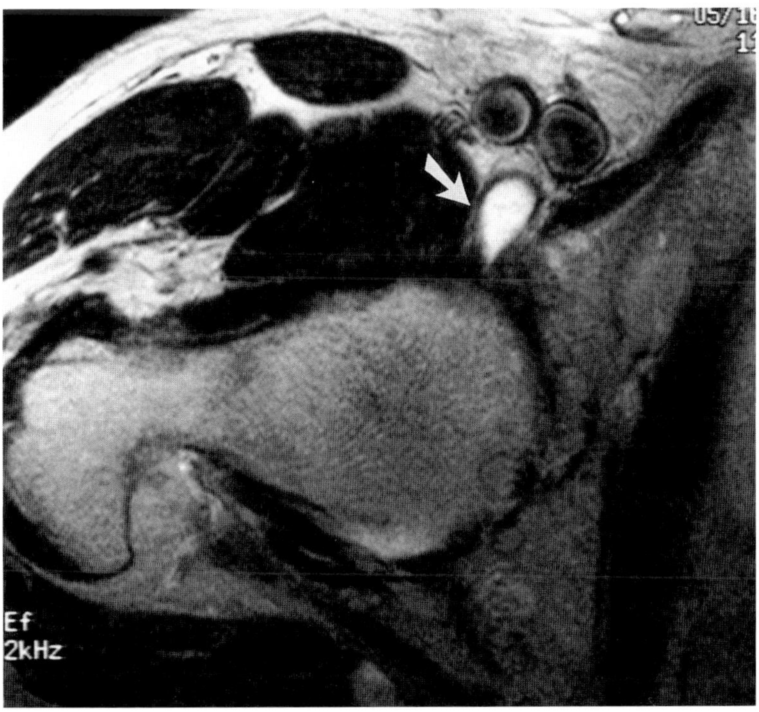

FIGURE 3.9 An 82-year-old woman with right hip pain. Axial FSE T2-weighted (3000/95) image with incomplete fat suppression shows a small, well-marginated, tear-drop shaped, hyperintense lesion (arrow) abutting the anterior acetabular labrum. Although it was felt that this finding could represent a small amount of fluid within the iliopsoas bursa, a labral cyst was favored due to the presence of prominent adjacent labral degeneration. (Courtesy of Phillip Tirman, MD).

4 Fluid-Filled Bursae

Popliteal Cyst (Baker's Cyst)

Definition. A popliteal (Baker's) cyst is a synovial cyst consisting of fluid accumulation within the gastrocnemiosemimembranosus bursa, which communicates with the knee joint through a weak point or tear in the posterior capsule. There may be a ball-valve mechanism with one-way directional flow from the joint space into the bursa. Any condition causing a knee joint effusion may result in popliteal cyst formation. Underlying etiologies include internal derangement/trauma, inflammatory disorders, degenerative joint disease, and neoplastic/proliferative processes.

Clinical Features. Popliteal cysts are very common and usually incidental findings. These lesions are seen on 5 to 41% of knee MRI examinations, with an increasing prevalence with age. They are rare in children. These cysts may become quite large, producing a palpable mass with or without pain. Hemorrhage into a popliteal cyst or rupture of a popliteal cyst may mimic thrombophlebitis clinically. A popliteal cyst may also be confused clinically with a soft tissue neoplasm, popliteal artery aneurysm, hematoma, or varicose vein.

Location. Popliteal cysts arise posterior to the medial femoral condyle between the tendons of the semimembranosus and medial head of the gastrocnemius muscles.

Implications. Popliteal cysts are usually incidental findings not requiring therapy. These lesions may rupture or hemorrhage. Very large lesions may cause mass effect on adjacent structures.

MRI Findings. Fluid accumulation is identified within the gastrocnemiosemimembranosus bursa. The signal intensity is typically isointense with adjacent joint fluid demonstrating homogeneously hypointense signal on T1-weighted images and very bright signal on T2-weighted sequences. Internal septations, debris, hemorrhage, or osteochondral bodies may be identified within a popliteal cyst. The cyst may be multiloculated. Typically, a thin neck of fluid is seen between the medial head of the gastrocnemius and semimembranosus tendons leading into a more prominent posterior component. Popliteal cysts may extend or dissect into the adjacent soft tissues.

Differential Diagnosis. Based upon fluid signal characteristics, an uncomplicated popliteal cyst should be readily differentiated from a neoplasm, popliteal aneurysm, varix, or hematoma. By knowing the precise anatomic position of a popliteal cyst, it is possible to differentiate other isolated fluid collections and cystic masses such as a meniscal cyst, ganglion cyst, pes anserine bursitis, tibial collateral ligament bursitis, and semimembranosus-tibial collateral ligament bursitis.

References

Fielding J, Franklin P, Kustan J. Popliteal cysts: A reassessment using magnetic resonance imaging. *Skeletal Radiol* 20:433–435, 1991.

Janzen D, Peterfy C, Forbes J, et al. Cystic lesions around the knee joint: MR imaging findings. *AJR* 163:155–161, 1994.

Lenchik L, Kier R. Popliteal cysts on MR imaging: Valve as an ancillary sign of meniscal tears. *AJR* 166:1232, 1996.

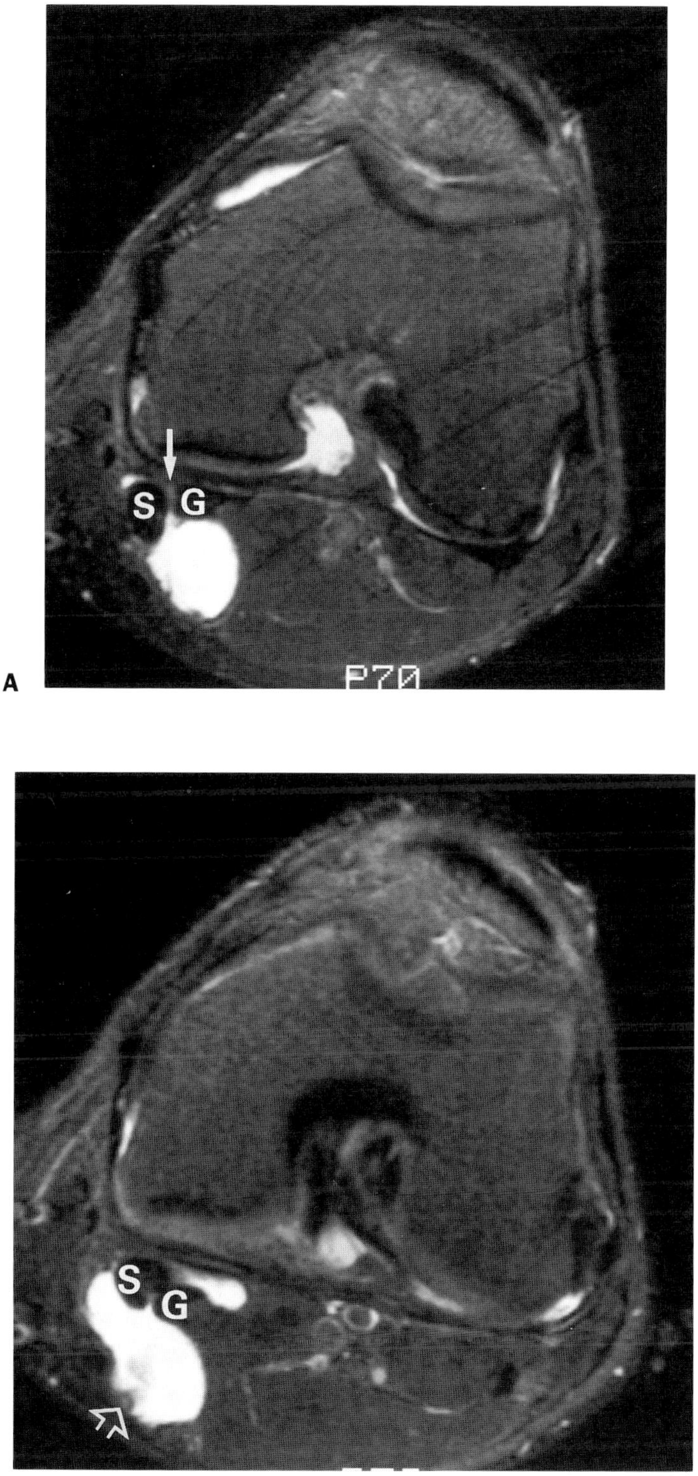

A

B

FIGURE 4.1 Popliteal cyst in a 36-year-old male. (A), (B) Axial FSE T2-weighted fat suppression images (3400/54) reveal fluid accumulation within the gastrocnemiosemimembranosus bursa. Note the thin neck of fluid (arrow) between the medial head of the gastrocnemius (G) and semimembranosus (S) tendons. Some internal debris is present (open arrow).

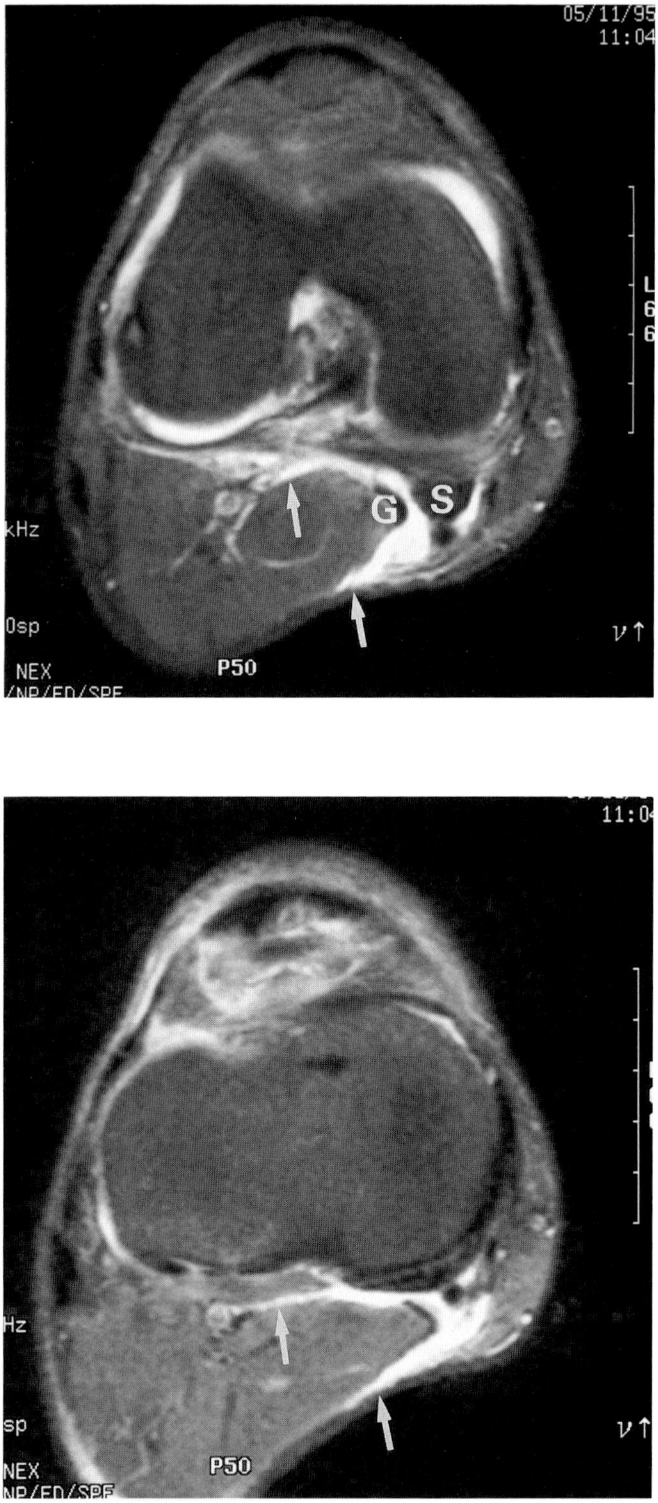

A

B

Figure 4.2 Ruptured popliteal cyst in a 37-year-old male. (A), (B) Axial FSE T2-weighted fat suppression images (3200/51) demonstrate fluid between and posterior to the gastrocnemius (G) and semimembranosus (S) tendons consistent with a popliteal cyst. Fluid is seen extending laterally and posteriorly (arrows) from the lesion consistent with rupture of the popliteal cyst.

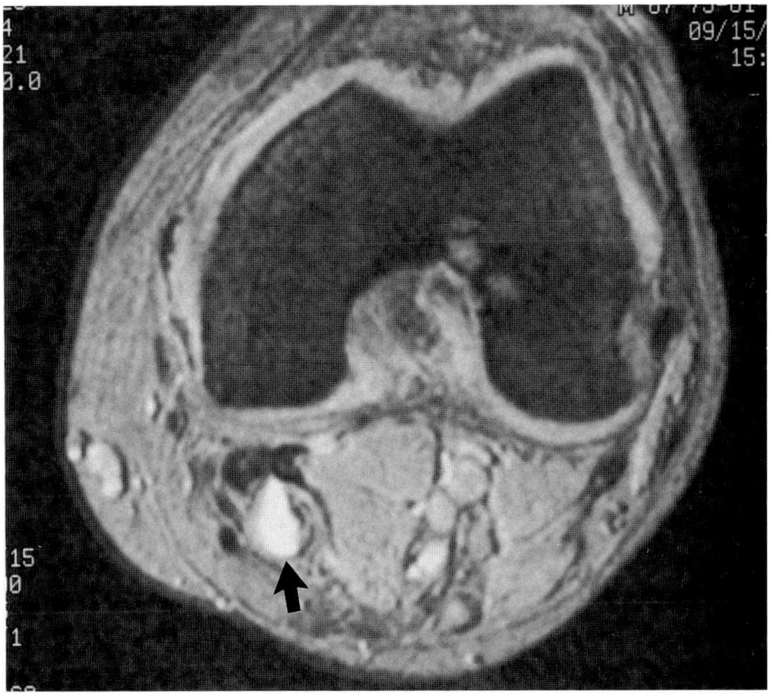

A

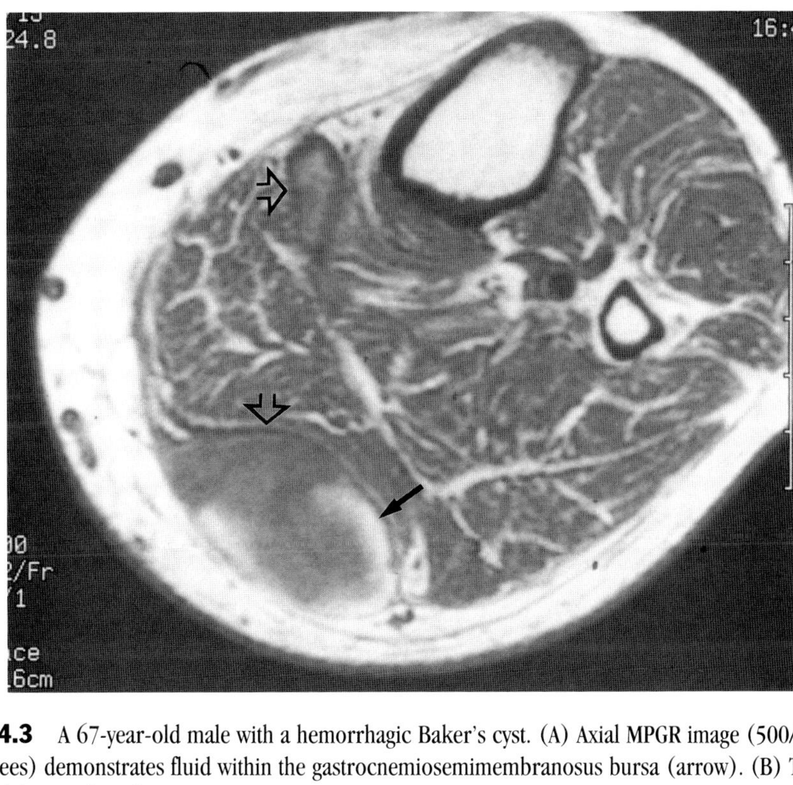

B

Figure 4.3 A 67-year-old male with a hemorrhagic Baker's cyst. (A) Axial MPGR image (500/15, 15 degrees) demonstrates fluid within the gastrocnemiosemimembranosus bursa (arrow). (B) T1-weighted (500/12) and

(continued)

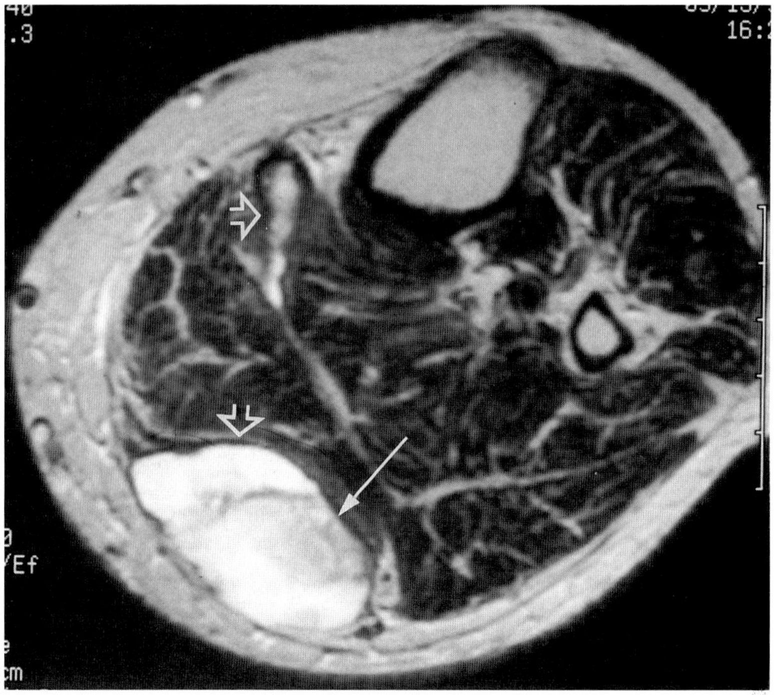

C

FIGURE 4.3 (continued) (C) FSE T2-weighted (3000/102) axial images of the calf demonstrate inferior dissection of the Baker's cyst (open arrows). Note the presence of bright signal within the lesion with T1-weighting (thin arrow) and heterogeneous signal on the T2-weighted image (long thin arrow) consistent with hemorrhage within the dissected Baker's cyst.

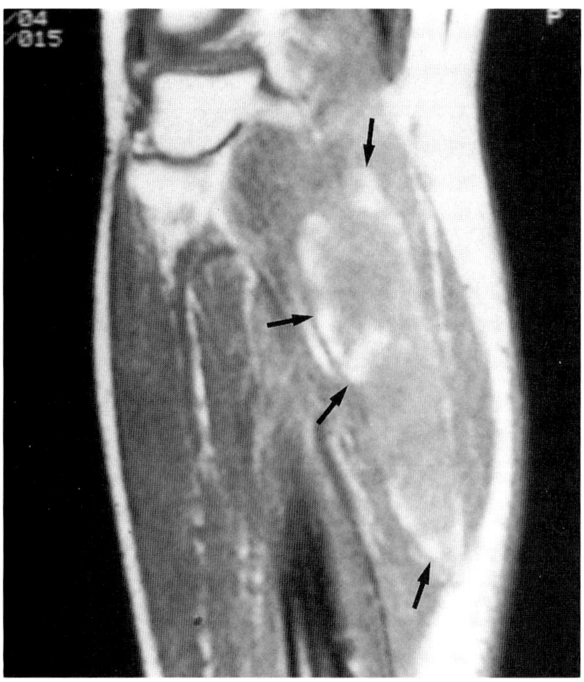

A

FIGURE 4.4 Hemorrhagic Baker's cyst in a 49-year-old male. (A) Sagittal T1-weighted image (617/11) demonstrates a dissected popliteal cyst within the posteromedial aspect of the upper calf. Areas of bright signal within the lesion (arrows) are consistent with hemorrhage. (B) Proton density (2000/18) and (C) T2-weighted (2000/80) axial images reveal heterogeneous areas of low signal intensity within the lesion (white arrows) due to hemorrhage.

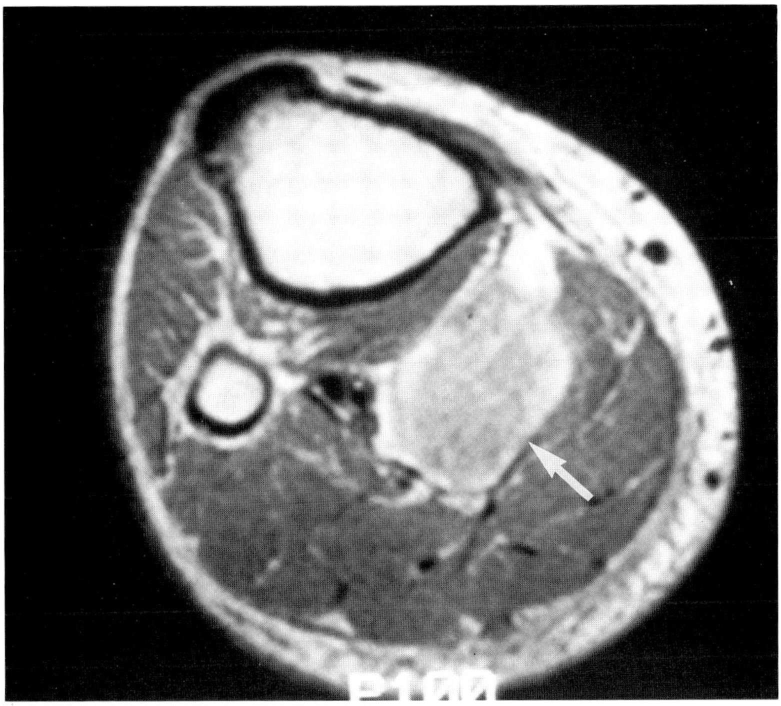

B

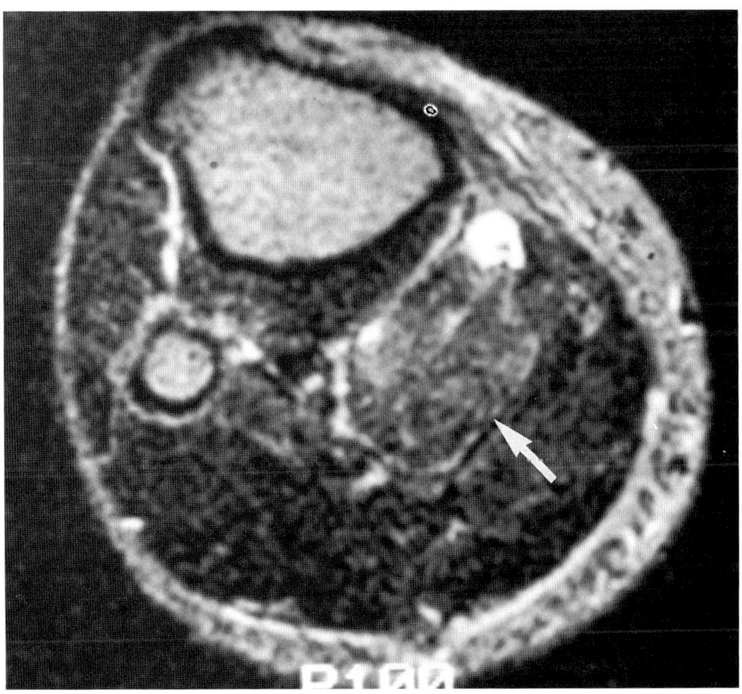

C

Pes Anserine Bursitis

Definition. This entity represents inflammation of the bursa beneath the pes anserinus tendons which may result from repetitive trauma. The term pes anserinus refers to the anatomic "goose's foot" appearance of the sartorius, gracilis, and semitendinosus tendons as they cross the proximal aspect of the tibia to insert on its medial surface. The bursa does not communicate with the knee joint.

Clinical Features. Patients of all ages may be affected. Chronic pes anserine bursitis seems to occur more frequently in patients with underlying osteoarthritis or rheumatoid arthritis. Most of these reported cases have also involved middle-aged to elderly women who are overweight. Acute pes anserine bursitis may occur more commonly in active, young to middle-aged patients. Patients may present with the classic symptoms of tenderness and swelling along the proximal tibia anteromedially or may complain of nonspecific medial knee pain which can mimic internal derangement of the knee. Symptoms may be exacerbated when ascending or descending stairs. A chronically inflamed bursa can present as a palpable mass lesion.

Location. The bursa is located immediately deep to the pes anserinus tendons near the insertion on the proximal tibia anteromedially. The proximal end of the pes anserine bursa is located 3–4 cm distal to the joint space. With inflammation and distension of the bursa, there may be extension of fluid around the tendons or along the tendons proximally.

Implications. Pes anserine bursitis is an important cause of medial knee pain which may mimic other causes of pain such as medial meniscal tear or cyst, medial collateral ligament injury, and medial patellar plica thickening. Once the diagnosis is suggested, the clinician may correlate the MRI findings with the physical examination findings to determine if pes anserine bursitis is causing the patient's symptoms. If other internal derangements of the knee are excluded, arthroscopy can be avoided and the patient may be treated conservatively with rest and nonsteroidal anti-inflammatory drugs. Refractory cases may respond to intrabursal steroid injection.

MRI Findings. One or more collections of fluid, which may be multiloculated, are seen beneath the pes anserinus tendons below the level of the knee joint. These fluid collections may track around the tendons or along the tendons proximally to a level at or above the knee joint line. The fluid collections are typically isointense with joint fluid on all pulse sequences, showing hypointense signal on T1-weighted images and very bright signal intensity with T2-weighting. The fluid collections are typically homogeneous, although internal debris, septations, or hemorrhage may be present.

Differential Diagnosis. The imaging differential diagnosis includes other isolated fluid collections and cystic masses such as meniscal cyst with parameniscal component, ganglion cyst, and semimembranosus-tibial collateral ligament bursitis. A meniscal cyst may be excluded by the absence of a meniscal tear extending into the fluid collection. The diagnosis of pes anserine bursitis would be preferred over ganglion cyst upon identification of the precise anatomic relationship of the fluid collection with the tendons. Semimembranosus-tibial collateral ligament bursitis appears as a fluid collection draped around the semimembranosus tendon at the level of the joint line. Differentiation from the latter entity can still occasionally be difficult, since overlap often occurs and it is not unusual to have fluid in the pes anserine and semimembranosus-tibial collateral ligament bursae concomitantly.

References

Forbes J, Helms C, Janzen D. Acute pes anserine bursitis: MR imaging. *Radiology* 194:525–527, 1995.

Zeiss J, Coombs R, Booth R, et al. Case report. Chronic bursitis presenting as a mass in the pes anserine bursa: MR diagnosis. *JCAT* 17:137–140, 1993.

A

B

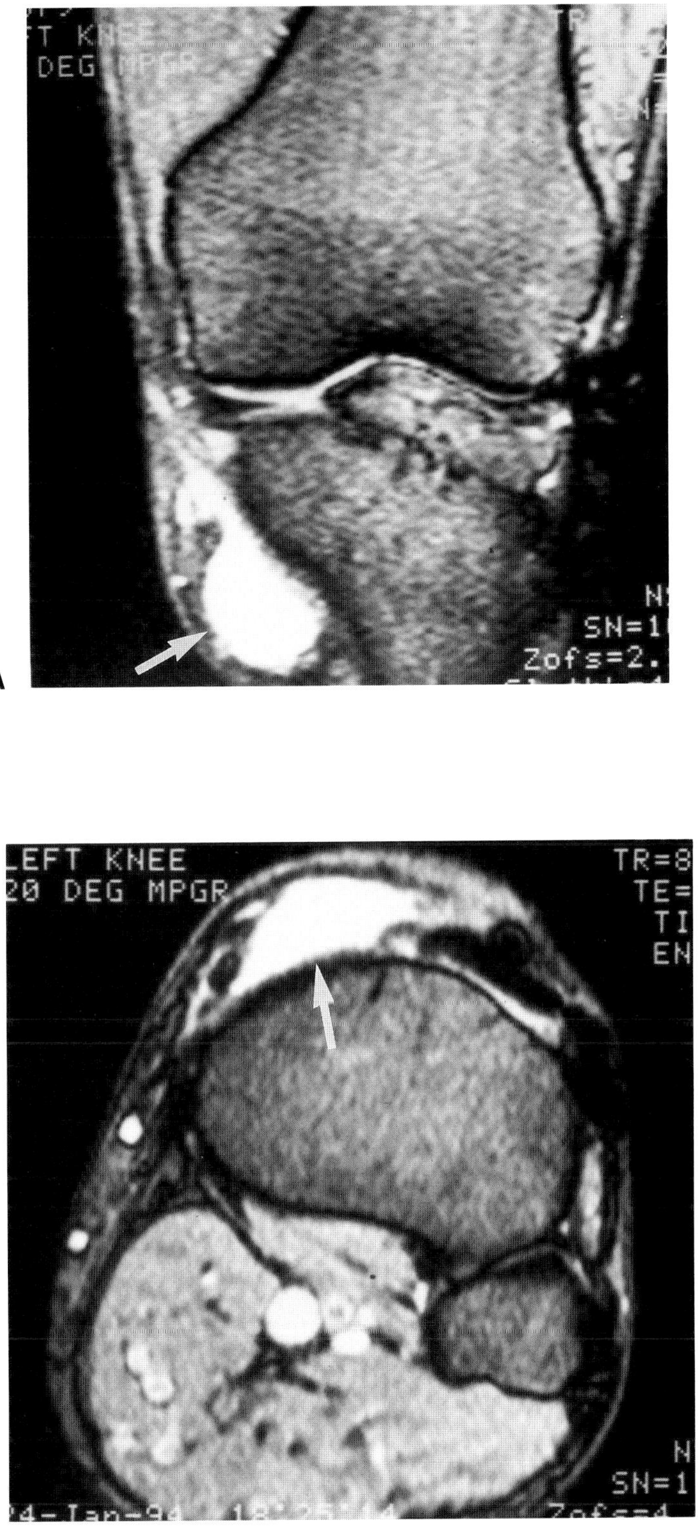

FIGURE 4.5 Pes anserinus bursitis in a patient with left knee pain and anteromedial swelling. MPGR (A) coronal (1000/27, 20 degrees) and (B) axial (800/18, 20 degrees) images demonstrate accumulation of fluid (arrows) near the anteromedial tibial insertion of the pes anserine tendons.

Semimembranosus-Tibial Collateral Ligament Bursitis

Definition. This entity is defined as inflammation of the bursa which drapes over the semimembranosus tendon as it crosses the knee joint line posteromedially. During extension, external rotation, and valgus stress of the knee, the semimembranosus tendon is "scissored" between the tibial collateral ligament and the medial tibial condyle. The semimembranosus-tibial collateral ligament bursa protects the tendon under these circumstances. Repetitive or acute trauma of this nature may result in bursitis.

Clinical Features. This entity seems to have a peak incidence in middle age. Patients usually present clinically with medial knee pain and tenderness, which may be acute or chronic. The symptoms can subside with conservative treatment and rest, but often return when normal activity is resumed. This bursitis can mimic other internal derangements of the knee.

Location. This bursa is shaped like an inverted U with a proximal deep pocket and a distal superficial pocket making up the two arms of the U. The proximal deep pocket lies between the semimembranosus tendon and the medial tibial condyle, whereas the distal superficial pocket lies between the semimembranosus tendon and the tibial collateral ligament. The two pockets are joined superiorly along the anterosuperior margin of the semimembranosus tendon. The bursa is located between the more superior semimembranosus-gastrocnemius bursa and the more inferior pes anserine bursa. It does not communicate with either of these bursae or the knee joint. The proximal end of the normal semimembranosus-tibial collateral ligament bursa is located where the semimembranosus tendon crosses the knee joint line posteromedially. The distal end of the bursa extends 1–2 cm below the joint line.

Implications. Once the MR diagnosis is suggested, the referring clinician can determine if the bursitis explains the patient's symptomatology. It is important not to misdiagnose this lesion as pes anserine bursitis which typically has pain and tenderness more anteroinferior to semimembranosus-tibial collateral ligament bursitis. If the MRI diagnosis does not match the clinical findings, unnecessary arthroscopy might be performed. A careful search should be performed for other causes of medial knee pain such as medial meniscal tear or cyst, medial collateral ligament injury, and medial patellar plica thickening. If these lesions and other internal derangements are excluded, the patient may be treated conservatively. Therapy consists of nonsteroidal anti-inflammatory agents and cessation of the offending activity either through immobilization or rest. Refractory cases can be treated with intrabursal steroid injection.

MRI Findings. The characteristic MRI features consist of fluid draped over the semimembranosus tendon in the shape of an inverted U. On coronal and sagittal images, the proximal-most portion of the semimembranosus-tibial collateral ligament bursa is seen adjacent to the posterior horn of the medial meniscus. The fluid collection should remain isointense to joint fluid on all pulse sequences, demonstrating low signal on T1-weighted images and hyperintense signal with T2-weighting. The signal intensity is typically homogeneous.

Differential Diagnosis. The imaging differential diagnosis consists of other isolated fluid collections and cystic masses, such as medial meniscal cyst with parameniscal component, ganglion cyst, popliteal cyst, pes anserine bursitis, and tibial collateral ligament bursitis. A meniscal cyst can be excluded by the absence of a meniscal tear extending into the fluid collection. Knowledge of the anatomy of this bursa should permit differentiation from a popliteal cyst, tibial collateral ligament bursitis, and pes anserine bursitis. The semimembranosus-gastrocnemius bursa (popliteal cyst) normally ends 1 cm proximal to the joint space. The proximal end of the pes anserine bursa is 3–4 cm distal to the joint space. Differentiation can still occasionally be difficult, however, as fluid can dissect into adjacent anatomic regions. Also, it is not unusual to have fluid in the pes anserine, tibial collateral ligament, or semimembranosus-gastrocnemius bursae concomitantly with semimembranosus-tibial collateral ligament bursitis. A ganglion cyst would not be expected to have the typical inverted U shape or precise anatomic location as the semimembranosus-tibial collateral ligament bursa.

References

Rothstein C, Laorr A, Helms C, et al. Semimembranosus-tibial collateral ligament bursitis: MR imaging findings. *AJR* 166:875–877, 1996.

Hennigan S, Schneck C, Mesgarzadeh M, et al. The semimembranosus-tibial collateral ligament bursa. *J of Bone Joint Surg* 76A:1322–1327, 1994.

A

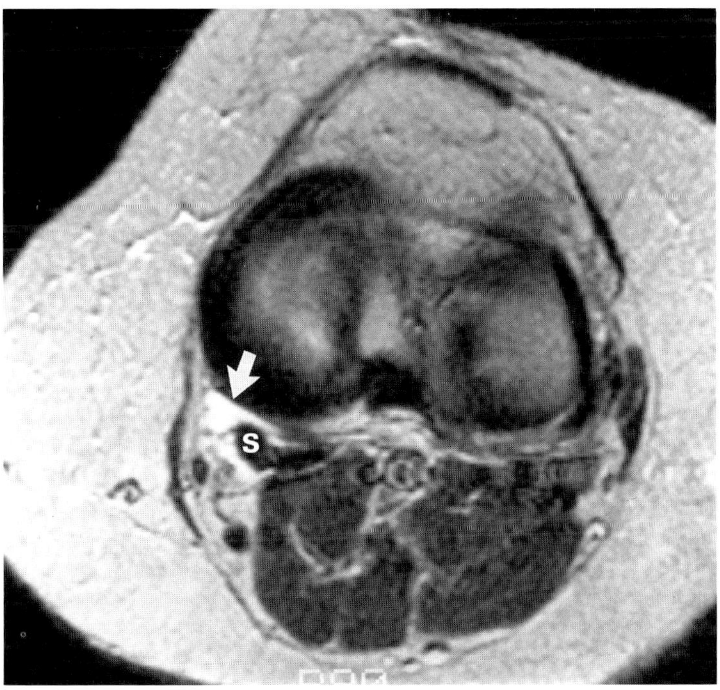

FIGURE 4.6 A 57-year-old woman with pain, tenderness, and swelling involving the medial left knee just below the joint line. (A) Axial T2-weighted image (2800/70) demonstrates an isolated collection of fluid (arrow) surrounding the semimembranosus tendon (S).

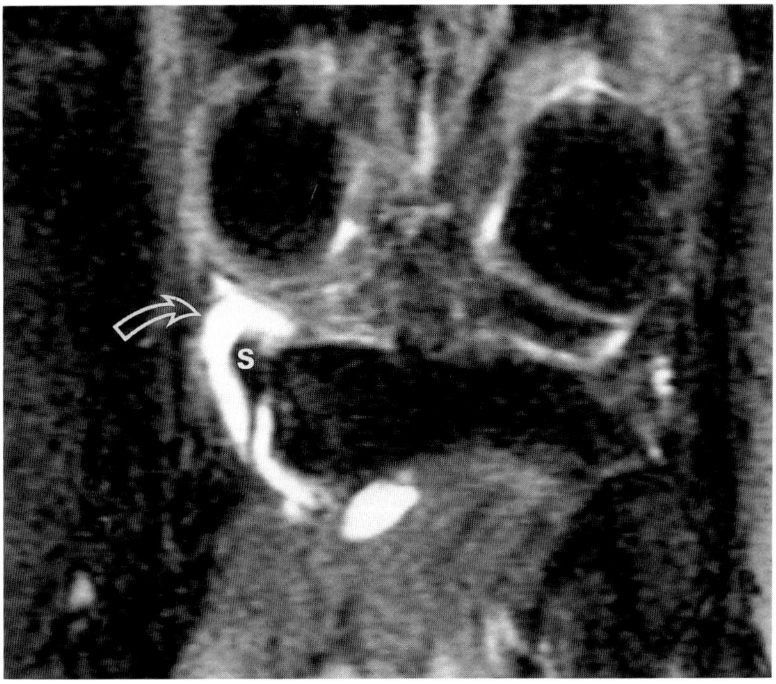

B

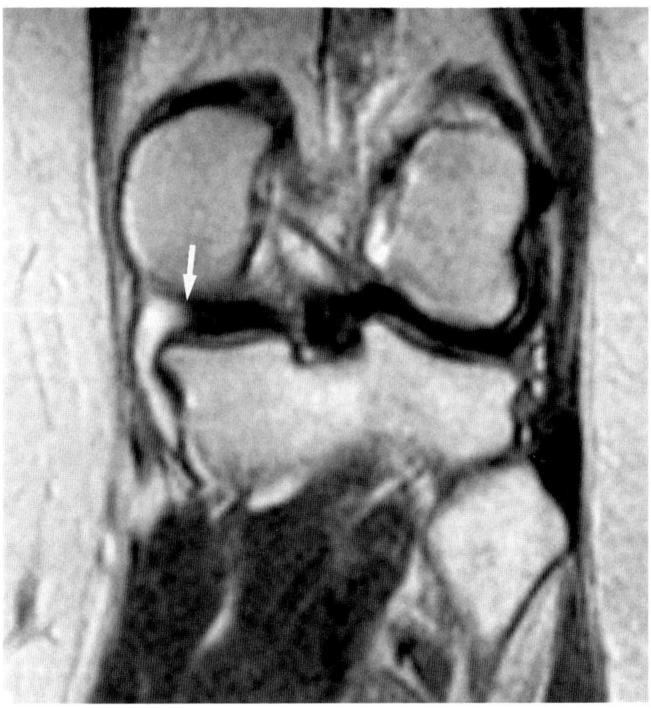

C

Figure 4.6 (continued) (B) Coronal FMPIR image (3733/28, TI-150) reveals a fluid collection in the shape of an inverted U (curved open arrow) draped over the semimembranosus tendon (S). (C) Coronal T2-weighted image (2000/70) shows the proximal portion of the fluid collection adjacent to the posterior horn of the medial meniscus (thin arrow).

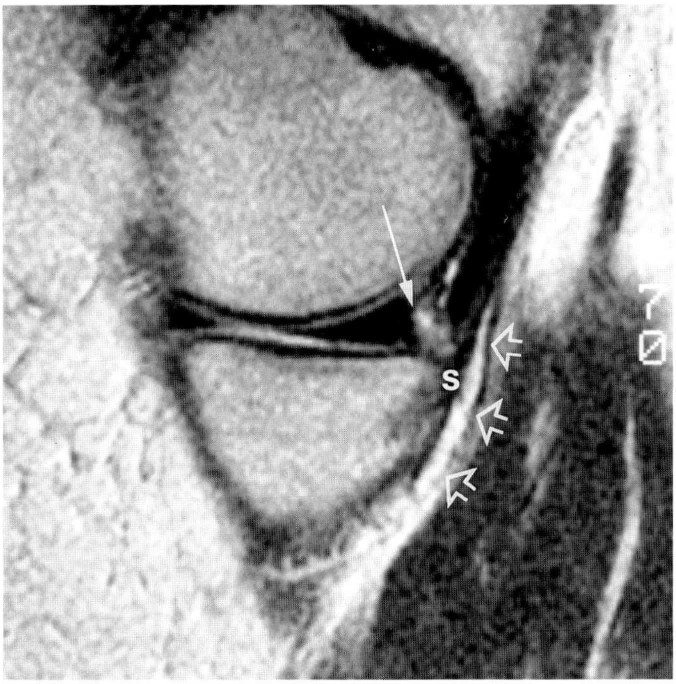

D

FIGURE 4.6 (continued) (D) Sagittal T2-weighted image (2000/70) depicts the proximal pole of the fluid collection adjacent to the posterior horn of the medial meniscus (long thin arrow) and the distal portion of the fluid collection (open arrows) extending along the semimembranosus tendon (S). These findings are diagnostic of semimembranosus-tibial collateral ligament bursitis.

Tibial Collateral Ligament Bursitis

Definition. Inflammation results in fluid accumulation within the tibial collateral ligament bursa. It is postulated that marginal osteophytes may deform the deep joint capsule and predispose to tibial collateral ligament bursitis.

Clinical Features. Tibial collateral ligament bursitis may be as common as inflammation of the pes anserine and prepatellar bursae. Patients typically present with isolated medial joint line pain in the absence of mechanical symptoms. A major criterion for the clinical diagnosis is prolonged pain relief following intrabursal steroid injection.

Location. The tibial collateral ligament bursa, which is variable in size, is interposed between the tibial collateral ligament (medial collateral ligament) and the deep joint capsule. This bursa has been identified in 93% of cadaveric knees.

Implications. This bursa must be distended with fluid in order to be visualized with MR imaging. Fluid may accumulate as a result of bursal inflammation, but may also result from acute injury of the tibial collateral ligament. If there is evidence of acute injury of the tibial collateral ligament, the diagnosis of tibial collateral ligament bursitis should probably be avoided because in these instances distension of the bursa most likely results from local hemorrhage or leakage of joint fluid through a ruptured deep capsule. Tibial collateral ligament bursitis can mimic other causes of medial knee pain such as medial meniscal tear or cyst, tibial collateral ligament injury, and medial patellar plica thickening. Once the diagnosis is suggested and other internal derangements of the knee are excluded, arthroscopy can be avoided and the patient may be treated with rest, nonsteroidal anti-inflammatory drugs, or intrabursal steroid injection.

MRI Findings. One or more well-defined fluid collections, which may be septated, are seen immediately deep to the tibial collateral ligament. The fluid may span the joint line or be located predominantly inferior to the joint line. In general, the fluid collection appears vertically elongated. The signal intensity is typically isointense with the adjacent joint fluid on all pulse sequences, demonstrating homogeneous low signal on T1-weighted images and bright signal intensity with T2-weighting.

Differential Diagnosis. The differential diagnosis of a fluid collection seen immediately deep to the tibial collateral ligament also includes meniscal cyst, ganglion cyst, and meniscocapsular separation. A meniscal cyst may be excluded by the absence of a meniscal tear seen extending into the fluid collection. A ganglion cyst may have a similar appearance, but is typically not associated with pain and should not be in the precise anatomic position of the tibial collateral ligament bursa, which is interposed between the tibial collateral ligament and the deep joint capsule. Meniscocapsular separation appears as fluid between the tibial collateral ligament and medial meniscus, but this fluid does not typically appear as a discrete fluid collection. Additionally, medial pain associated with meniscocapsular separation would be expected to have an abrupt onset following an injury. Pes anserine bursitis and semimembranosus-tibial collateral ligament bursitis are also causes of medial knee pain, but should be distinguishable from tibial collateral ligament bursitis on anatomic grounds. The pes anserine bursa is located more anterior and inferior to the tibial collateral ligament bursa. The semimembranosus-tibial collateral ligament bursa typically appears as a fluid collection in the shape of an inverted U, which is draped over the semimembranosus tendon. Either of these two entities may be seen concomitantly with tibial collateral ligament bursitis.

References

Lee J, Yao L. Tibial collateral ligament bursa: MR imaging. *Radiology* 178:855–857, 1991.

Rothstein C, Laorr A, Helms C, et al. Semimembranosus-tibial collateral ligament bursitis: MR imaging findings. *AJR* 166:875–877, 1996.

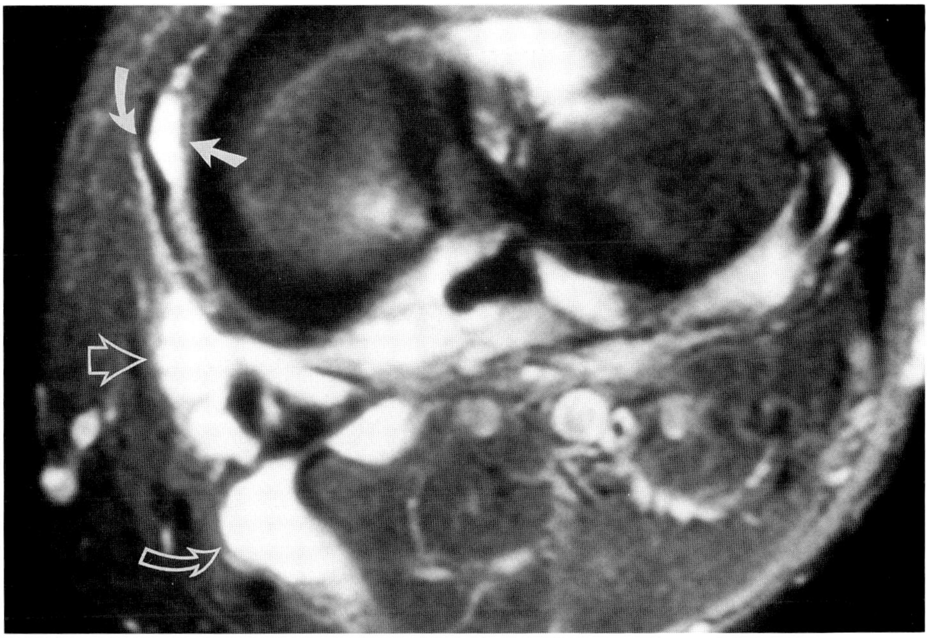

FIGURE 4.7 A 51-year-old male with medial knee pain. Axial FSE T2-weighted fat suppression image reveals a fluid collection (arrow) immediately deep to the medial collateral ligament (curved arrow) consistent with tibial collateral ligament bursitis. In addition, fluid is seen within the semimembranosus-tibial collateral ligament bursa (open arrow) and the gastrocnemiosemimembranosus bursa (curved open arrow). (Rothstein C, Laorr A, Helms C, et al. Semimembranosus-tibial collateral ligament bursitis: MR imaging findings. *AJR* 166:875–877, 1996. Reprinted with permission.)

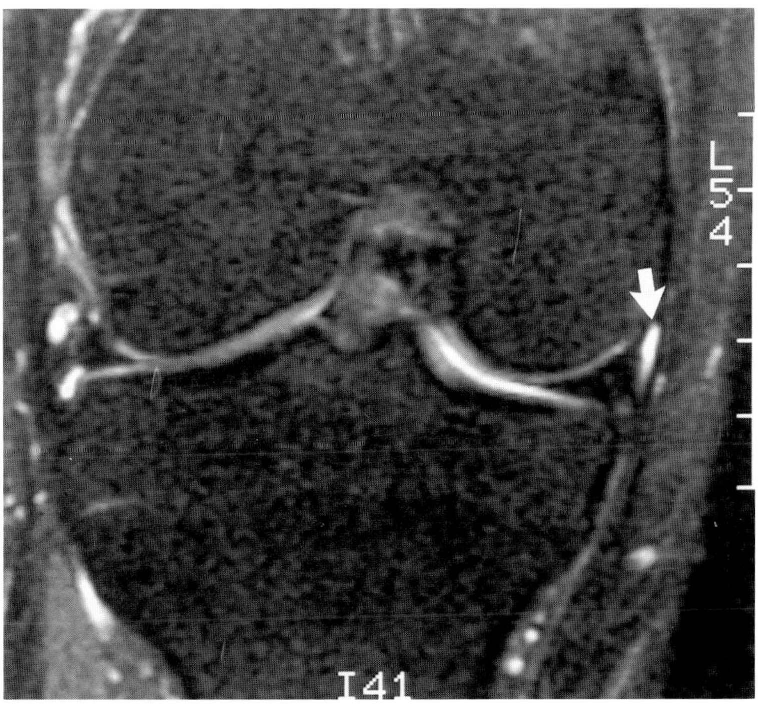

FIGURE 4.8 Coronal FSE T2-weighted fat suppression image (4150/54) of a 37-year-old man demonstrates a small amount of fluid within the tibial collateral ligament bursa (arrow).

Prepatellar Bursitis

Definition. The prepatellar bursa is a synovium-lined potential space anterior to the patella. This bursa normally contains only a minimal amount of fluid, which is not detected on imaging studies. Inflammation of this bursa results from chronic trauma to the prepatellar soft tissues, which are compressed between the patella and a hard surface during such activities as kneeling or crawling. Prepatellar bursitis has also been termed "housemaid's knee" or "carpet-layer's knee."

Clinical Features. Patients present with pain, swelling, and tenderness over the patella. Infectious bursitis may result from penetrating trauma.

Location. The prepatellar bursa is located between the patella and the overlying skin.

Implications. Symptoms typically subside following cessation of the offending activity. Infectious bursitis may require drainage.

MRI Findings. With inflammation, the prepatellar bursa becomes distended with fluid and typically appears as an elliptical fluid collection located anterior to the patella and patellar tendon. The fluid collection demonstrates hypointense signal intensity on T1-weighted images and bright signal intensity on T2-weighted sequences. The signal intensity is often heterogeneous and poorly defined due to the presence of internal debris and hemorrhage.

Differential Diagnosis. Prepatellar bursitis should usually be distinguishable from other fluid collections in this area such as a hematoma or abscess on the basis of clinical history.

References

Munk P, Helms C. *MRI of the Knee*. Gaithersburg, MD; Aspen Publishers; 1992, pp 53–54.

Janzen D, Peterfy C, Forbes J, et al. Cystic lesions around the knee joint: MR imaging findings. *AJR* 163:155–161, 1994.

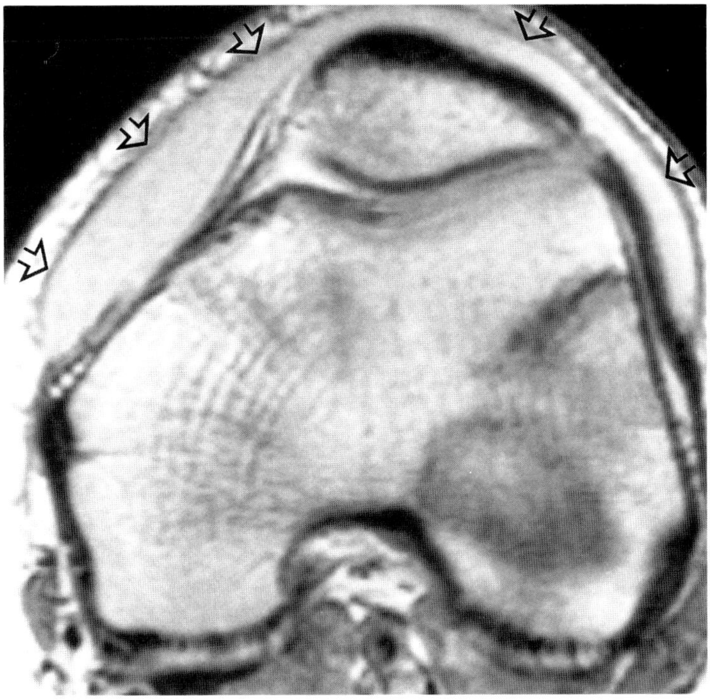

A

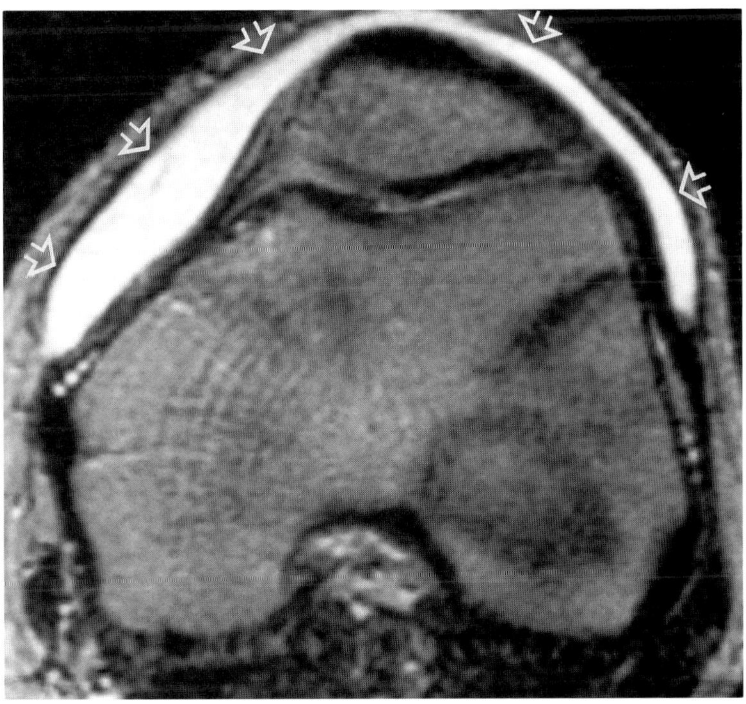

B

FIGURE 4.9 A 17-year-old male with prepatellar bursitis. (A) Proton density (2000/20) and (B) T2-weighted (2000/70) axial scans demonstrate an elongated fluid collection (open arrows) extending across the anterior aspect of the knee at the level of the patella.

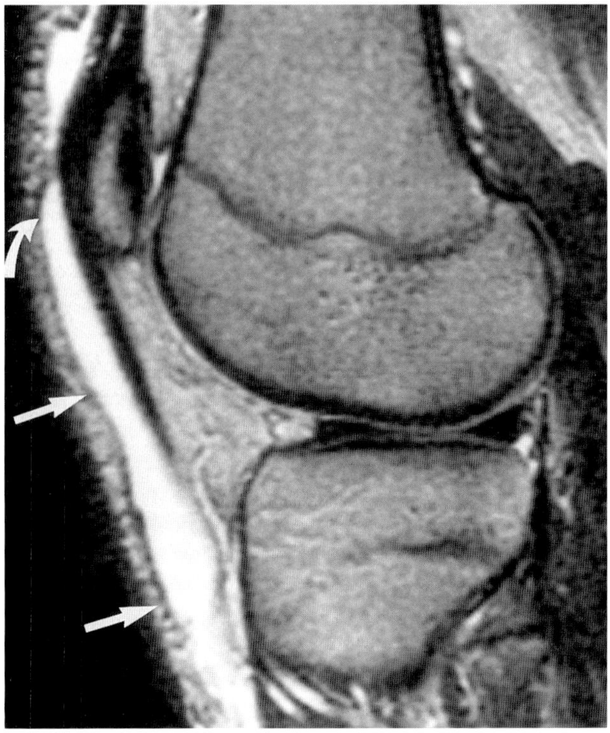

C

FIGURE 4.9 (continued) (C) Sagittal T2-weighted image (2000/70) reveals extension of bursal fluid (arrows) along the anterior aspects of the patella and patellar tendon.

Trochanteric Bursitis

Definition. The trochanteric bursa consists anatomically of three distinct bursae around the greater trochanter of the femur. Trochanteric bursitis consists of fluid accumulation within the bursa as a result of inflammation or infection. Repetitive sliding of the tensor fascia lata over the greater trochanter may cause inflammation of this bursa. The trochanteric bursa may also become inflamed or infected following total hip arthroplasty. The inflamed bursa frequently communicates with the hip joint space in patients with prior hip surgery or disease of the hip joint, but this communication is rare in those without these conditions.

Clinical Features. Predisposing factors for trochanteric bursitis include hip joint abnormality, previous hip surgery, altered gait, obesity, and trauma (acute or chronic/repetitive in nature). Trochanteric bursitis is a frequent cause of hip pain and typically affects middle-aged and older individuals. Women are more commonly affected. This condition is common in runners and racquet sport players. Patients typically complain of pain at the lateral aspect of the hip or thigh. Physical examination reveals point tenderness near the inferior portion of the greater trochanter. Fluid distension of the trochanteric bursa may also be seen in asymptomatic individuals.

Location. The three discrete bursae comprising the trochanteric bursa are the gluteus maximus, medius, and minimus bursae which are located between the respective tendons and the greater trochanter. The gluteus maximus bursa is the largest of the three and is located posteriorly, whereas the gluteus medius and minimus bursae are located anterior to the greater trochanter.

Implications. Treatment consists principally of activity modification, nonsteroidal anti-inflammatory medications, and physical therapy. Refractory cases may be treated with intrabursal steroid injection.

MRI Findings. The MRI appearance consists of a fluid collection intimately associated with the greater trochanter. The signal is typically hypointense on T1-weighted sequences and markedly hyperintense on T2-weighted sequences, similar to that of joint fluid. The signal is generally homogeneous in appearance, but may appear heterogeneous if there is internal debris or associated infection. MRI cannot reliably differentiate between an inflamed and infected bursa.

Differential Diagnosis. The MRI differential diagnosis consists principally of other fluid collections such as iliopsoas bursitis, hematoma, and abscess. Iliopsoas bursitis can be distinguished with knowledge of the anatomic sites of these two bursae. A hematoma should be distinguishable based upon clinical grounds and would also typically demonstrate heterogeneous signal intensity. A hematoma may also contain areas of bright signal on T1-weighted sequences due to the presence of methemoglobin. An abscess would not be expected to precisely correspond to the anatomic position of the trochanteric bursa. Most soft tissue tumors do not exhibit signal intensity as high as fluid on T2-weighted sequences, although there are exceptions (i.e., myxoma). In addition, knowledge of the exact anatomic location of this bursa should enable differentiation from the vast majority of soft tissue tumors about the hip. Intravenous gadolinium may also be helpful in difficult cases since a distended bursa would exhibit only peripheral rim enhancement.

References

Varma D, Parihar A, Richli W. CT appearance of the distended trochanteric bursa. *JCAT* 17:141–143, 1993.

Mink J, Deutsch A. *MRI of the Musculoskeletal System. A Teaching File.* New York, NY; Raven Press; 1990, pp 228–229.

Stoller D. *Magnetic Resonance Imaging in Orthopaedics and Sports Medicine*. Philadelphia, PA; J.B. Lippincott Company; 1993, pp 98, 101.

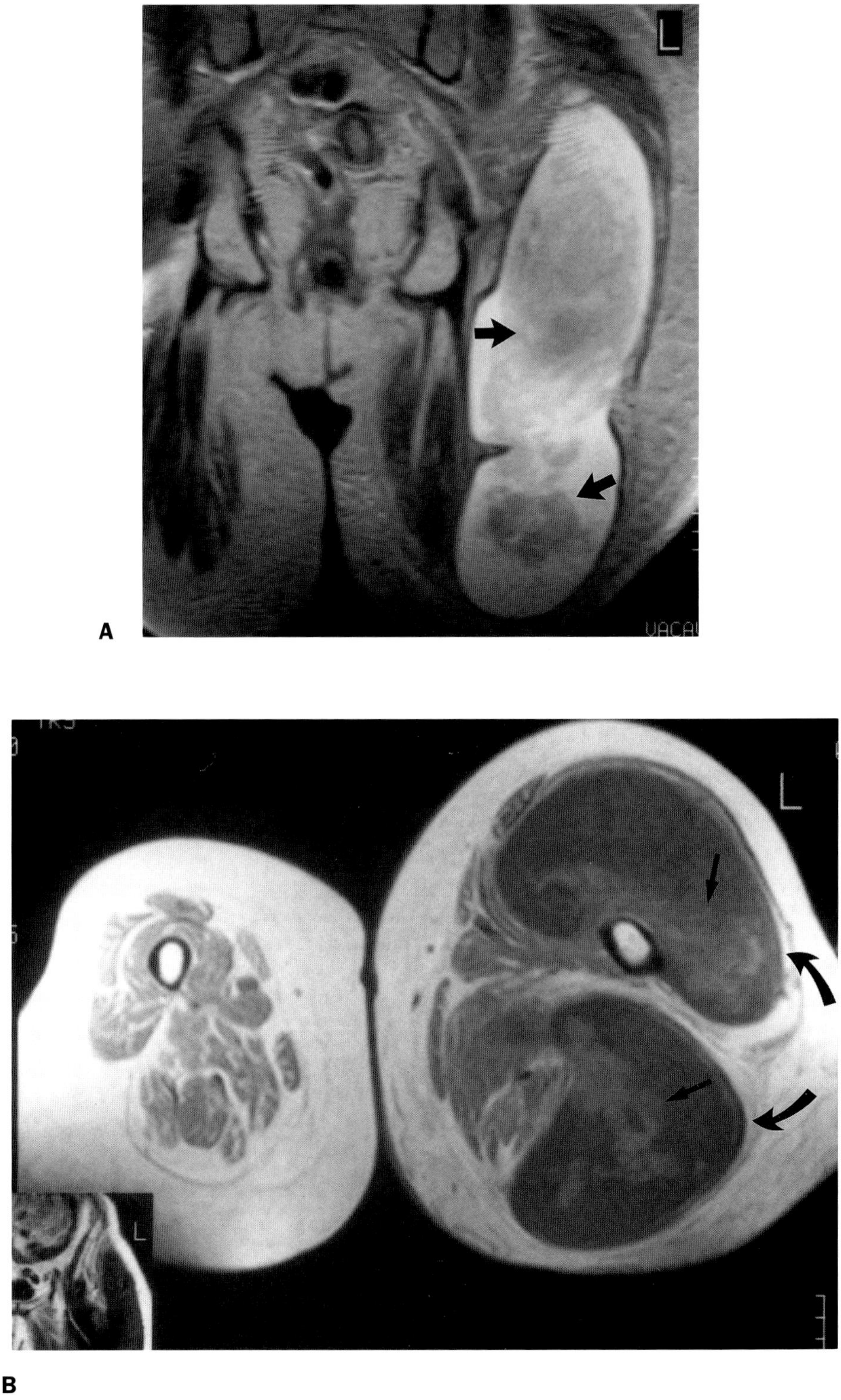

FIGURE 4.10 A 78-year-old woman status post total left hip arthroplasty presented with a large palpable mass lesion around the left hip and upper thigh. (A) Coronal T2-weighted image (3620/80) posterior to the left hip joint reveals a portion of the markedly distended greater trochanteric bursa. Note the relatively hypointense signal centrally (arrows) consistent with internal debris. (B) Axial T1-weighted image (800/25) of the upper thighs reveals a bilobed configuration of the prominently distended bursa with anterior and posterior components (curved arrows). There are internal areas of intermediate signal intensity consistent with debris (thin arrows).

Iliopsoas Bursitis

Definition. The iliopsoas bursa is the largest bursa around the hip joint, measuring approximately 4×7 cm. This bursa is found in approximately 98% of individuals and communicates with the hip joint space in about 15% of patients. The normal bursa is collapsed. Fluid accumulation within this bursa may result from various disease processes of the hip which lead to increased intra-articular pressure and extension of synovial fluid into the bursa. The most commonly associated disease entity of the hip is osteoarthritis, but numerous other associated processes including rheumatoid arthritis, pigmented villonodular synovitis, synovial chondromatosis, trauma, surgery, gout, osteonecrosis, and septic arthritis have been reported. Age-related synovial proliferation within the bursa itself may result in overproduction of bursal fluid and distention of the bursa.

Clinical Features. Iliopsoas bursitis typically occurs in patients over the age of 50. It is extremely rare in children. Affected patients often have associated disease of the hip joint, frequently long-standing. The clinical features are variable and patients may present with pain, a mass lesion, symptoms related to compression of adjacent structures, or secondary infection. Patients may also be asymptomatic. Pain (present in about 40% of cases) may be localized or referred to the lower extremity, hip, or abdomen. A palpable groin mass is present in approximately 40% of cases. Neuropathy may result from compression of the femoral nerve. Compression of the femoral or iliac veins may result in lower extremity edema. There may also be symptoms related to compression of the bladder, ureter, or bowel. In addition, a distended iliopsoas bursa may rupture or dissect into adjacent soft tissues.

Location. The iliopsoas bursa is interposed between the iliopsoas muscle and the anterior hip joint capsule and is located lateral to the femoral vessels.

Implications. For those cases associated with hip joint abnormality, treatment should be directed toward the articular process. Cases of isolated iliopsoas bursitis may be treated with nonsteroidal anti-inflammatory medications and possibly intrabursal steroid injection.

MRI Findings. On MRI, iliopsoas bursitis appears as a well-marginated single or multiloculated mass which exhibits hypointense signal on T1-weighted images and markedly hyperintense signal on T2-weighted sequences. The signal intensity should parallel adjacent joint fluid on all pulse sequences. There may be solid components contained within the distended bursa representing cellular debris, fibrin, hemorrhage, loose bodies, or synovial proliferation. The signal intensity of these internal components is variable depending on the composition, but is most often hypointense on T2-weighted sequences. The bursal fluid may dissect anteriorly between the iliopsoas tendon and the pectineus muscle and extend inferiorly toward the lesser trochanter or superiorly as far as the pelvic cavity. Changes of associated hip joint space abnormality and joint effusion are frequently seen.

Differential Diagnosis. Based upon signal characteristics and knowledge of the anatomic position of this bursa, iliopsoas bursitis should be readily distinguished from other mass lesions in this area including soft tissue tumors, inguinal hernia, adenopathy, aneurysm, hematoma, and undescended testis. If distinction is still not possible, gadolinium administration may be helpful for differentiation since the distended bursa should exhibit only peripheral rim enhancement. MRI cannot reliably distinguish between an inflamed and an infected bursa.

References

Varma D, Richli W, Charnsangavej C, et al. MR appearance of the distended iliopsoas bursa. *AJR* 156:1025–1028, 1991.

Meaney J, Cassar-Pullicino V, Etherington R, et al. Iliopsoas Bursa Enlargement. *Clin Radiol* 45:161–168, 1992.

Pritchard R, Shah H, Nelson C, et al. MR and CT appearance of iliopsoas bursal distension secondary to diseased hips. *JCAT* 14:797–800, 1990.

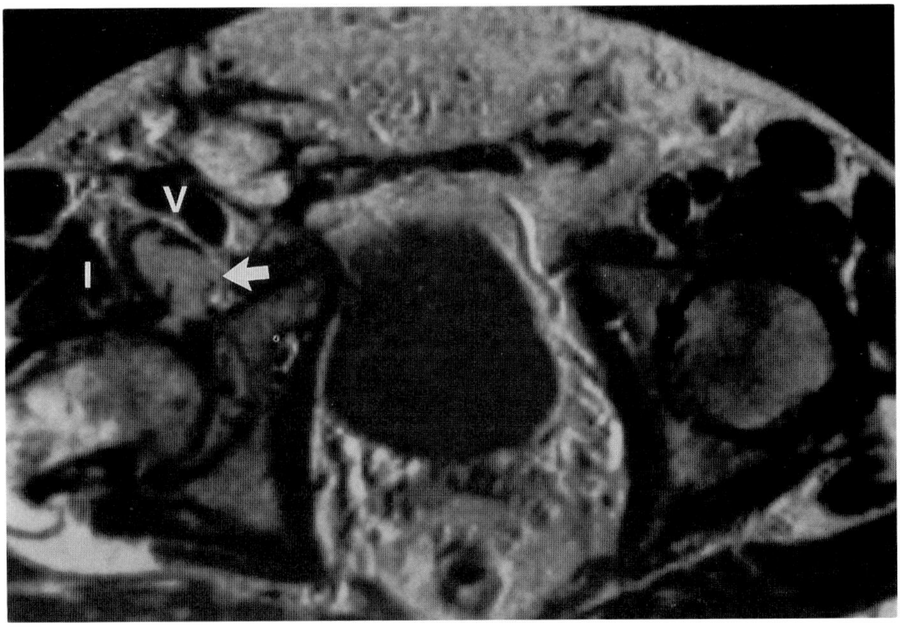

A

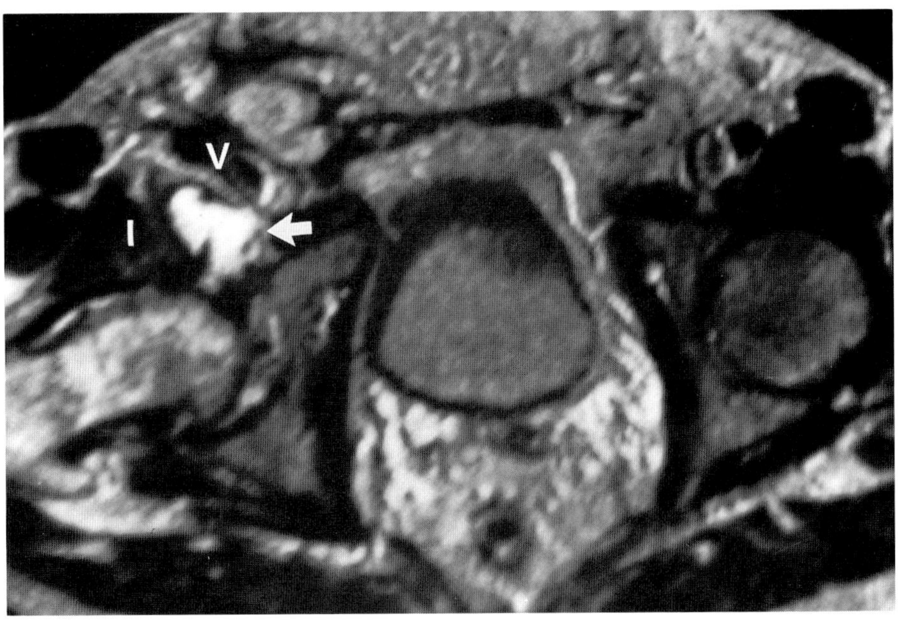

B

FIGURE 4.11 Iliopsoas bursitis. (A) Proton density and (B) T2-weighted axial images demonstrate fluid accumulation within the iliopsoas bursa (arrows). It is located between the anterior hip joint and the iliopsoas muscle (I) and is lateral to the femoral vessels (V). Note the associated right hip pathology.

5 Vascular Lesions

Hemangioma of Soft Tissue

Definition. Soft tissue hemangiomas are benign vascular neoplasms which are composed of cavernous, capillary, or venous vascular channels. Histologic examination demonstrates endothelial-lined vascular channels of variable diameter, which are separated by fibrous and/or fatty linear strands. The vascular channels are oriented in a parallel or striated configuration. In any particular lesion, the fatty or fibrous component may be prominent. Frequently, fatty tissue is present in the margins. These lesions are histopathologically identical to hemangiomas of bone.

Clinical Features. Hemangioma is the most common vascular tumor of the soft tissues. In addition, it is the most common soft tissue tumor in infants and children. Most cutaneous hemangiomas are asymptomatic and rarely evaluated radiographically. The majority of deeper soft tissue hemangiomas remain asymptomatic until late childhood or early adulthood, when they may present as palpable masses with pain or swelling. Frequently, these lesions are accompanied by overlying skin changes such as reddish-blue discoloration or enlarged veins. Rarely, they may be associated with pulsation or bruit on physical examination. Young women are most frequently affected, but hemangiomas may occur at any age.

Location. Hemangiomas may arise in any tissue but are particularly common in the skin. They may have a regional distribution such as an entire extremity, but are far more commonly localized. Deeper soft tissue hemangiomas may involve muscle, tendon, connective tissue, or fat. A relatively common location involves skeletal muscle in the lower extremities.

Implications. Cutaneous lesions that present early in life have a favorable prognosis and typically regress spontaneously. Other lesions are cured with surgical excision. They may hemorrhage considerably with percutaneous biopsy or open biopsy. Hemangiomas may be associated with consumption coag ulopathy or cardiac decompensation, if large. Growth disturbances may occur including overgrowth of the involved extremity or less commonly shortening of the involved extremity.

MRI Findings. Hemangiomas less than 2 cm in size are typically homogeneously bright on T2-weighted sequences. Lesions larger than 2 cm usually show a characteristic striated-septated appearance on T2-weighted images. In this configuration, serpiginous high-signal zones (which represent stagnant blood in vascular channels) are seen with intervening low signal intensity linear or round areas (which correspond to fibrofatty septa and thrombosed vascular channels). Marginal fat in these lesions appears hyperintense on T1-weighted images. The shape of the mass is often multilobulated or tubular. Calcification within hemangiomas is common, appearing as hypointense foci on all pulse sequences. Phleboliths are a specific type of calcification which may be identified and are highly suggestive of the diagnosis. However, identification of phleboliths is easier with plain radiographs. Fluid-fluid levels, which are nonspecific, may be seen within the lesion. Associated muscle atrophy or overgrowth of the adjacent bone and soft tissue may be present.

Differential Diagnosis. The differential diagnosis of soft tissue hemangiomas includes other fat-containing masses such as lipoma, atypical lipoma, and well-differentiated liposarcoma. A hemangioma may be distinguished from these lesions by the identification of the distinctive striated-septated appearance or by the presence of phleboliths on MRI or plain radiography.

References

Cohen E, Kressel H, Perosio T, et al. MR imaging of soft-tissue hemangiomas: Correlation with pathologic findings. *AJR* 150:1079–1081, 1988.

Suh J, Hwang G, Hahn S. Soft tissue hemangiomas: MR manifestations in 23 patients. *Skeletal Radiol* 23:621–625, 1994.

Nelson M, Stull M, Teitelbaum G, et al. Magnetic resonance imaging of peripheral soft tissue hemangiomas. *Skeletal Radiol* 19:477–482, 1990.

Hawnaur J, Whitehouse R, Jenkins J, et al. Musculoskeletal haemangiomas: Comparison of MRI with CT. *Skeletal Radiol* 19:251–258, 1990.

Madewell J, Sweet D. Tumors and tumor-like lesions in or about joints. In Resnick D: *Bone and Joint Imaging*. Philadelphia, PA; W.B. Saunders Co; 1989: p 1184.

Ehara S, Sone M, Tamakawa Y, et al. Fluid-fluid levels in cavernous hemangioma of soft tissue. *Skeletal Radiol* 23:107–109, 1994.

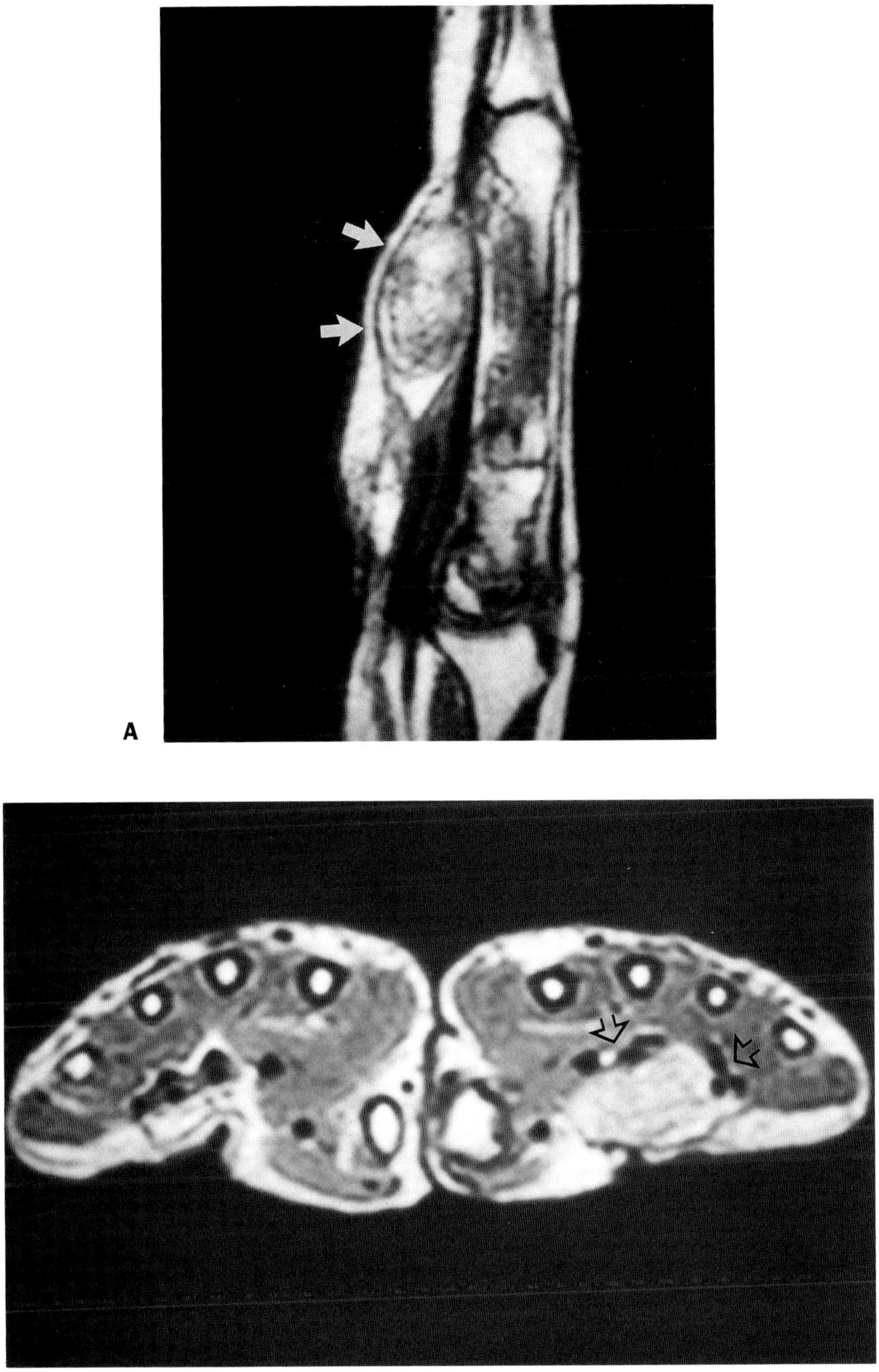

A

B

FIGURE 5.1 A 58-year-old woman with a hemangioma of the left hand. (A) Sagittal T1-weighted image reveals an oval mass (arrows) involving the volar soft tissues of the hand. Note the extensive hyperintense signal within the lesion, likely reflecting a predominant fatty component. (B) Proton density and

(continued)

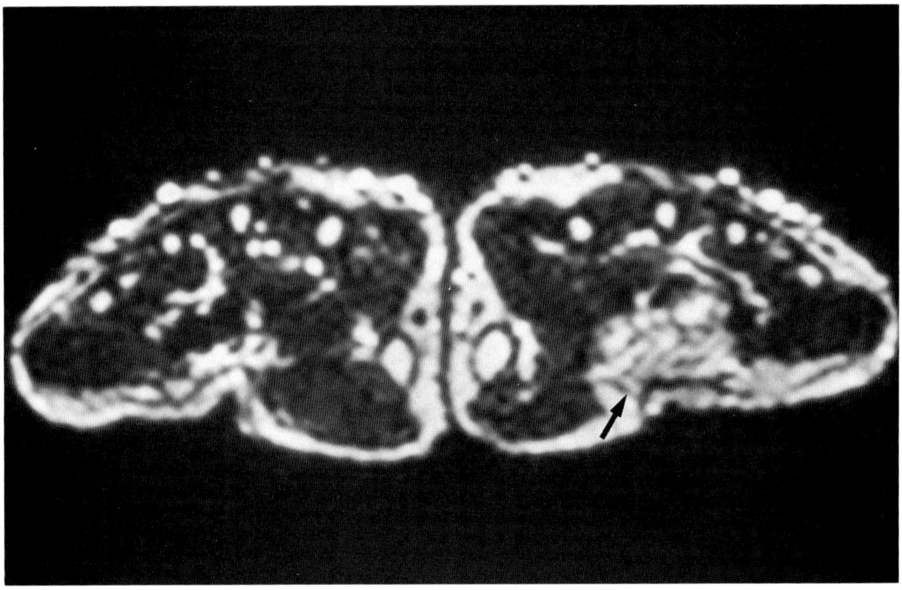

C

FIGURE 5.1 (continued) (C) T2-weighted axial images demonstrate mass effect on the flexor tendons (open arrows). Note the characteristic striated-septated appearance on the T2-weighted image (thin arrow).

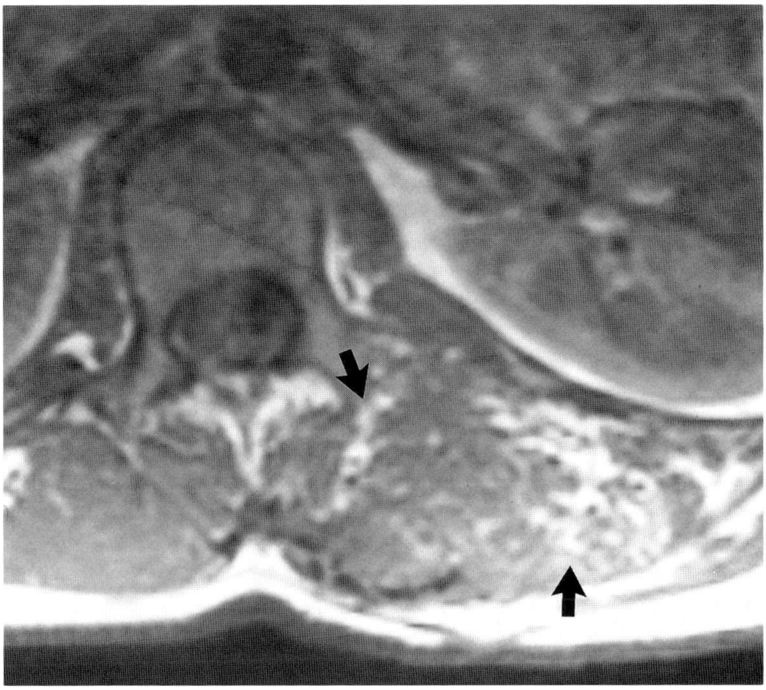

A

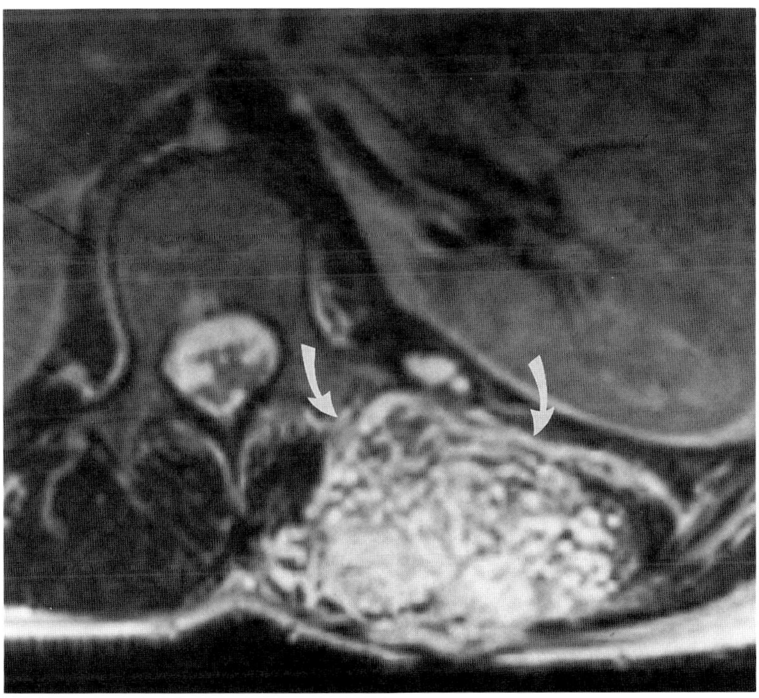

B

FIGURE 5.2 A 30-year-old woman with a soft tissue hemangioma of the upper lumbar paraspinous region. (A) T1-weighted (600/11) and (B) FSE T2-weighted (3700/102) axial scans demonstrate a hemangioma which is partially ill-defined. Note the bright areas within the lesion with T1-weighting (arrows) likely corresponding to fat, as well as the characteristic striated-septated appearance with T2-weighting (curved arrows).

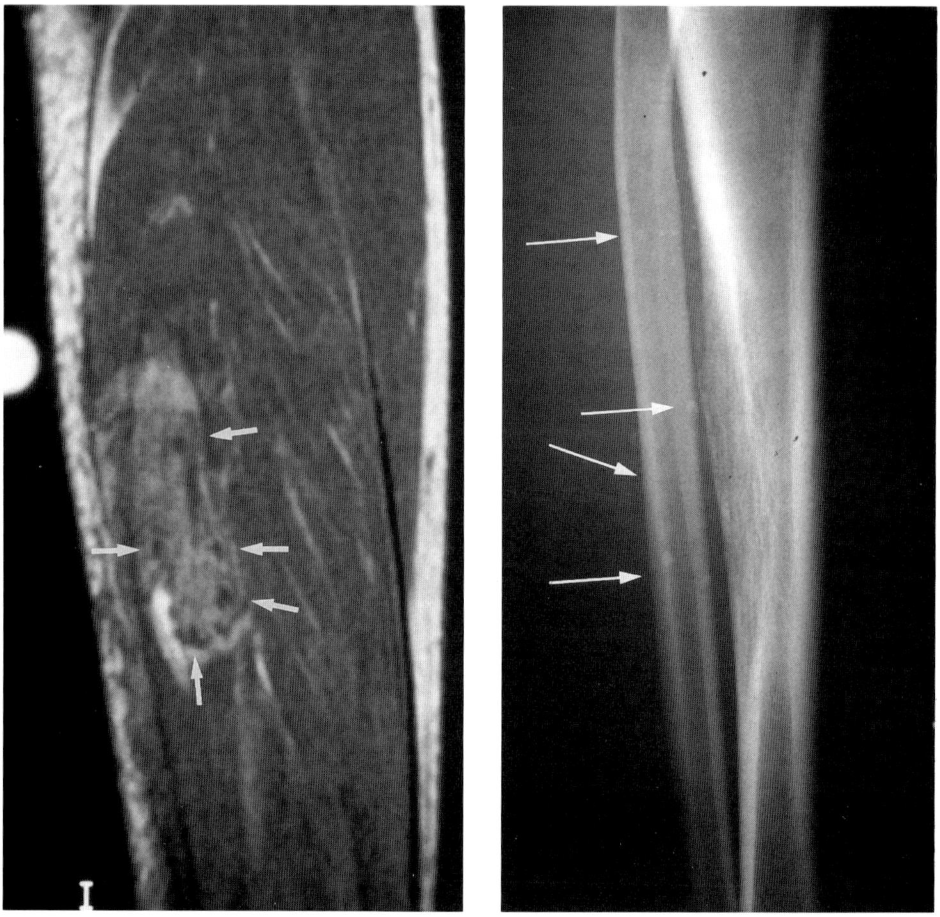

A **B**

Figure 5.3 A 41-year-old male with a hemangioma of the left calf with osseous involvement. (A) Sagittal T1-weighted image (750/30) reveals a poorly-marginated hemangioma. Note the hyperintense signal of the lesion corresponding to the presence of fat. Also note the round foci of signal void (arrows) corresponding to phleboliths (long thin arrows) seen on the accompanying radiograph (B). Radiograph also reveals erosion of the posterior tibial cortex. (C), (D) Axial FSE dual-echo T2-weighted scans (3000/50,100) depict the posterior cortical involvement (curved arrows). The striated-septated appearance is much less pronounced than in Figures 5.1 and 5.2.

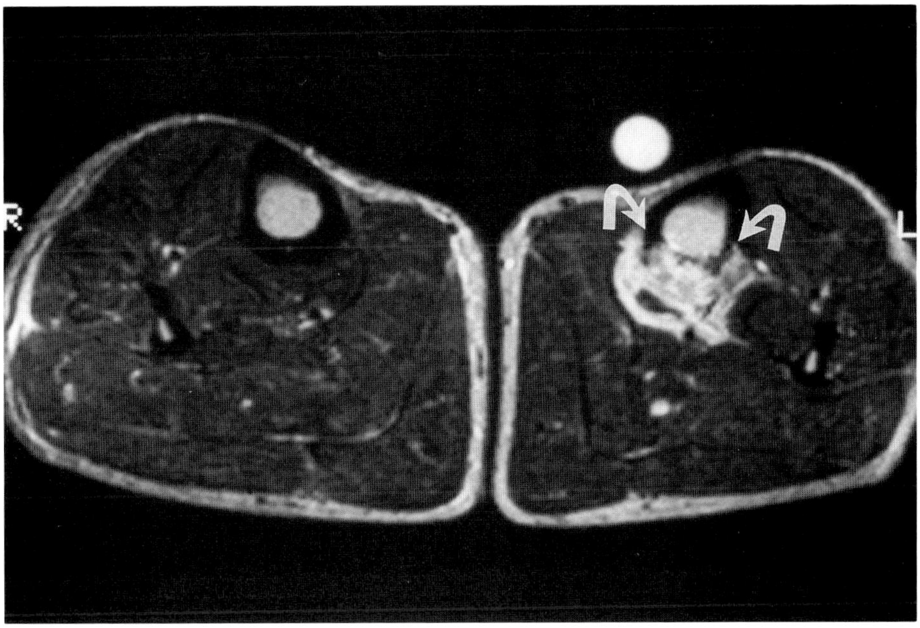

C

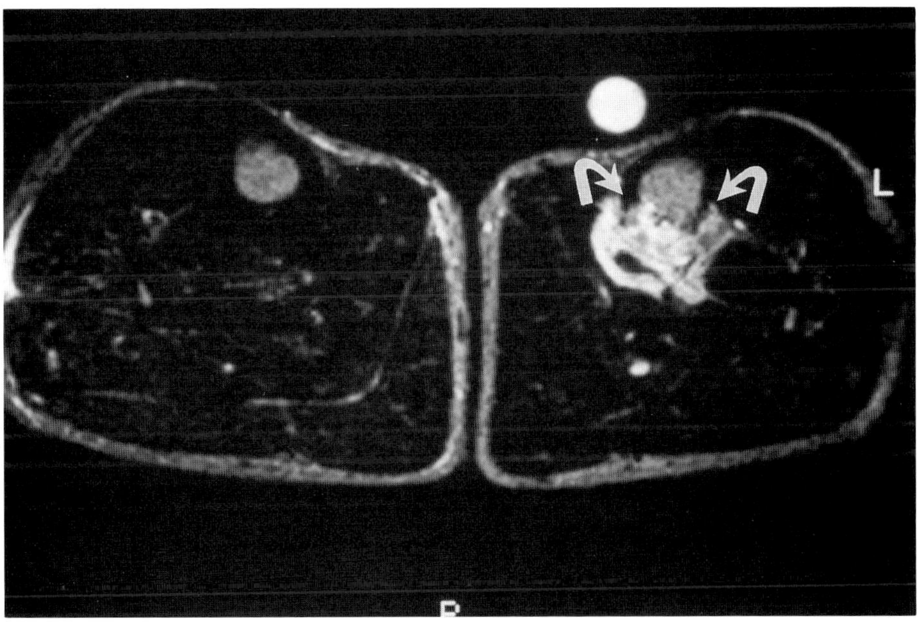

D

Soft Tissue Vascular Anomalies

Definition. For simplicity, vascular anomalies will be considered in two general categories: (1) vascular malformations and (2) acquired vascular pathology that results in a mass lesion. Vascular malformations may contain high flow (arteriovenous malformation) or slow flow (venous, capillary, or lymphatic malformations). Of these, arteriovenous malformations (AVMs) are most noteworthy due to the high blood flow state. AVMs consist of enlarged and tortuous feeding arteries and draining veins with early filling of these veins due to arteriovenous shunting. Although the exact cause of vascular malformations is unclear, a congenital etiology is suspected. The second category consists of vascular anomalies that are acquired and includes aneurysm, pseudoaneurysm, and varix. An aneurysm refers to focal dilatation of an artery in which all three layers of the vessel wall (intima, media, and adventitia) are involved and intact. Aneurysms usually occur secondary to atherosclerotic disease. A pseudoaneurysm results from a disruption or tear of the arterial wall which may involve only the intima or all vessel wall layers. Pseudoaneurysms may occur following blunt or penetrating trauma, percutaneous needle or catheter placement, or surgery. A varix (varicosity, varicose vein) is defined as dilatation of a vein. Varices may arise in association with chronic venous disease or may be primary in nature.

Clinical Features. Vascular malformations may present with symptoms related to blood flow through the lesion or symptoms related to compression of adjacent structures. They may also present for cosmetic reasons or may be asymptomatic. Of the vascular malformations, AVMs are the most clinically significant. The symptoms of an AVM are related to the amount of blood flow through the lesion. There may be a thrill or bruit on physical examination as well as elevated skin temperature over the lesion. In addition, there may be associated bone and soft tissue overgrowth or atrophy of the distally located structures. Severe pain may be present from compression on adjacent structures. Ischemic symptoms from a steal phenomenon may be present. Soft tissue ulceration may occur. Large lesions may be associated with high-output cardiac failure. Aneurysms, pseudoaneurysms, and varices may be asymptomatic or may present as palpable lesions or with symptoms related to mass effect on adjacent structures. Aneurysms and pseudoaneurysms may be pulsatile or be associated with bruit on auscultation.

Location. Vascular malformations may occur throughout the soft tissues. Aneurysms, pseudoaneurysms, and varices occur in a vascular distribution.

Implications. Treatment of vascular malformations is generally reserved for symptomatic lesions. Therapeutic options include percutaneous or transcatheter embolization, or surgery. Sequential embolizations are frequently necessary. Vascular malformations commonly recur following therapy. Amputation may eventually be required for large lesions. Aneurysms should be treated surgically if symptomatic or if at risk for rupture. Pseudoaneurysms are at significant risk for rupture. Extremity pseudoaneurysms can often be treated effectively with sonographically guided compression repair. If this is unsuccessful, they may be treated with transcatheter embolization or surgical repair. Varices can be treated surgically if symptomatic.

MRI Findings. The MR appearance of vascular anomalies is highly variable and dependent principally on the amount and velocity of blood flow through the lesion. Various flow sensitive MR sequences can be utilized in depicting vascular anomalies including gradient-recalled echo (GRE) and MR angiography techniques (phase contrast, time-of-flight). If in doubt, intravenous gadolinium could be administered to confirm the vascular nature of a mass lesion. Due to high velocity flow, AVMs typically appear as numerous tubular/serpiginous areas of signal void on conventional spin-echo pulse sequences. Venous malformations contain slow flow and tend to appear intermediate in signal intensity on T1-weighted images. An aneurysm appears as focal arterial dilatation. Associated mural thrombus is common and may exhibit variable signal intensity. A true aneurysm is continuous with the arterial lumen. A pseudoaneurysm consists of a collection of blood outside the vessel lumen and communicates with the arterial lumen via a neck or tract. Variable amounts of blood flow and thrombus are present within pseudoaneurysms and they may be completely thrombosed. Pseudoaneurysms can be multilobulated. A varix consists of focal venous dilatation. It may be round, oval, or tubular in shape and is continuous with the venous lumen. It may resemble a cyst or fluid collection on spin-echo, fast spin-echo, and gradient-recalled echo sequences.

Differential Diagnosis. In general, the diagnosis of a vascular anomaly can be confirmed by demonstrating blood flow through the lesion. Vascular malformations have no appreciable solid mass component, which differentiates these lesions from other vascular lesions such as hemangioma and alveolar soft part sarcoma. A completely thrombosed pseudoaneurysm cannot be reliably differentiated from a perivascular hematoma on MRI. Although a varix may resemble a cyst or fluid collection on various pulse sequences, it can usually be distinguished by connecting it with a vein on adjacent images. If the distinction is not straightforward, flow sensitive pulse sequences or intravenous gadolinium can be used to make the distinction.

References

Meyer J, Hoffer F, Barnes P, et al. Pictorial essay. Biological classification of soft-tissue vascular anomalies: MR correlation. *AJR* 157:559–564, 1992.

Kransdorf M, McFarland D, Moser R, et al. Case report 649. *Skeletal Radiol* 20:63–65, 1991.

Gould E, Potter H, Huvos A, et al. Case report 671. *Skeletal Radiol* 20:303–305, 1991.

Recht M, Sachs P, LiPuma J, et al. Case report. Popliteal artery pseudoaneurysm in a patient with hereditary multiple exostoses: MRI and MRA diagnosis. *JCAT* 17:300–302, 1993.

Paulson E, Kliewer M, Hertzberg B, et al. Pictorial Essay. Color doppler sonography of groin complications following femoral artery catheterization. *AJR* 165:439–444, 1995.

Hilborn M, Munk P, Miniaci A, et al. Case Report. Pseudoaneurysm after therapeutic knee arthroscopy: Imaging findings. *AJR* 163:637–639, 1994.

A

B

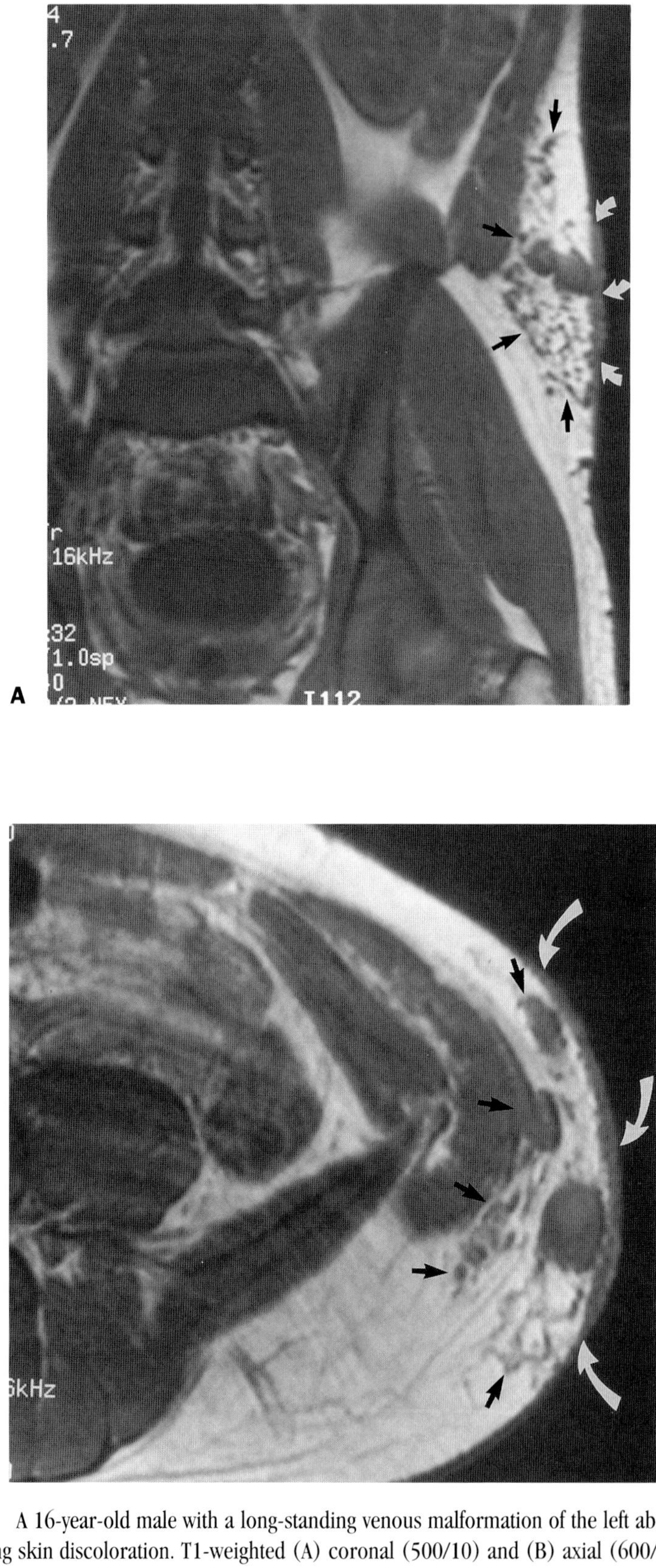

FIGURE 5.4 A 16-year-old male with a long-standing venous malformation of the left abdominal wall with overlying skin discoloration. T1-weighted (A) coronal (500/10) and (B) axial (600/11) images demonstrate numerous tubular and serpiginous structures of intermediate signal intensity within the subcutaneous tissues (arrows). Absence of signal void within the structures is consistent with slow flow. Note the overlying cutaneous involvement (curved arrows).

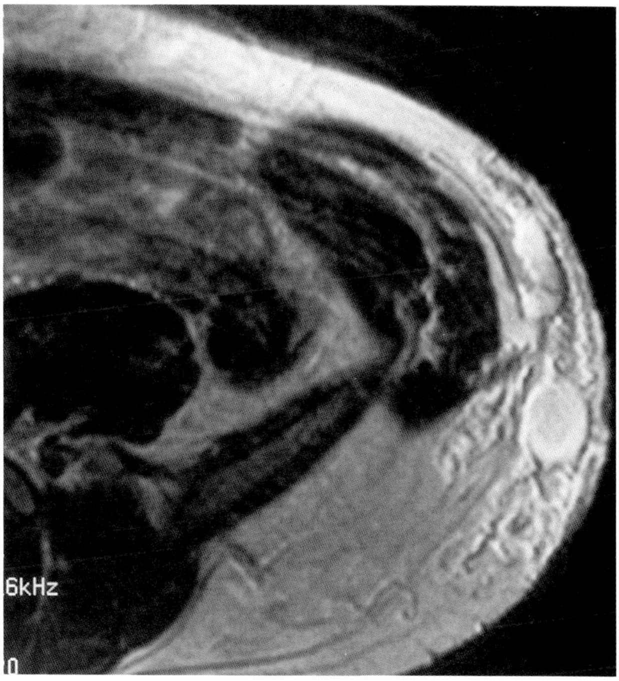

C

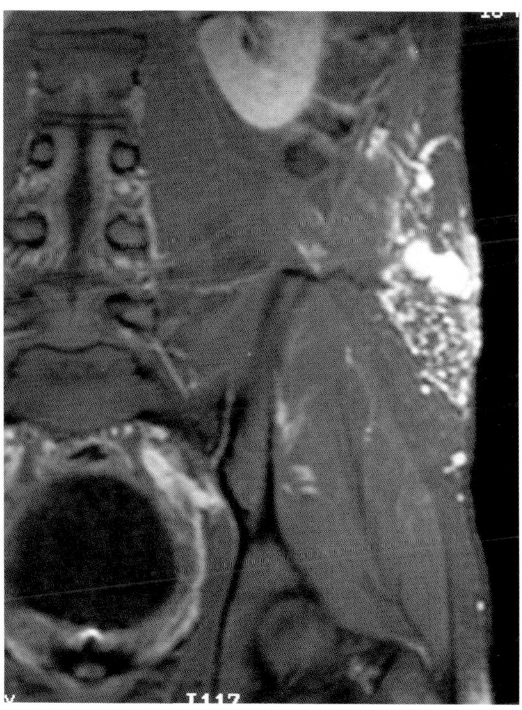

D

FIGURE 5.4 (continued) (C) The lesion becomes bright with FSE T2-weighting (3500/96). Intravenous gadolinium can be used to better define the lesion. There is improved delineation of the vascular structures on the contrast-enhanced coronal T1-weighted fat suppression (700/10) image (D).

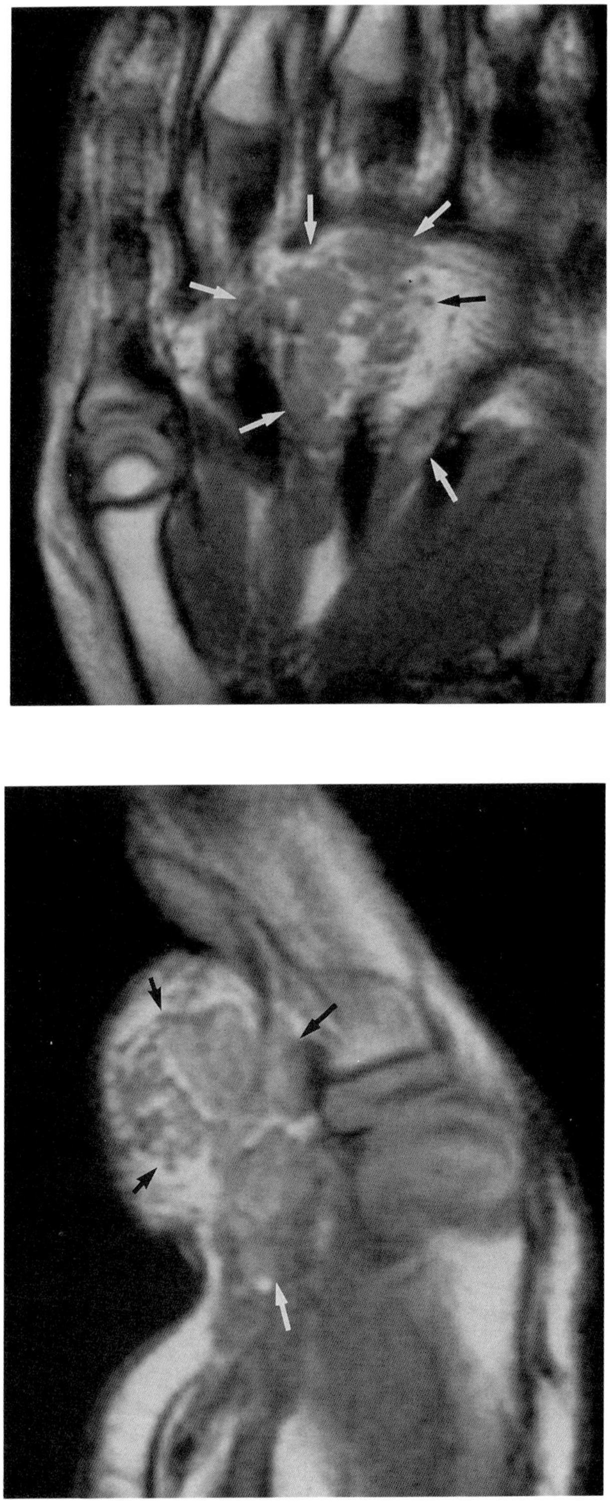

A

B

FIGURE 5.5 A 5-year-old male with a two-year history of swelling in the 2nd-3rd and 3rd-4th web spaces of the right hand. T1-weighted (A) coronal (550/30) and (B) sagittal (750/30) images demonstrate multiple round and tubular structures of intermediate signal intensity (arrows) involving the volar soft tissues.

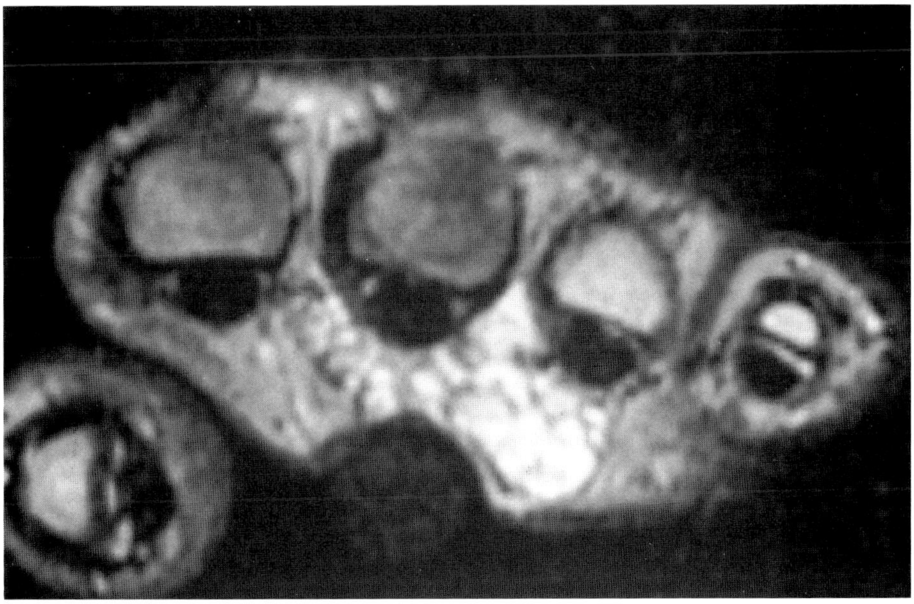

C

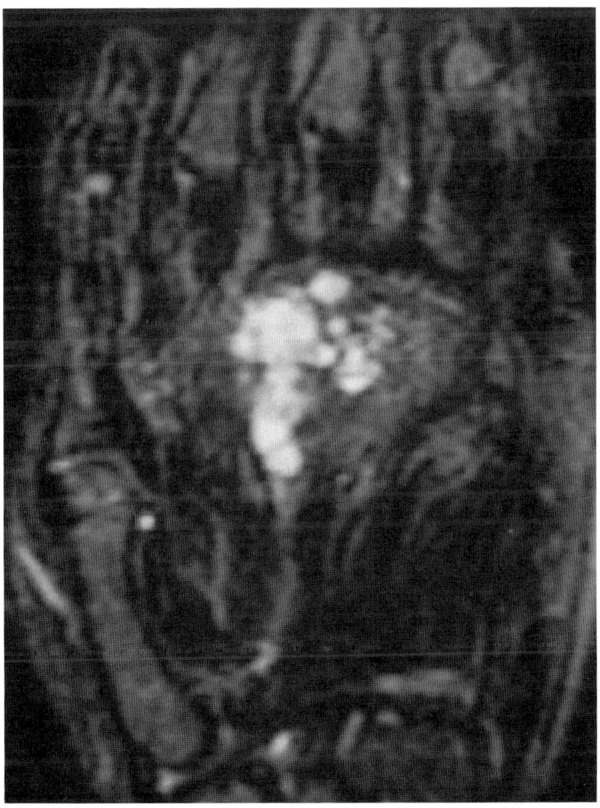

D

FIGURE 5.5 (continued) These areas become hyperintense on (C) axial T2-weighted (1700/70) and (D) coronal FSE T2-weighted fat suppression (2317/126) scans. The appearance is consistent with a vascular lesion. The absence of signal void indicates slow flow within the lesion, which could represent a venous, capillary, or lymphatic malformation based upon the MR appearance.

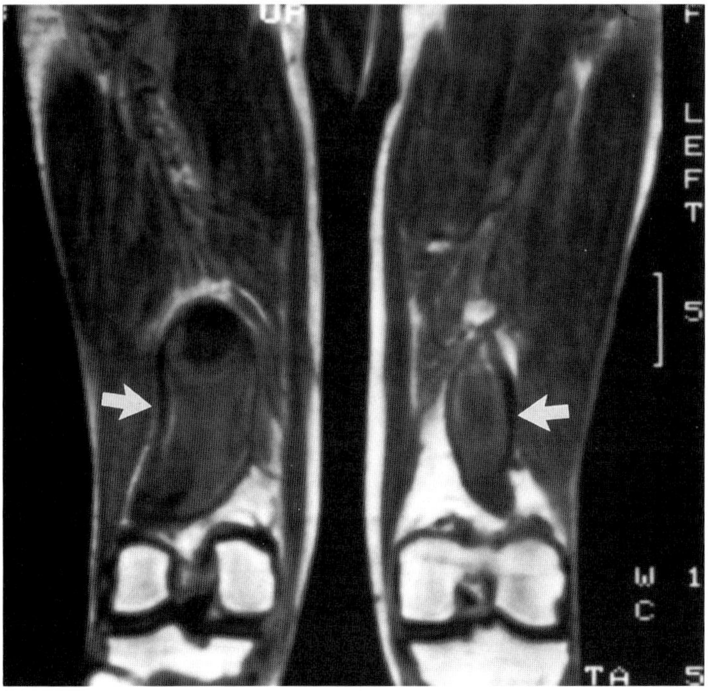

A

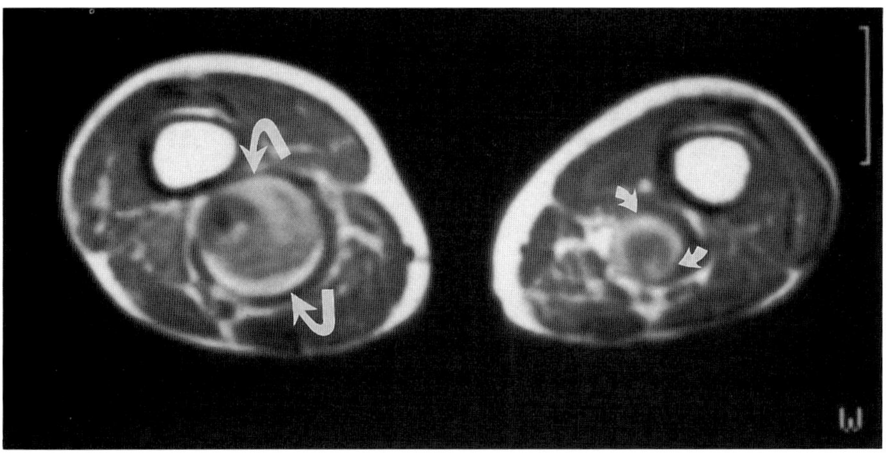

B

FIGURE 5.6 A 75-year-old male with bilateral lower extremity aneurysms. T1-weighted (A) coronal (600/15) and (B) axial (700/15) images reveal fusiform aneurysms (arrows) involving the distal portions of both superficial femoral arteries at the level of the adductor hiatus. Areas of increased signal within the aneurysms may be due to blood products within mural thrombus or flow-related enhancement from low-velocity blood flow (curved arrows). (C) Coronal T2-weighted scan (2500/90) demonstrates heterogeneous signal intensity within both aneurysms which may represent blood products versus turbulent or slow blood flow. Note the horizontal pulsation artifacts (open arrows).

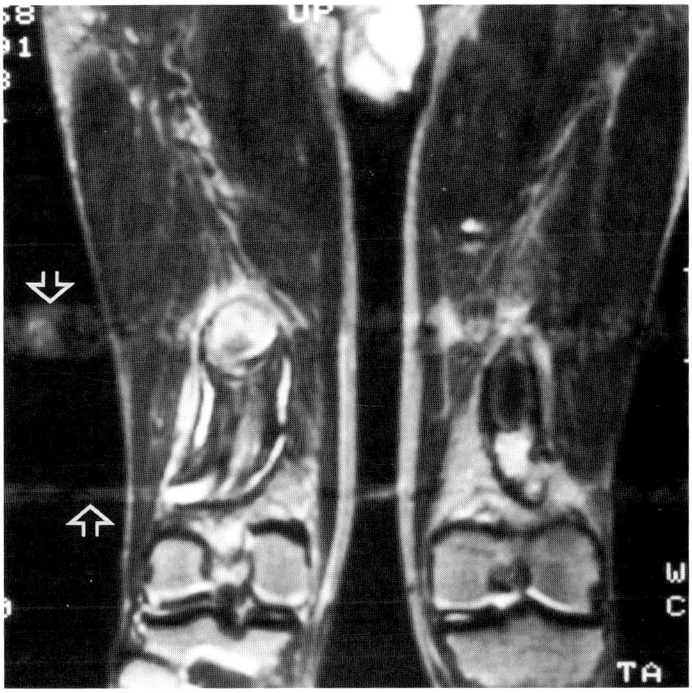

C

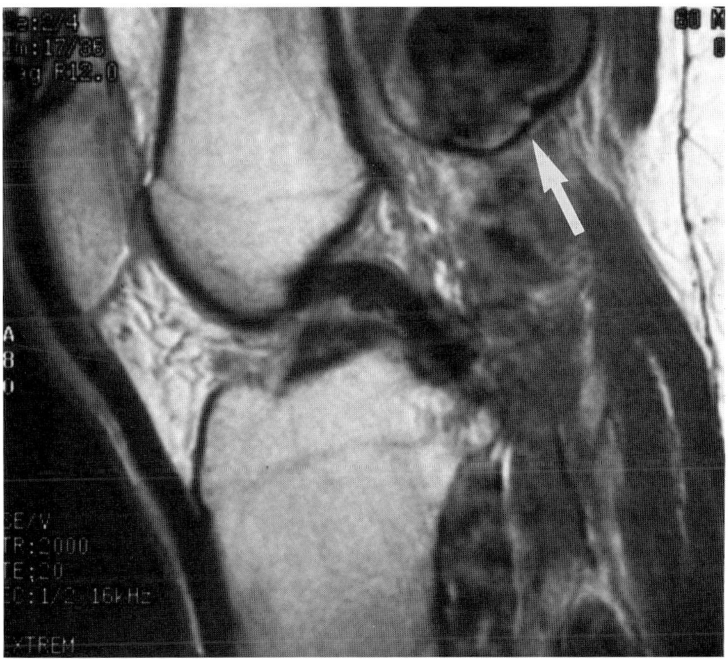

A

Figure 5.7 A 60-year-old male with a pseudoaneurysm of the popliteal artery. (A) Sagittal proton density image (2000/20) demonstrates a prominent pseudoaneurysm (arrow) involving the proximal popliteal artery.

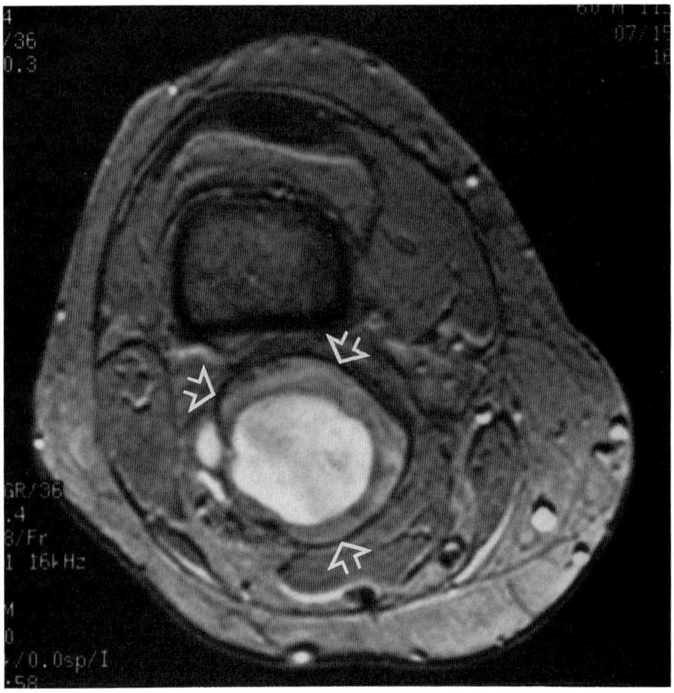

B

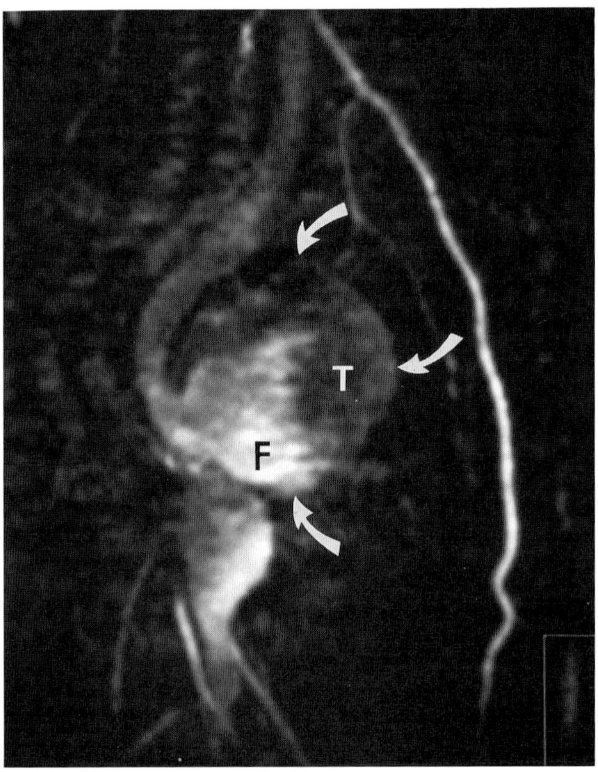

C

FIGURE 5.7 (continued) (B) Axial gradient-recalled echo image reveals hyperintense signal centrally (from blood flow) and peripheral mural thrombus (open arrows). (C) MR angiography scan nicely depicts the relationship of the pseudoaneurysm (curved arrows) to the popliteal artery and differentiates flow (F) within the lesion from mural thrombus (T). (Courtesy of Larry Cohan, MD).

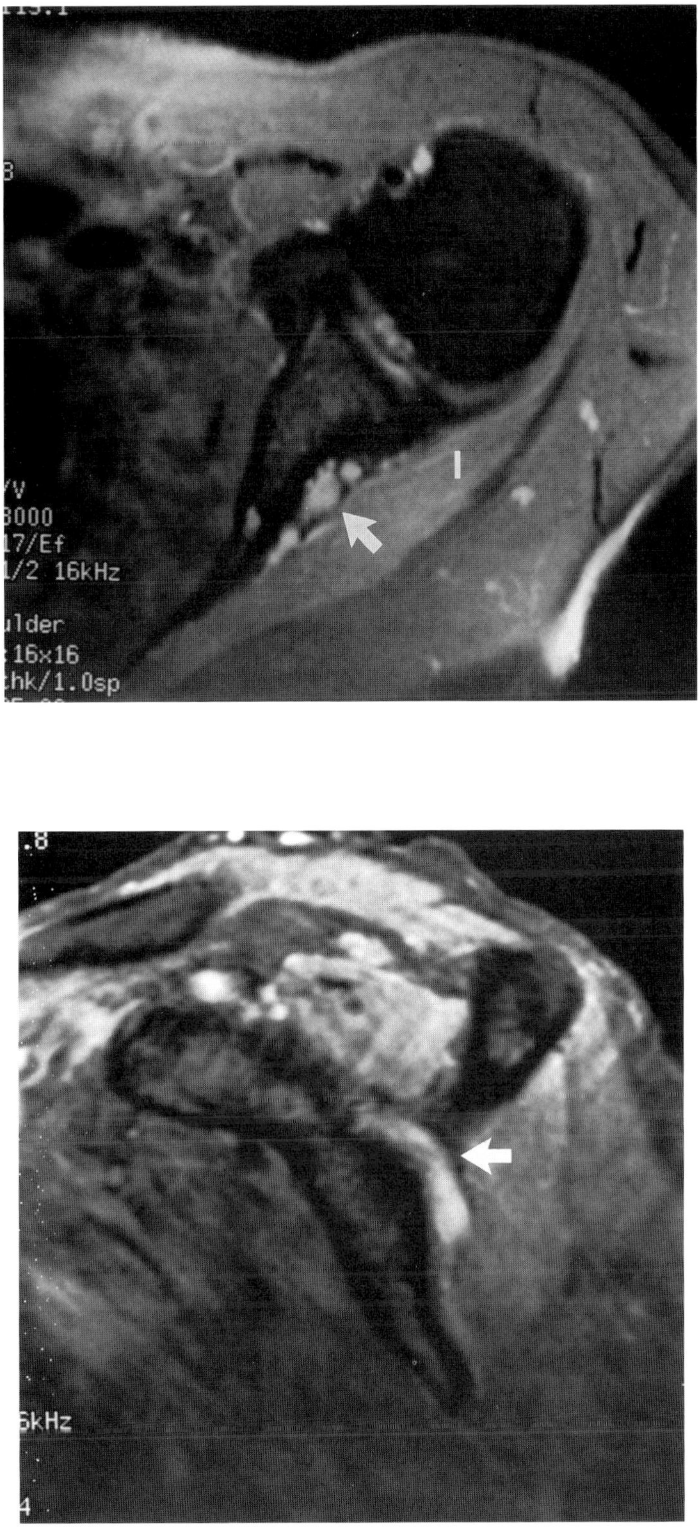

A

B

FIGURE 5.8 A 58-year-old male with suprascapular nerve impingement. FSE proton density with fat suppression (A) axial (3000/17) and (B) sagittal (3600/23) images demonstrate a hyperintense tubular structure (arrows) within the spinoglenoid notch. This lesion could represent a ganglion cyst or varix, which could be distinguished by the use of intravenous gadolinium or a flow-sensitive pulse sequence. Note the relative increased signal within the infraspinatus muscle (I) resulting from compression of the distal suprascapular nerve.

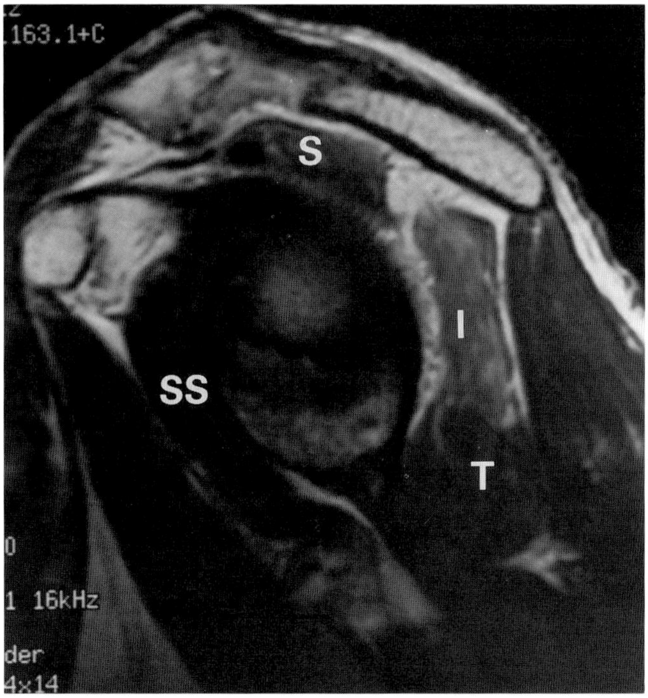

C

FIGURE 5.8 (continued) (C) Contrast-enhanced sagittal T1-weighted scan (550/17) demonstrates atrophy of the infraspinatus muscle (I) related to denervation. At surgery, a varix was found in the spinoglenoid notch. Subscapularis (SS), Supraspinatus (S), Teres Minor (T). (Courtesy of Regina Robinson, M.D.).

A

B

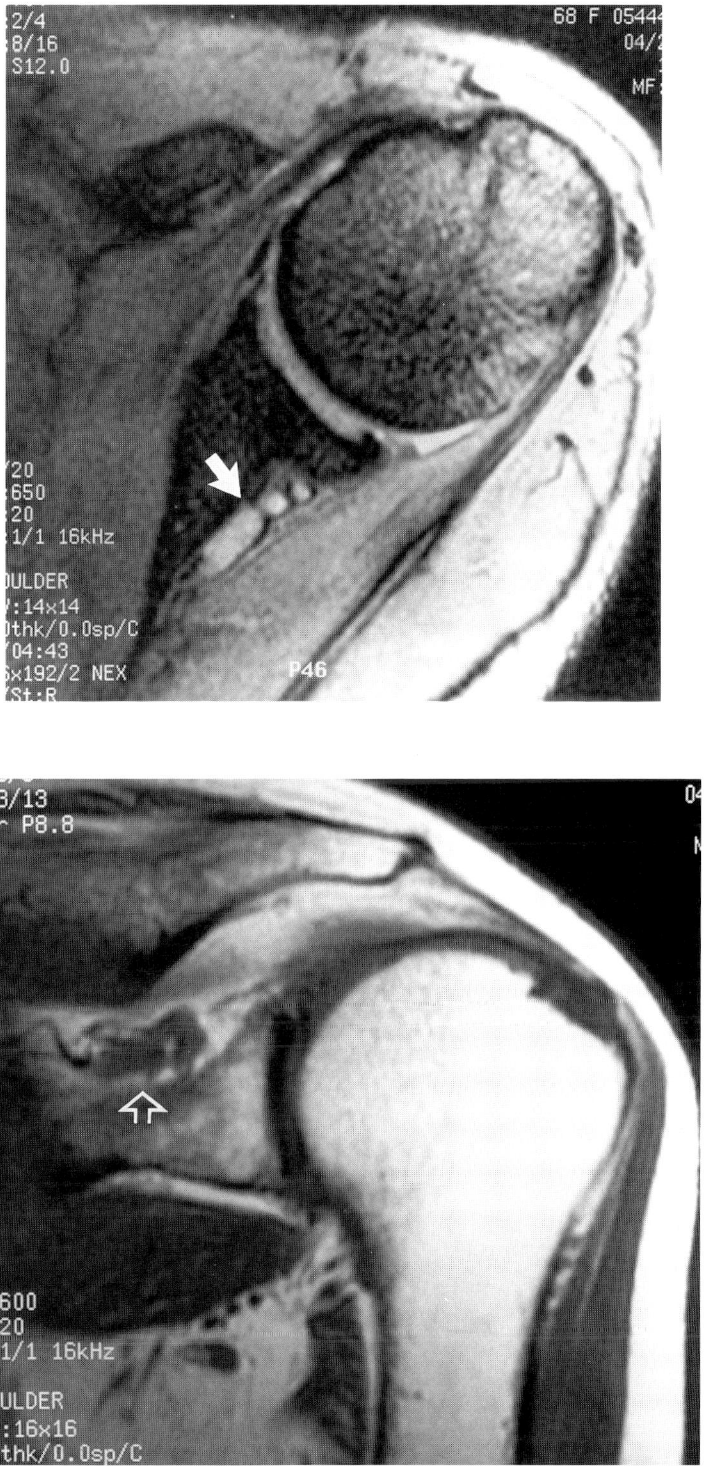

FIGURE 5.9 A 68-year-old woman with a spinoglenoid notch varix. (A) Axial MPGR image (650/20,20 degrees) demonstrates a lobulated hyperintense lesion within the spinoglenoid notch (arrow). This appearance could represent a ganglion cyst or varix. (B) Coronal T1-weighted image (600/20) demonstrates a tubular configuration most consistent with a varix (open arrow). Distinction between a varix and cyst could be achieved with the use of intravenous gadolinium or a flow-sensitive sequence. The patient had no associated infraspinatus signal abnormality.

Hemangiopericytoma of Soft Tissue

Definition. Hemangiopericytoma of soft tissue is a hypervascular malignant mesenchymal neoplasm that is thought to arise from pericytes, which are cells surrounding capillaries and postcapillary venules. This lesion typically consists of elongated cells surrounding a network of variably sized thin-walled vessels.

Clinical Features. Hemangiopericytomas are uncommon tumors, accounting for less than 2% of all soft tissue sarcomas. They may affect all age groups, but occur most commonly in the 5th and 6th decades of life. These lesions generally present as masses, with or without associated pain. Due to hypervascularity, there may occasionally be clinically significant arteriovenous shunting.

Location. Hemangiopericytomas may occur throughout the body, but the most common locations (in descending frequency) are the lower extremity, pelvis/retroperitoneum, head and neck region, trunk, and upper extremity.

Implications. The prognosis for these lesions is variable. Local recurrence is associated with a poor prognosis and often precedes distant metastasis. Surgery may be complicated by severe hemorrhage and preoperative arterial embolization may be helpful for large lesions. Hemangiopericytomas may be associated with various paraneoplastic syndromes such as hypoglycemia, hypophosphatemic osteomalacia, and hypertrophic osteoarthropathy.

MRI Findings. These lesions typically appear as well-circumscribed masses on MRI. They are isointense to moderately hyperintense compared with muscle on T1-weighted images and may be isointense to fat or of very bright signal intensity on T2-weighted sequences. These lesions may contain calcification (appearing as signal void on all pulse sequences) or central areas of necrosis (appearing hypointense with T1-weighting and markedly hyperintense with T2-weighting). Erosion of the adjacent bone is uncommon.

Differential Diagnosis. The MR signal characteristics of hemangiopericytoma are nonspecific and may be seen with any of the soft tissue sarcomas as well as numerous benign soft tissue lesions.

References

Lorigan J, David C, Evans H, et al. The clinical and radiologic manifestations of hemangiopericytoma. *AJR* 153:345–349, 1989.

Kransdorf M, Jelinek J, Moser R, et al. Soft-tissue masses: Diagnosis using MR imaging. *AJR* 153:541–547, 1989.

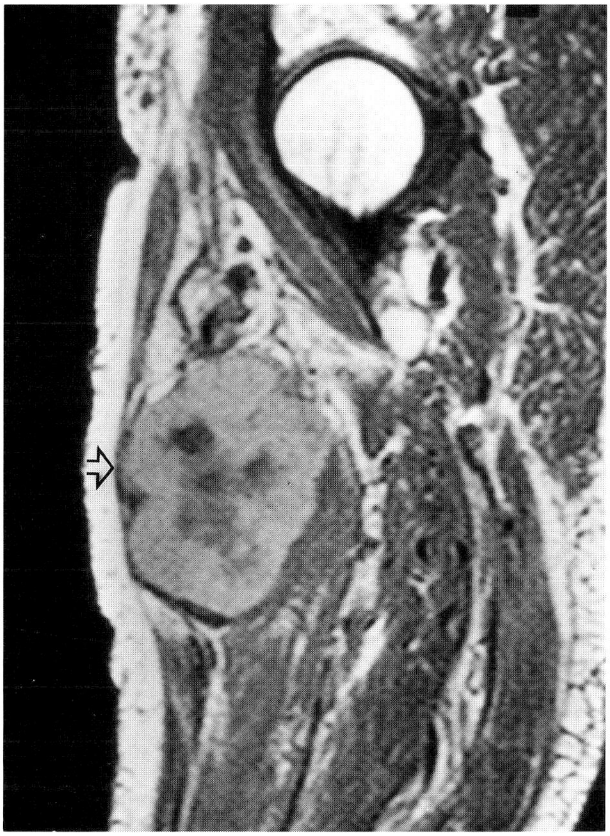

A

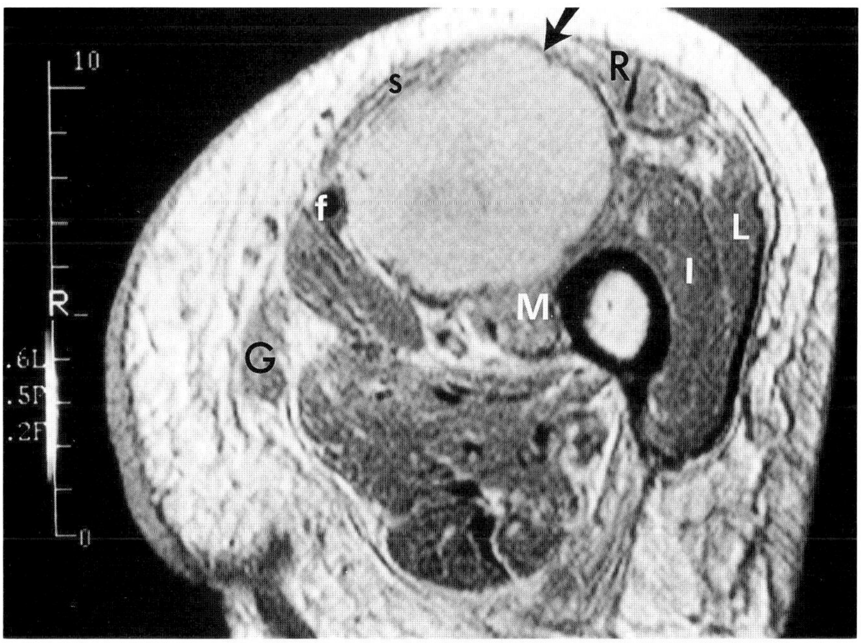

B

FIGURE 5.10 Hemangiopericytoma of the thigh in an 87-year-old woman. (A) Sagittal T1-weighted image demonstrates a slightly lobulated, well-marginated mass (open arrow) in the anterior aspect of the upper thigh. The predominant signal intensity is between that of muscle and fat. The central areas of low signal intensity likely represent necrosis. (B) Axial proton density image defines the anteromedial position of the tumor (arrow). There is mass effect on the sartorius (S), rectus femoris (R), and vastus medialis (M) muscles as well as medial displacement of the femoral artery (f). Vastus intermedius (I), Vastus lateralis (L). (Courtesy of James O. Johnston, MD).

6 Masses Arising from Nerves

Schwannoma

Definition. The two types of benign peripheral nerve sheath tumors are schwannoma and neurofibroma. A schwannoma (which has also been termed neurilemoma and neurinoma) is an encapsulated neoplasm arising from the Schwann cells of a peripheral nerve sheath. It consists of two distinct histologic components, an ordered hypercellular area and a loose myxoid area. In addition, there may be areas of hemorrhage, cystic degeneration, and necrosis.

Clinical Features. Schwannomas are uncommon tumors which typically occur between 20 and 50 years of age, although all age groups may be affected. Schwannomas typically present as slowly growing, painless masses. They can be associated with pain, tenderness, and neurologic symptoms (typically paresthesias in the distribution of the involved peripheral nerve). These lesions can be quite large at the time of presentation. Multiple lesions are occasionally present, especially in association with neurofibromatosis.

Location. Schwannomas tend to arise along major nerve trunks in the extremities, especially the peroneal and ulnar nerves. Upper extremity lesions tend to be anterior (flexor areas), where the larger nerves are present.

Implications. Surgery is the treatment of choice and most schwannomas can be resected without resultant neurologic deficit. Recurrence following surgery is unusual. Malignant transformation is extremely rare.

MRI Findings. On MRI, schwannomas typically appear as smooth, well-marginated masses in the distribution of a major nerve trunk. The mass may appear connected to the nerve bundle at its proximal and distal aspects. Lobulation may be present. Schwannomas generally exhibit hypointense signal (approximately isointense to muscle) on T1-weighted images and bright signal intensity on T2-weighted sequences. The signal intensity may be homogeneous or heterogeneous. The inhomogeneous appearance may reflect hypocellularity, hypercellularity, xanthomatous change, cystic degeneration, necrosis, or hemorrhage. In about half of cases, there is a "target" pattern on T2-weighted sequences with a high signal peripheral rim and a central zone of lower signal intensity. This pattern corresponds histologically to peripheral myxomatous tissue surrounding a central area of fibrocollagenous tissue. Mild muscle atrophy of the surrounding or distally innervated musculature may be seen.

Differential Diagnosis. Many schwannomas demonstrate nonspecific signal characteristics that can be seen with numerous benign and malignant lesions. The diagnosis of schwannoma should be considered if a mass is intimately associated with a large nerve trunk, especially if there is a "target" signal pattern or muscle atrophy in the nerve distribution. MRI is not reliable in differentiating a schwannoma from a neurofibroma or in distinguishing benign from malignant peripheral nerve sheath tumors.

References

Stull M, Moser R, Kransdorf M, et al. Magnetic resonance appearance of peripheral nerve sheath tumors. *Skeletal Radiol* 20:9–14, 1991.

Suh J, Abenoza P, Galloway H, et al. Peripheral (extracranial) nerve tumors: Correlation of MR imaging and histologic findings. *Radiology* 183:341–346, 1992.

Schultz E, Sapan M, McHeffey-Atkinson B, et al. Case report 872. *Skeletal Radiol* 23:593–595, 1994.

Varma D, Moulopoulos A, Sara A, et al. MR imaging of extracranial nerve sheath tumors. *JCAT* 16:448–453, 1992.

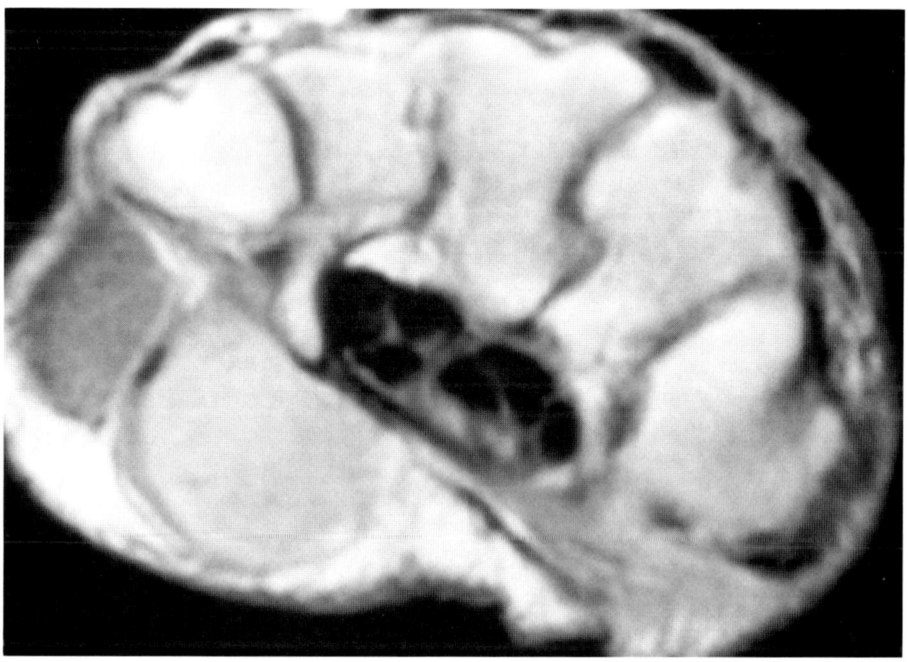

A

FIGURE 6.1 A 70-year-old woman with a palpable mass at the ulnar aspect of the left wrist associated with weakness, numbness, and tingling. The lesion was excised and diagnosed as a schwannoma on pathologic examination. Axial (A) proton density (1700/30) and

(continued)

B

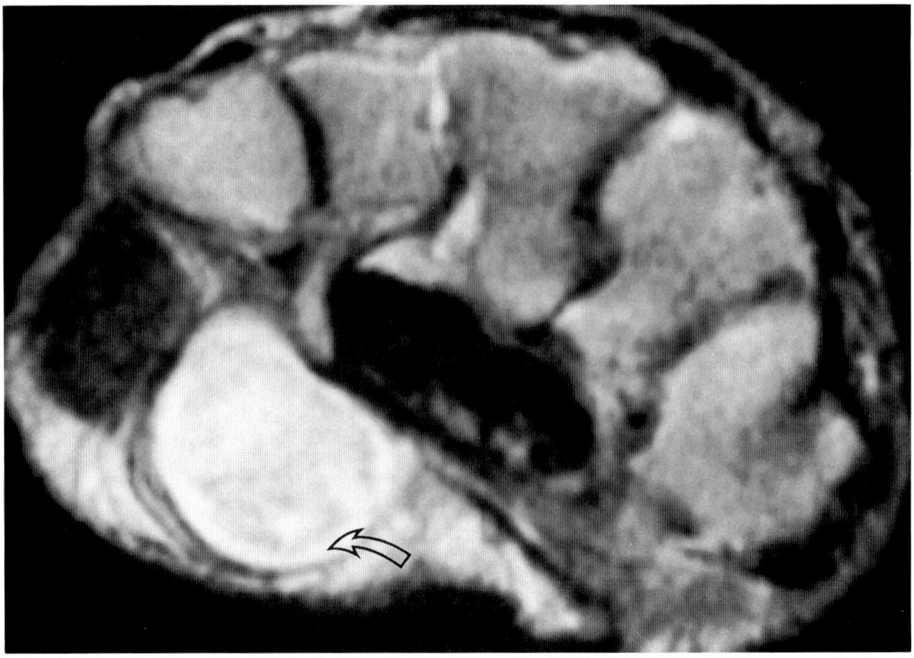

C

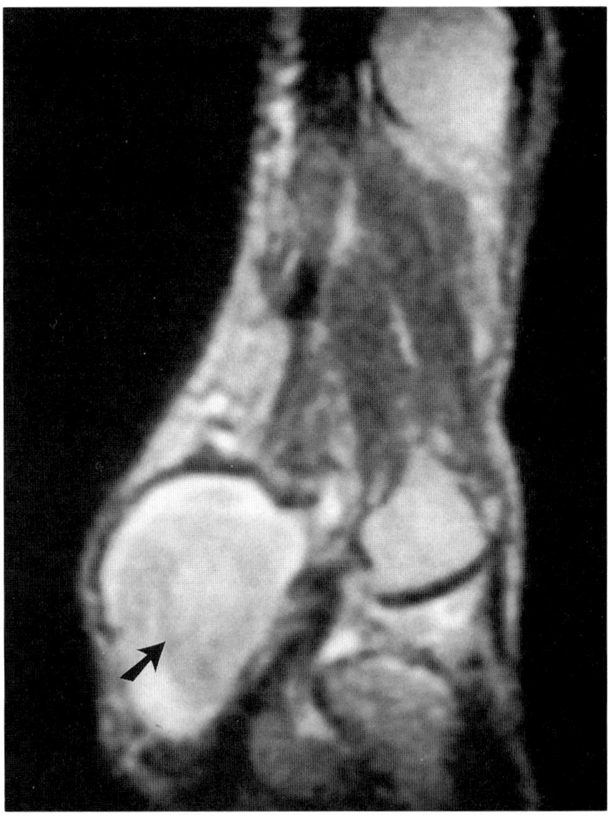

FIGURE 6.1 (continued) (B) T2-weighted (1700/80) images reveal a well-marginated mass in the region of the ulnar nerve. Note the characteristic "target" appearance with a peripheral rim of bright signal (open arrow) surrounding a central area of lower signal intensity. (C) Sagittal T2-weighted image (1700/80) again demonstrates the characteristic "target" appearance that is present in about half of all lesions. The central zone of relatively lower signal intensity (arrow) corresponds to fibrocollagenous tissue.

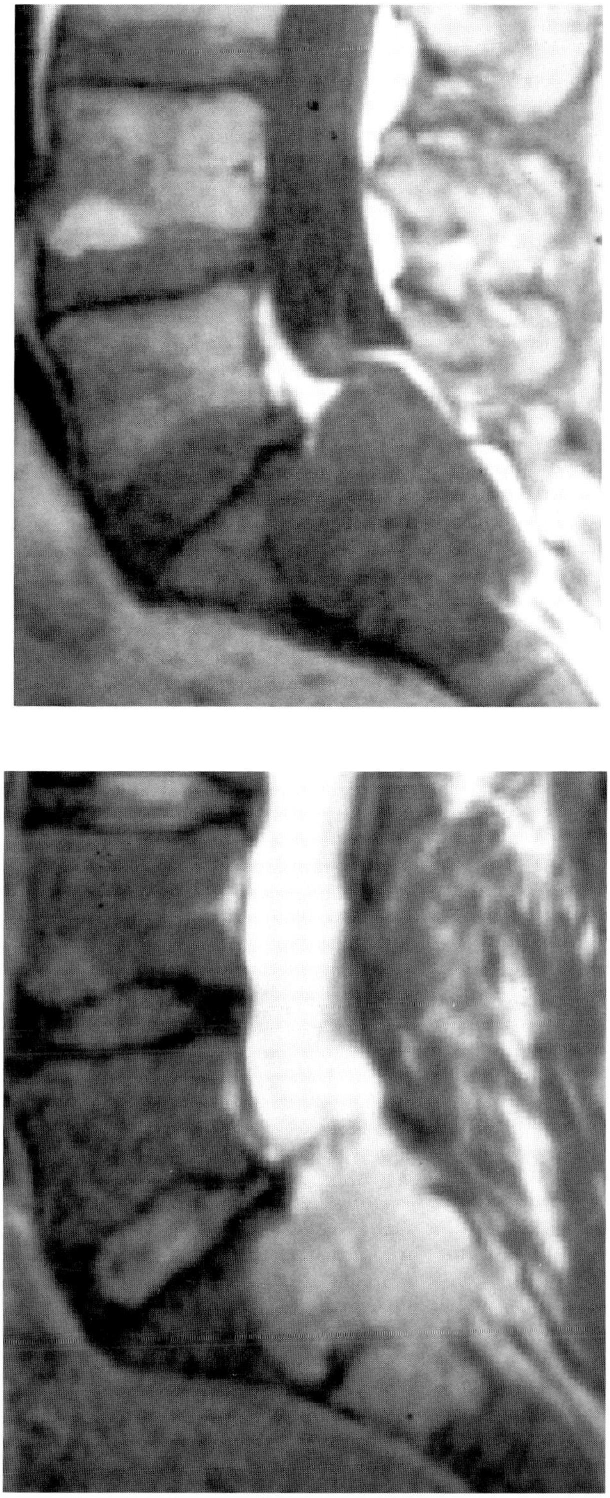

A

B

FIGURE 6.2 A 38-year-old male with a pathologically-proven schwannoma arising from a sacral nerve. Sagittal (A) T1-weighted (500/16) and (B) T2-weighted (1800/80) images demonstrate a lobulated mass within the upper sacrum and spinal canal. Note the absence of a "target" appearance on the T2-weighted image.

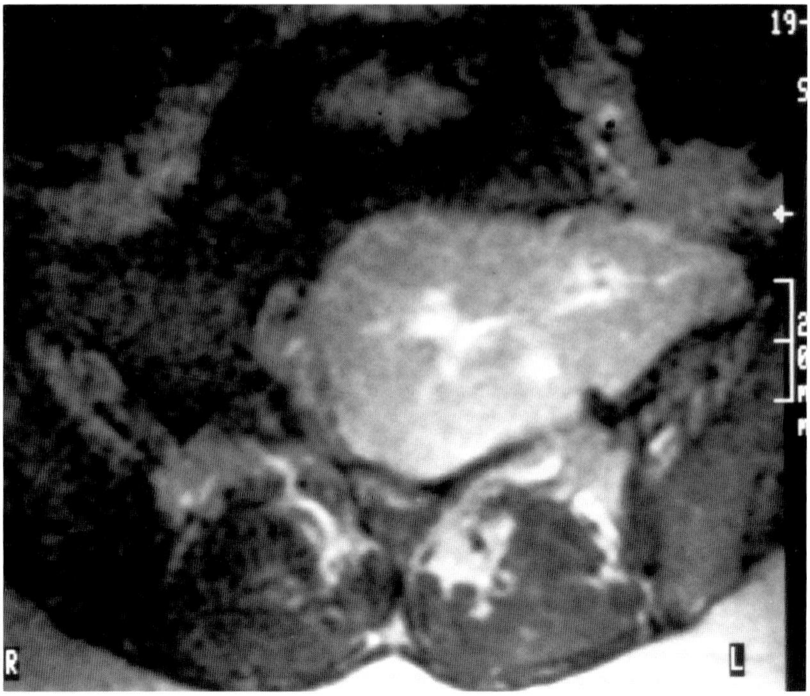

C

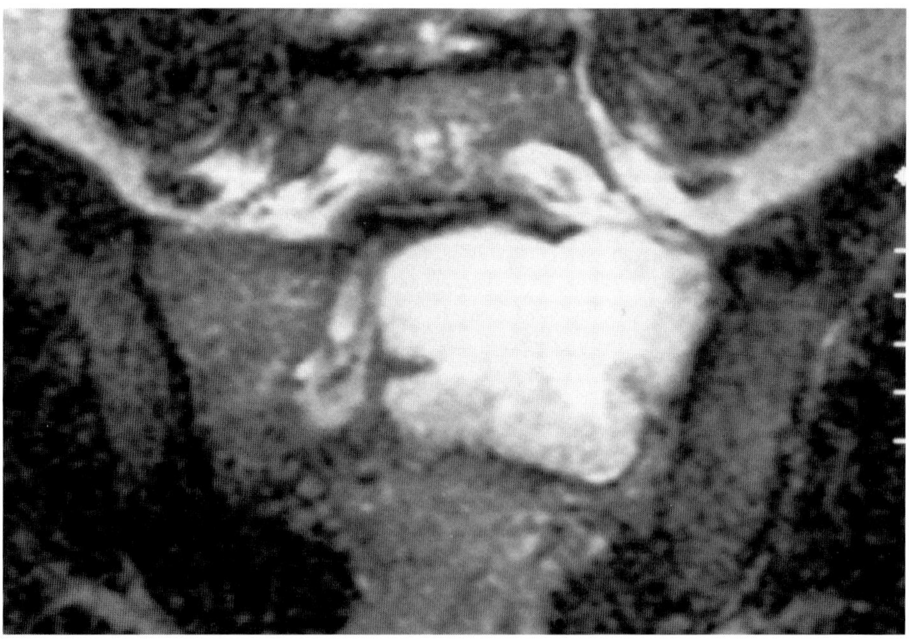

D

Figure 6.2 (continued) T2-weighted (C) axial (2617/80) and (D) oblique coronal (1800/80) images reveal that the mass is centered about the left S1 nerve. There is heterogeneous signal intensity, with the very bright areas likely representing cystic degeneration or necrosis.

Neurofibroma

Definition. The two types of benign peripheral nerve sheath tumors are neurofibroma and the more common schwannoma. Both arise from Schwann cells. Neurofibromas consist of elongated cells with a collagenous and mucoid matrix. There is a central hypercellular area and a peripheral zone of loose myxoid material. A specific type of neurofibroma is the plexiform neurofibroma, which is characteristic of neurofibromatosis type 1 (NF-1). Plexiform neurofibromas consist of multiple, tortuous masses ("bag of worms"), and histologically reveal a peripheral zone of myxoid material with a high fluid content and a central zone of fibrocollagenous tissue.

Clinical Features. Most solitary neurofibromas occur between the ages of 20 and 30 and present as slowly growing, painless masses. Neurofibromas may arise sporadically or in association with NF. In NF, the neurofibromas present during childhood or adolescence. The presence of multiple neurofibromas is characteristic for NF-1.

Location. Solitary neurofibromas most often arise from cutaneous nerves, with an equal distribution over the body.

Implications. A neurofibroma infiltrates the nerve bundle and separates nerve fascicles. It is therefore difficult to surgically remove the lesion without sacrificing the nerve. The presence of multiple neurofibromas is characteristic for NF-1, in which the lesions have an estimated 2% rate of malignant transformation. The presence of a plexiform neurofibroma is pathognomonic of NF-1. In NF-1, the sudden onset of pain or enlargement of a lesion is suspicious for malignant transformation. Solitary neurofibromas only rarely undergo malignant transformation.

MRI Findings. Neurofibromas typically appear as smooth, well-marginated masses in the distribution of a peripheral nerve. The mass may appear connected to the nerve bundle at its proximal and distal aspects. Neurofibromas generally exhibit hypointense signal (approximately isointense to muscle) on T1-weighted images and bright signal intensity on T2-weighted sequences. This signal intensity may be homogeneous or inhomogeneous. The inhomogeneity reflects areas of hypocellularity and hypercellularity within the tumor. In about half of cases, there is a "target" pattern on T2-weighted sequences with a high signal peripheral rim and a central zone of lower signal intensity. This pattern corresponds histologically to peripheral myxomatous tissue surrounding a central area of fibrocollagenous tissue. Plexiform neurofibromas typically appear as amorphous, lobulated masses ("bag of worms") with ill-defined margins and inhomogeneous signal intensity; these masses may have areas of high signal intensity on T1-weighted images due to a high mucinous content.

Differential Diagnosis. Many neurofibromas demonstrate nonspecific signal characteristics that can be seen with numerous benign and malignant lesions. The diagnosis of a neurofibroma should be considered if a mass is intimately associated with a peripheral nerve, especially if there is a "target" signal pattern. MRI is not reliable in differentiating a neurofibroma from a schwannoma or in distinguishing benign from malignant peripheral nerve sheath tumors.

References

Stull M, Moser R, Kransdorf M, et al. Magnetic resonance appearance of peripheral nerve sheath tumors. *Skeletal Radiol* 20:9–14, 1991.

Suh J, Abenoza P, Galloway H, et al. Peripheral (extracranial) nerve tumors: Correlation of MR imaging and histologic findings. *Radiology* 183:341–346, 1992.

Sullivan T, Seeger L, Doberneck S, et al. Case report 828. *Skeletal Radiol* 23:149–152, 1994.

Varma D, Moulopoulos A, Sara A, et al. MR imaging of extracranial nerve sheath tumors. *JCAT* 16:448–453, 1992.

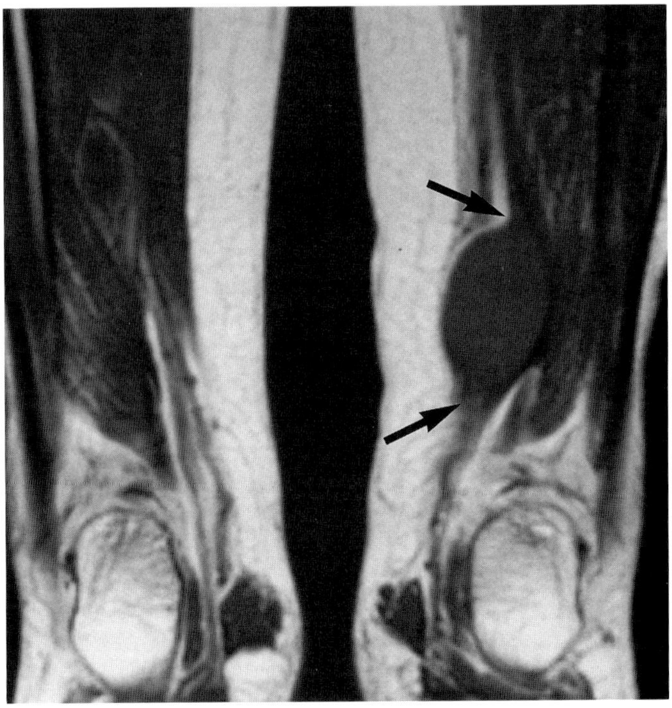

A

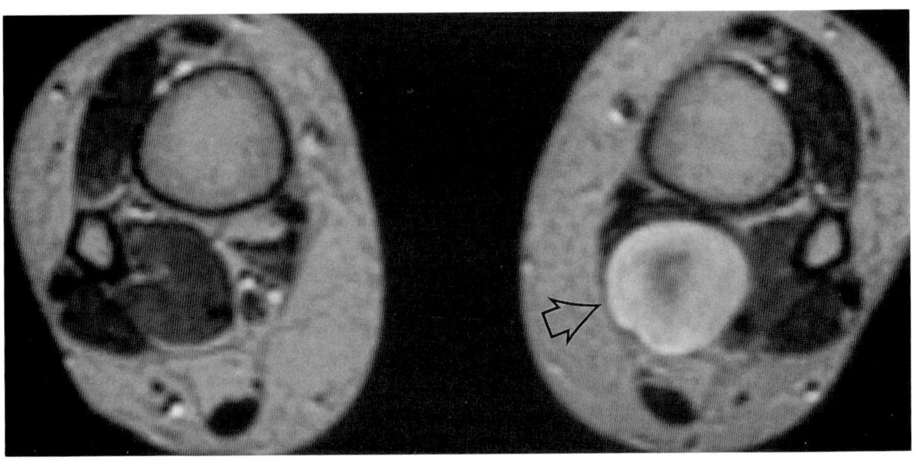

B

FIGURE 6.3 A 31-year-old woman with a three-month history of a palpable distal left calf mass. (A) Coronal T1-weighted image (600/20) reveals an oval-shaped mass which is isointense with adjacent muscle. This lesion appears to be connected to the posterior tibial nerve at its proximal and distal poles (arrows). (B) Axial T2-weighted image (2000/70) demonstrates the classic "target" appearance (open arrow), which is present in about half of peripheral nerve sheath tumors. Surgery confirmed the presence of a neurofibroma arising from the posterior tibial nerve.

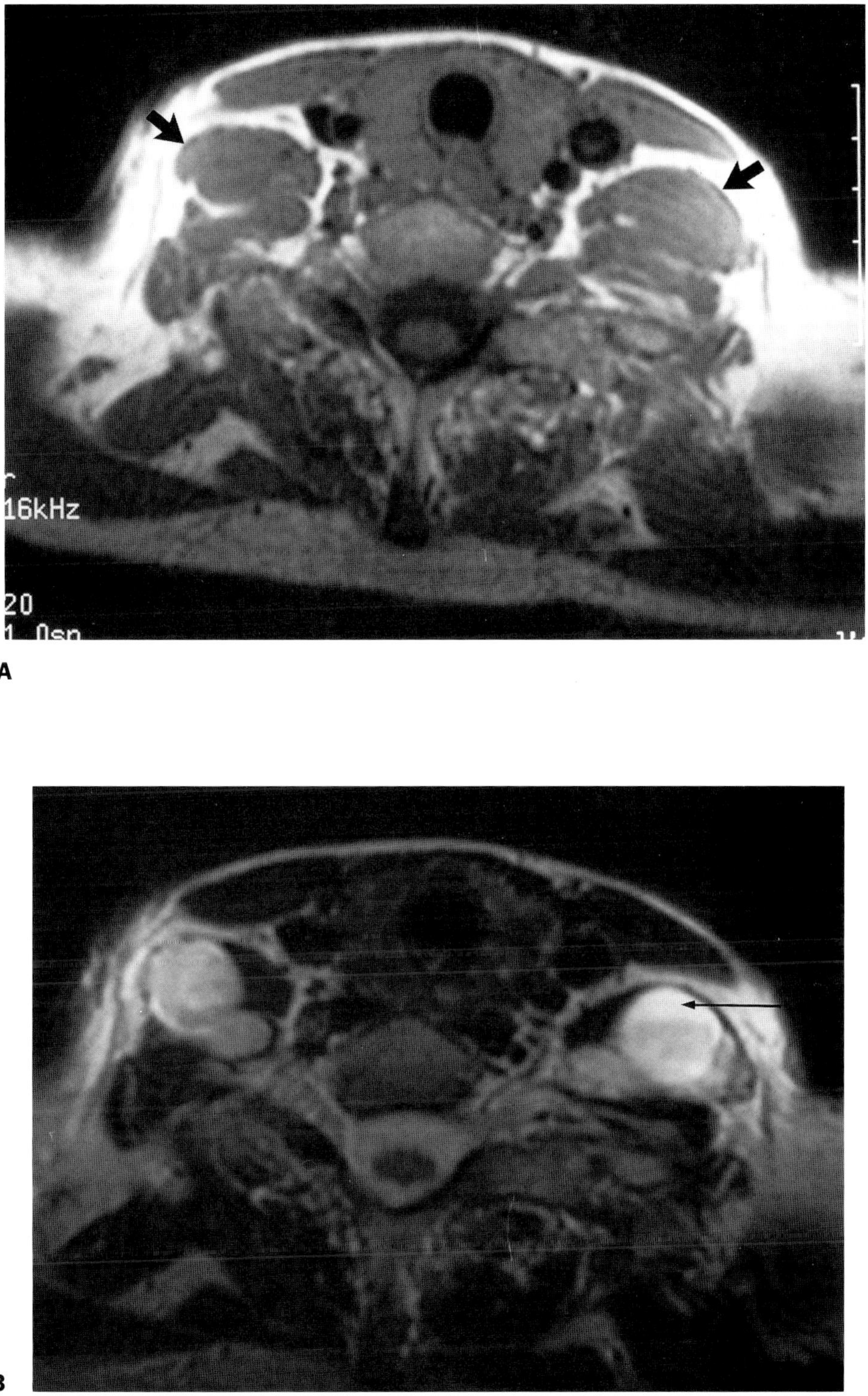

A

B

FIGURE 6.4 Bilateral neck neurofibromas in a patient with neurofibromatosis. (A) Axial T1-weighted image (583/11) demonstrates bilateral neck masses (arrows) which are isointense with surrounding muscle.

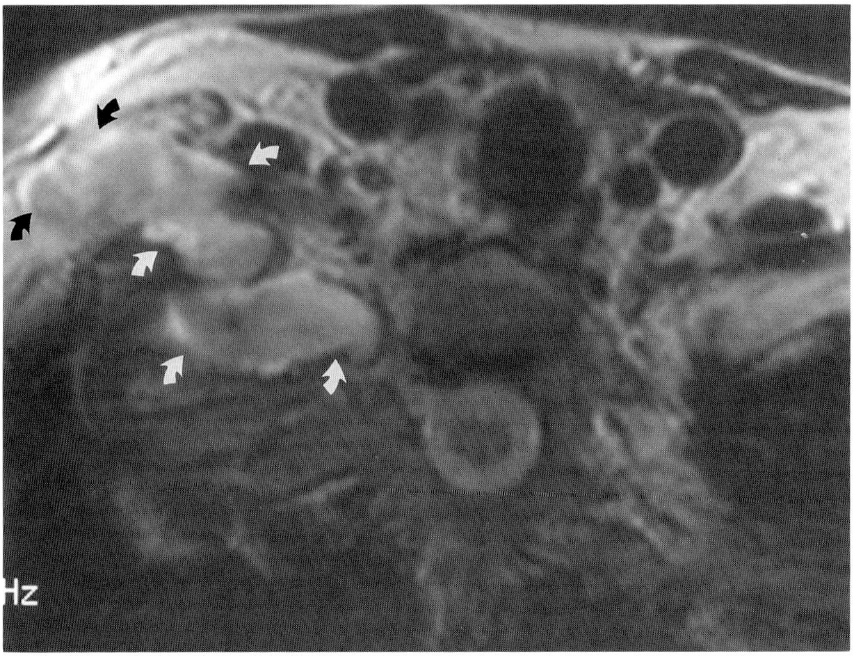

C

FIGURE 6.4 (continued) (B), (C) Axial FSE T2-weighted scans (4433/102) demonstrate the characteristic "target" appearance of both lesions, more pronounced on the left. The peripheral rim of high signal intensity (long thin arrow) corresponds to myxomatous tissue. Note the lobulated configuration of the lesion on the right extending along the nerve distribution (curved arrows).

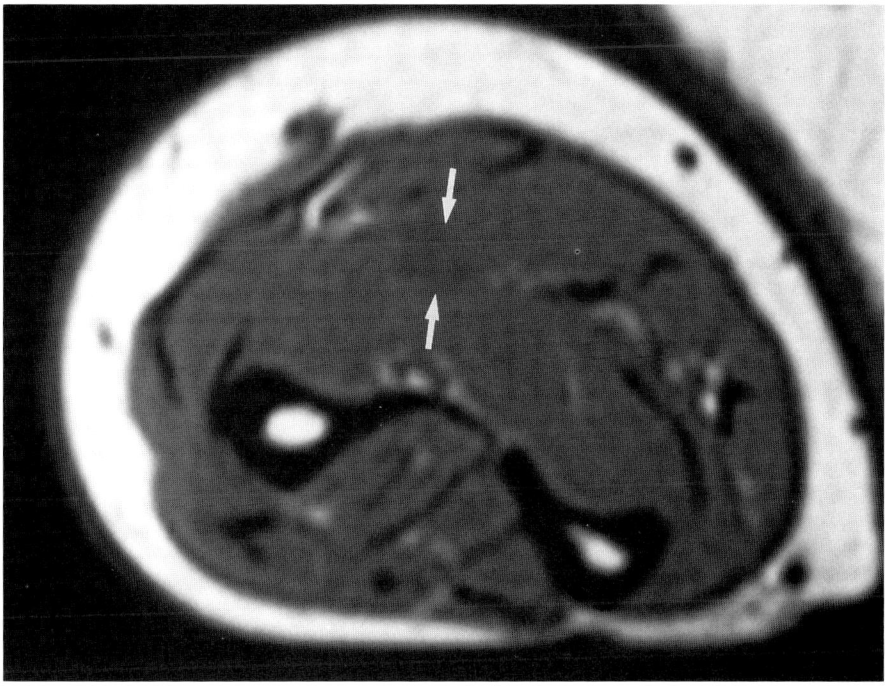

A

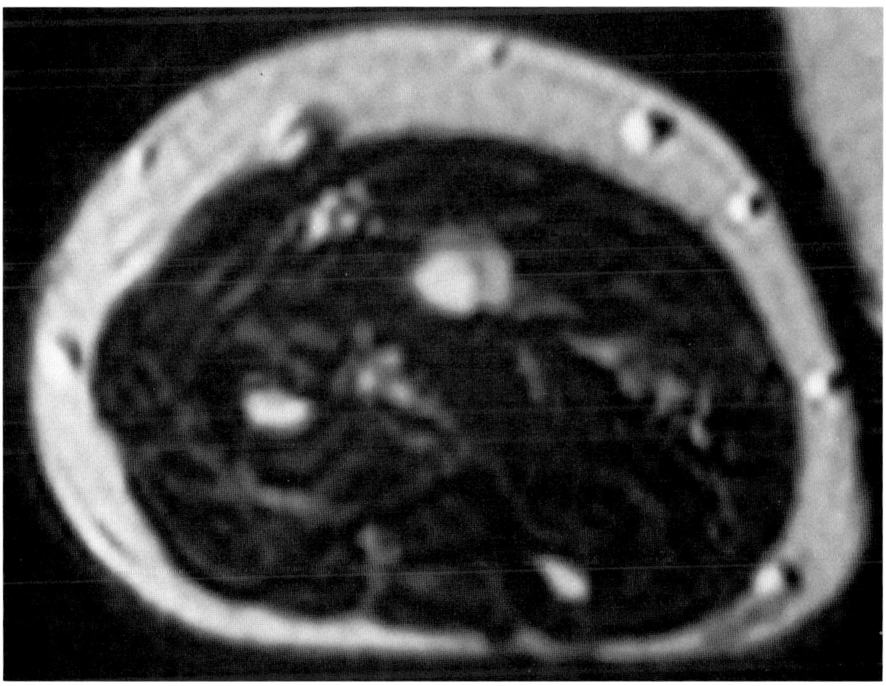

B

FIGURE 6.5 A 46-year-old woman with neurofibromatosis who presented with neuropathy in the median nerve distribution. (A) Axial T1-weighted image (800/14) demonstrates a barely-perceptible hypointense lesion (arrows). (B) Axial FSE T2-weighted image (5150/100) demonstrates hyperintensity of the lesion. Findings are consistent with a neurofibroma arising from the median nerve.

Malignant Peripheral Nerve Sheath Tumor

Definition. Malignant peripheral nerve sheath tumors most likely arise from multiple nerve sheath cells including fibroblasts, Schwann cells, and perineural cells. Various terminology has been used to refer to these lesions including neurofibrosarcoma, malignant schwannoma, malignant neurilemoma, nerve-sheath fibrosarcoma, and neurogenic sarcoma. Malignant peripheral nerve sheath tumors may arise de novo or from pre-existing neurofibromas. Origin from a pre-existing schwannoma is very rare.

Clinical Features. Malignant peripheral nerve sheath tumors comprise approximately 10% of all soft tissue sarcomas. They most often occur between 20 and 50 years of age and present as soft tissue masses, typically associated with pain and neurologic symptoms. Approximately 50% of lesions occur in patients with neurofibromatosis (NF) and 2–29% of NF patients will develop one of these lesions, typically at a younger age than the general population.

Location. These lesions tend to occur along major nerve trunks, most commonly in the extremities proximally and the trunk (associated with the sciatic nerve, brachial plexus, and sacral plexus). Most are located in the deep soft tissues.

Implications. Patients with NF tend to have larger, more aggressive lesions that tend to recur and metastasize. The poor prognosis in NF is partly related to the lesions developing in the deep soft tissues, thus inhibiting early detection. Malignant peripheral nerve sheath tumors are treated similarly to other aggressive soft tissue sarcomas.

MRI Findings. Malignant peripheral nerve sheath tumors typically appear as large masses with indistinct margins in the distribution of a major nerve trunk. These lesions tend to appear hypointense (isointense to muscle) or of intermediate intensity (between that of muscle and fat) on T1-weighted sequences and bright on T2-weighted sequences. The signal intensity is inhomogeneous and dependent upon the amount of hemorrhage and necrosis. Mild muscle atrophy of the surrounding or distally innervated musculature may be seen. Adjacent bone destruction may be present.

Differential Diagnosis. These lesions exhibit nonspecific signal characteristics that can be seen with numerous benign and malignant lesions. The diagnosis of a malignant peripheral nerve sheath tumor should be considered if a mass is intimately associated with a major nerve trunk, especially in the setting of neurofibromatosis. MRI is not reliable in distinguishing benign from malignant peripheral nerve sheath tumors, although marked inhomogeneity and poorly defined margins are more common in the malignant variety.

References

Stull M, Moser R, Kransdorf M, et al. Magnetic resonance appearance of peripheral nerve sheath tumors. *Skeletal Radiol* 20:9–14, 1991.

Levine E, Huntrakoon M, Wetzel L. Malignant nerve-sheath neoplasms in neurofibromatosis: Distinction from benign tumors by using imaging techniques. *AJR* 149:1059–1064, 1987.

Suh J, Abenoza P, Galloway H, et al. Peripheral (extracranial) nerve tumors: Correlation of MR imaging and histologic findings. *Radiology* 183:341–346, 1992.

Varma D, Moulopoulos A, Sara A, et al. MR imaging of extracranial nerve sheath tumors. *JCAT* 16:448–453, 1992.

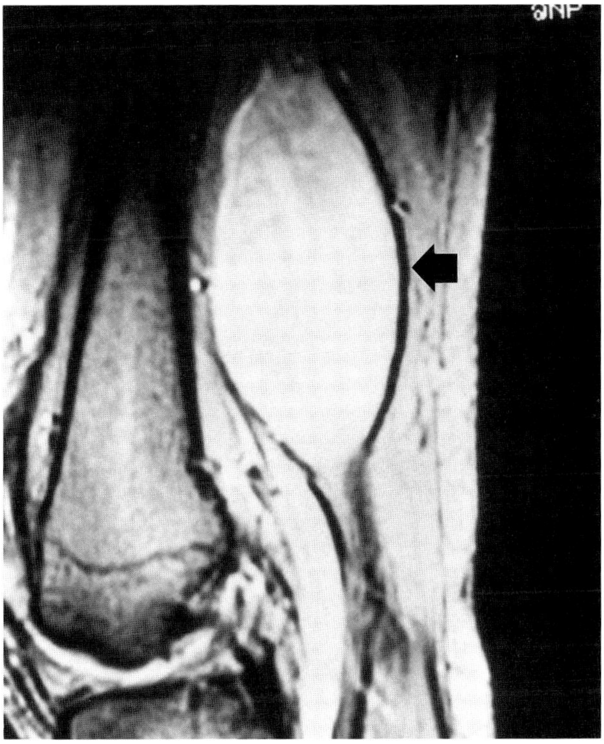

A

FIGURE 6.6 A 28-year-old woman with neurofibromatosis and a large distal thigh mass. (A) Sagittal gradient-recalled echo and

(*continued*)

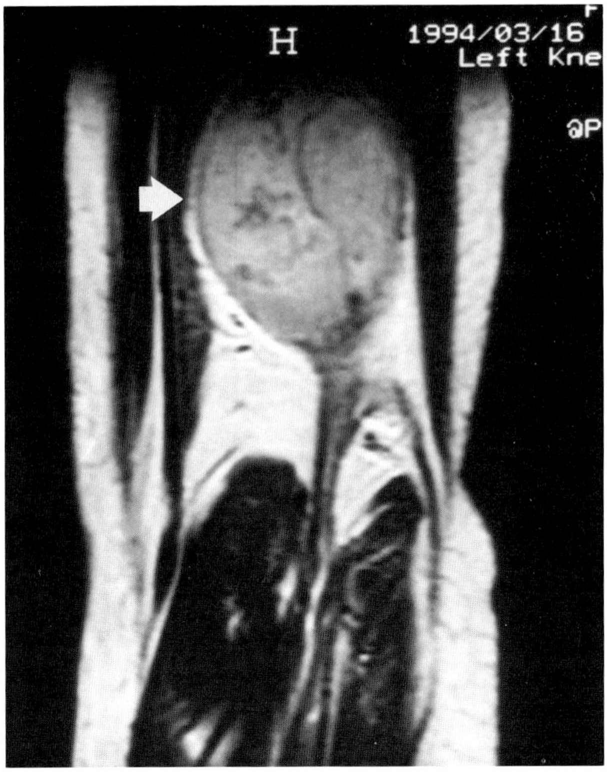

B

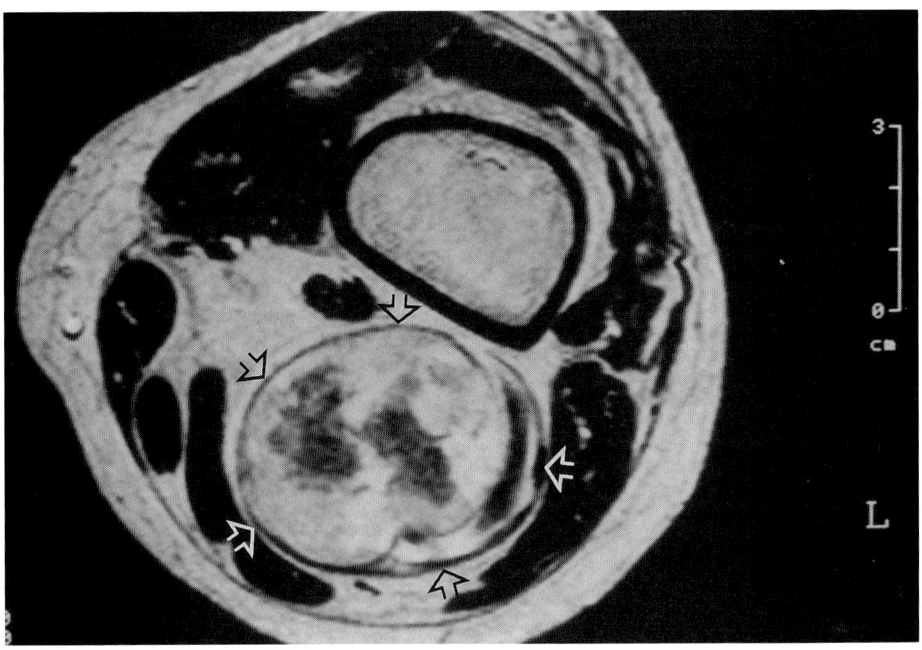

C

FIGURE 6.6 (continued) (B) coronal T2-weighted images demonstrate a large fusiform mass (arrows) arising from the distal sciatic nerve. (C) Axial T2-weighted image reveals heterogeneous signal intensity with areas of low, intermediate, and bright signal present within the lesion. Note that the mass appears well-marginated (open arrows). Pathologic examination confirmed the presence of a malignant peripheral nerve sheath tumor. (Courtesy of James O. Johnston, MD).

Fibrolipomatous Hamartoma of the Median Nerve

Definition. Various terms have been used to describe this lesion including fibrofatty overgrowth, lipomatous hamartoma, lipofibroma, fibrolipoma, lipofibromatous hamartoma, and fatty infiltration of the median nerve. Many consider this lesion to be congenital. Histologically, the lesion demonstrates abundant perineural and epineural fibrosis and infiltration of adipose cells in the interfascicular connective tissue. The nerve fascicles are typically normal in appearance, although atrophy has been reported as a late finding.

Clinical Features. Fibrolipomatous hamartoma is a rare lesion, occurring most commonly in infants and less often in children and young adults. Usually, the patient has been aware of the mass for many years. Early symptoms are often minimal or absent. Late symptoms include carpal tunnel syndrome, pain, motor deficit, and paresthesia. Macrodactyly of the involved extremity is present in approximately two-thirds of cases.

Location. More than 80% of these lesions arise in the median nerve. Cases involving the ulnar nerve, radial nerve, and dorsal foot have also been described.

Implications. Fibrolipomatous hamartomas are benign lesions. Surgical excision of these lesions is controversial with results varying from successful to major neurologic deficit. Treatment most often consists of surgical exploration, biopsy, and carpal tunnel release.

MRI Findings. The MRI findings are pathognomonic. Images reveal a clustered group of longitudinally oriented cylindrical structures measuring approximately 3 mm in diameter. These cylindrical structures demonstrate a signal void on all pulse sequences corresponding to nerve fascicles with accompanying epineural and perineural fibrosis. These cylindrical structures are separated by areas of fatty signal intensity, representing infiltrating adipose cells. If large enough, the mass displaces the flexor tendons and causes bulging of the flexor retinaculum.

Differential Diagnosis. If MR demonstrates a mass in the distribution of the median nerve with the characteristic cable-like appearance and signal characteristics described above, the diagnosis of fibrolipomatous hamartoma can be made. A hemangioma can sometimes have a similar appearance with fatty signal intensity and foci of hypointense signal representing vascular channels, calcification, or phleboliths. An arteriovenous malformation could also have a similar appearance with cylindrical areas of signal void from blood flow. Both of these lesions can be confidently differentiated from a fibrolipomatous hamartoma by the identification of a normal median nerve.

References

Cavallaro M, Taylor J, Gorman J, et al. Imaging findings in a patient with fibrolipomatous hamartoma of the median nerve. *AJR* 161:837–838, 1993.

Boren W, Henry R, Wintch K. MR diagnosis of fibrolipomatous hamartoma of nerve: Association with nerve territory-oriented macrodactyly (macrodystrophia lipomatosa). *Skeletal Radiol* 24:296–297, 1995.

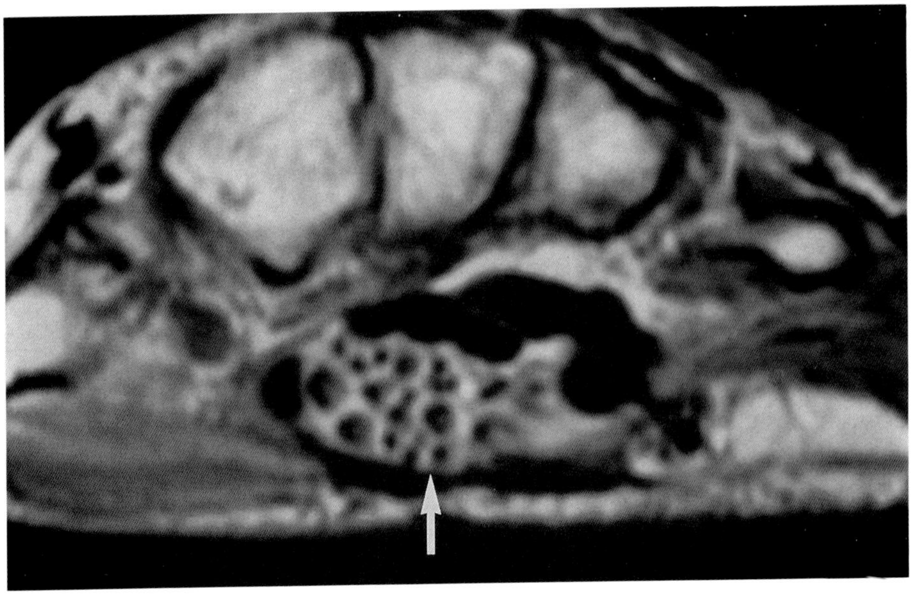

A

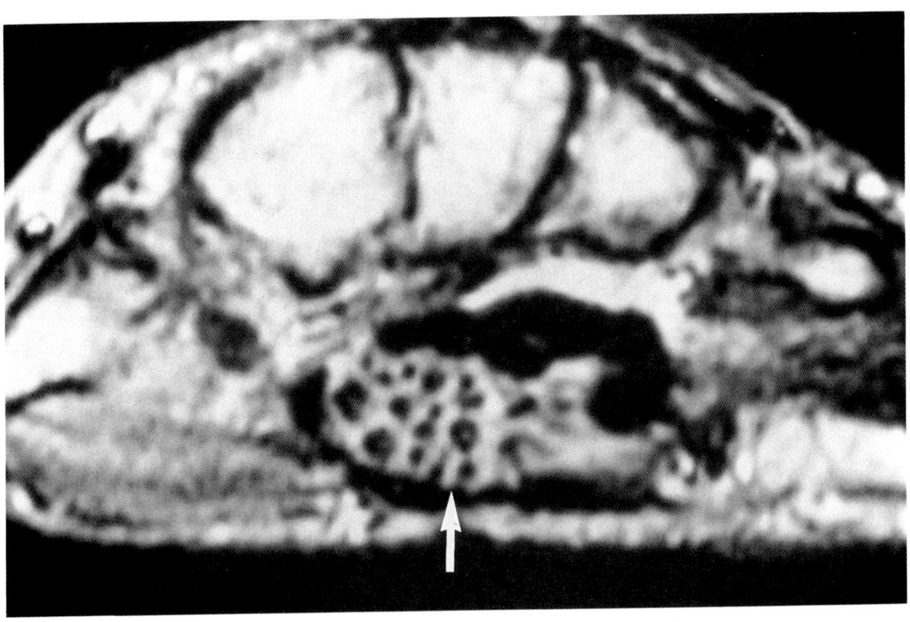

B

FIGURE 6.7 A 74-year-old woman with carpal tunnel syndrome. Axial (A) proton density and (B) T2-weighted images reveal a large fibrolipomatous hamartoma of the median nerve (arrows). Note the characteristic appearance of numerous foci of signal void surrounded by fatty signal intensity. (Courtesy of John Kirby, MD).

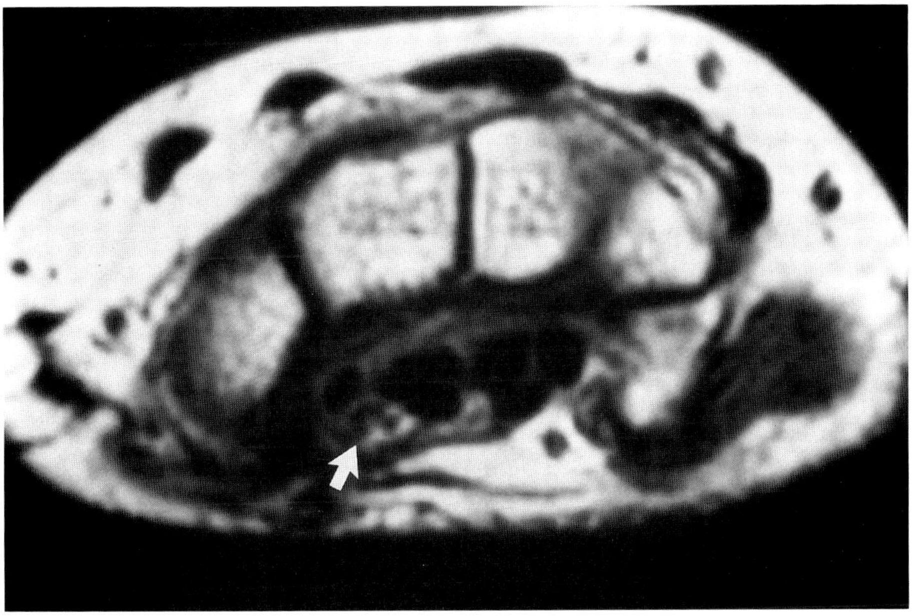

FIGURE 6.8 Axial proton density image (2000/20) demonstrates a small fibrolipomatous hamartoma of the median nerve (arrow) in a 21-year-old woman.

7 Inflammatory Lesions

Soft Tissue Infection

Definition. Infection of the soft tissues can have multiple forms including abscess, pyomyositis, fasciitis, and cellulitis. Soft tissue infection may result from various routes of contamination including hematogenous spread, direct extension of infection involving an adjacent bone or joint, and direct implantation from penetrating injury, surgery, or other intervention.

Clinical Features. All ages may be affected. Risk factors include diabetes, immunosuppression, and intravenous drug abuse. Staphylococcus aureus is a frequent responsible organism. Clinical manifestations include pain, swelling/mass, tenderness, warmth, erythema, fever, leukocytosis, and elevated sedimentation rate.

Location. Any musculoskeletal location may be affected. The foot is particularly vulnerable in diabetic patients.

Implications. Abscesses/infected fluid collections typically require surgical or percutaneous drainage in addition to antibiotic therapy. Necrotizing soft tissue infections are potentially fatal and require imminent surgical intervention. They may be associated with tissue destruction out of proportion to physical findings. Additionally, the clinical course may be rapidly progressive and high mortality rates have been reported.

MRI Findings. Abscesses and infected fluid collections typically appear hypointense to slightly hyperintense in relation to muscle on T1-weighted images and hyperintense on T2-weighted sequences. The signal intensity may be heterogeneous depending on the amount of debris and hemorrhage present. Peripheral rim enhancement following gadolinium administration typically occurs. This may be helpful in distinguishing these areas from simple soft tissue infection (such as cellulitis). Gadolinium may also be useful in distinguishing between viable and nonviable tissue prior to surgical debridement. Abscesses and infected fluid collections are associated with variable amounts of surrounding inflammation and edema, exhibiting hypointense signal (hypointense or isointense to muscle) with T1-weighting and hyperintense signal with T2-weighting. Adjacent bony structures should be carefully evaluated for evidence of associated osteomyelitis.

Differential Diagnosis. The MRI features of soft tissue infection are nonspecific and must be correlated with the clinical findings. Abscesses cannot be reliably differentiated from necrotic soft tissue neoplasms. Soft tissue hematomas can also have a similar appearance. Infected fluid collections cannot be distinguished from noninfected collections of fluid. Additionally, their signal characteristics are typically identical to those of synovial or ganglion cysts, fluid-filled bursae, and some soft tissue tumors (such as myxoma).

References

Munk P, Vellet A, Hilborn M, et al. Musculoskeletal infection: Findings on magnetic resonance imaging. *Can Assoc Radiol J* 45:355–362, 1994.

Applegate G, Cohen A. Pyomyositis: Early detection utilizing multiple imaging modalities. *MRI* 9:187–193, 1991.

Rahmouni A, Chosidow O, Mathieu D, et al. MR imaging in acute infectious cellulitis. *Radiology* 192:493–496, 1994.

Fleckenstein J, Burns D, Murphy F, et al. Differential diagnosis of bacterial myositis in AIDS: Evaluation with MR imaging. *Radiology* 179:653–658, 1991.

A

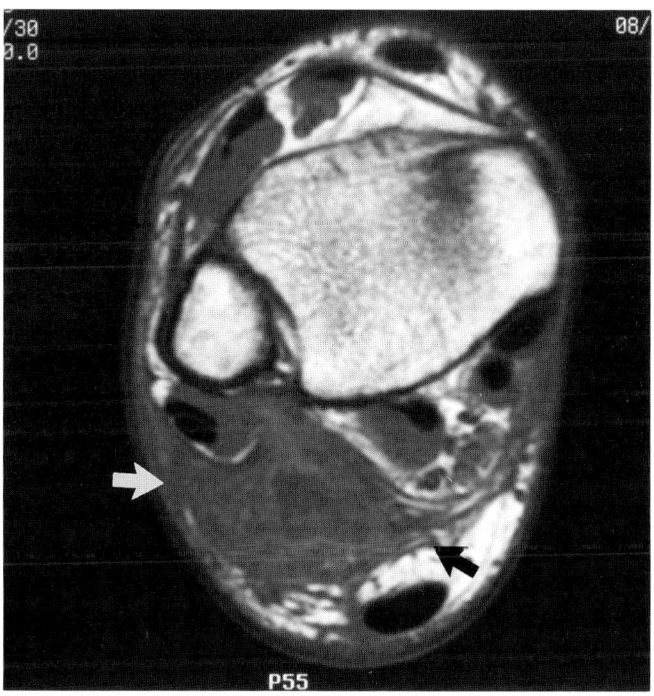

FIGURE 7.1 Ankle abscess in a 30-year-old male. (A) Axial T1-weighted image demonstrates an ill-defined abscess (arrows) centered in the lateral portion of the pre-Achilles (Kager's) fat pad.

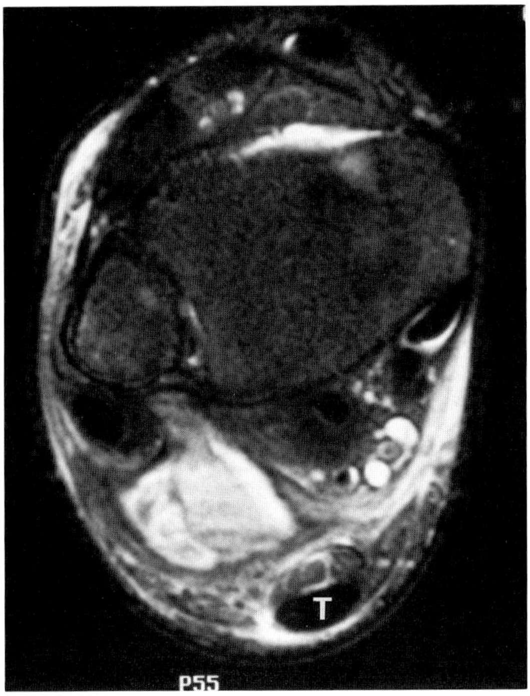

B

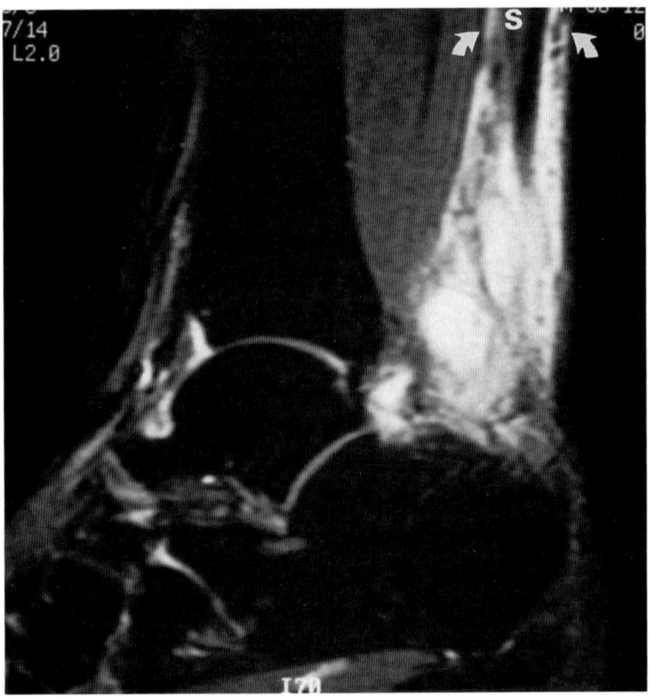

C

Figure 7.1 (continued) (B) Axial FSE T2-weighted fat suppression image highlights the abscess and associated edema including extension anterolaterally, medially, and around the Achilles tendon (T). (C) Sagittal FMPIR image demonstrates superior extension (curved arrows) around the Achilles tendon and soleus muscle (S).

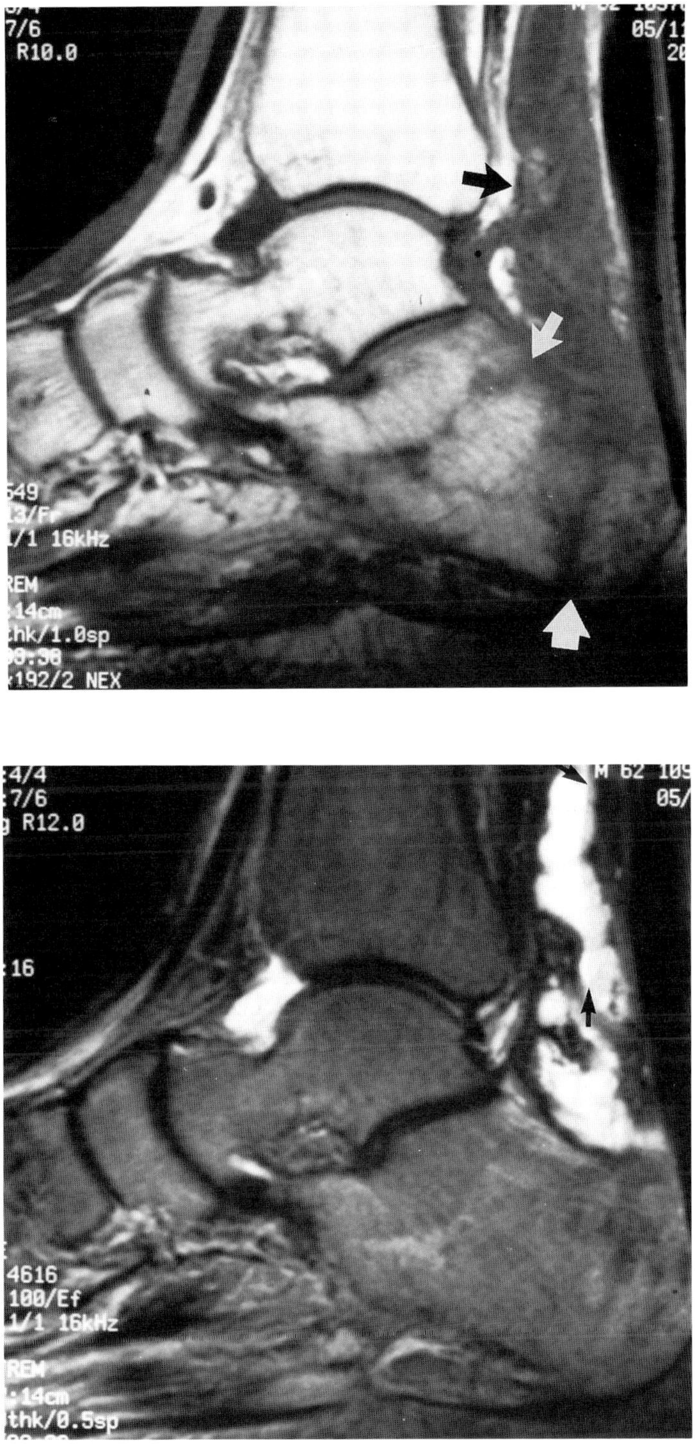

A

B

FIGURE 7.2 A 62-year-old male with an ankle abscess and associated calcaneal osteomyelitis. (A) Sagittal T1-weighted image (549/13) demonstrates an abscess in the pre-Achilles (Kager's) fat pad (arrow) and associated osteomyelitis involving the calcaneus (white arrows). Incidentally noted is fusiform Achilles tendon thickening consistent with chronic tendonitis. (B) Sagittal FSE T2-weighted fat suppression (4616/100) and

(*continued*)

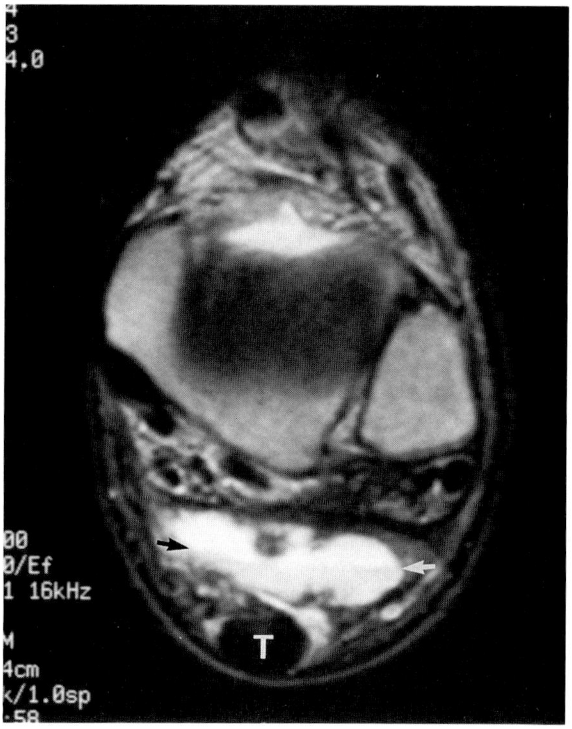

C

FIGURE 7.2 (continued) (C) axial FSE T2-weighted (3500/100) images demonstrate the lobulated nature of the abscess as well as a fluid-fluid level (small arrows). There is extension of fluid around a portion of the Achilles tendon (T).

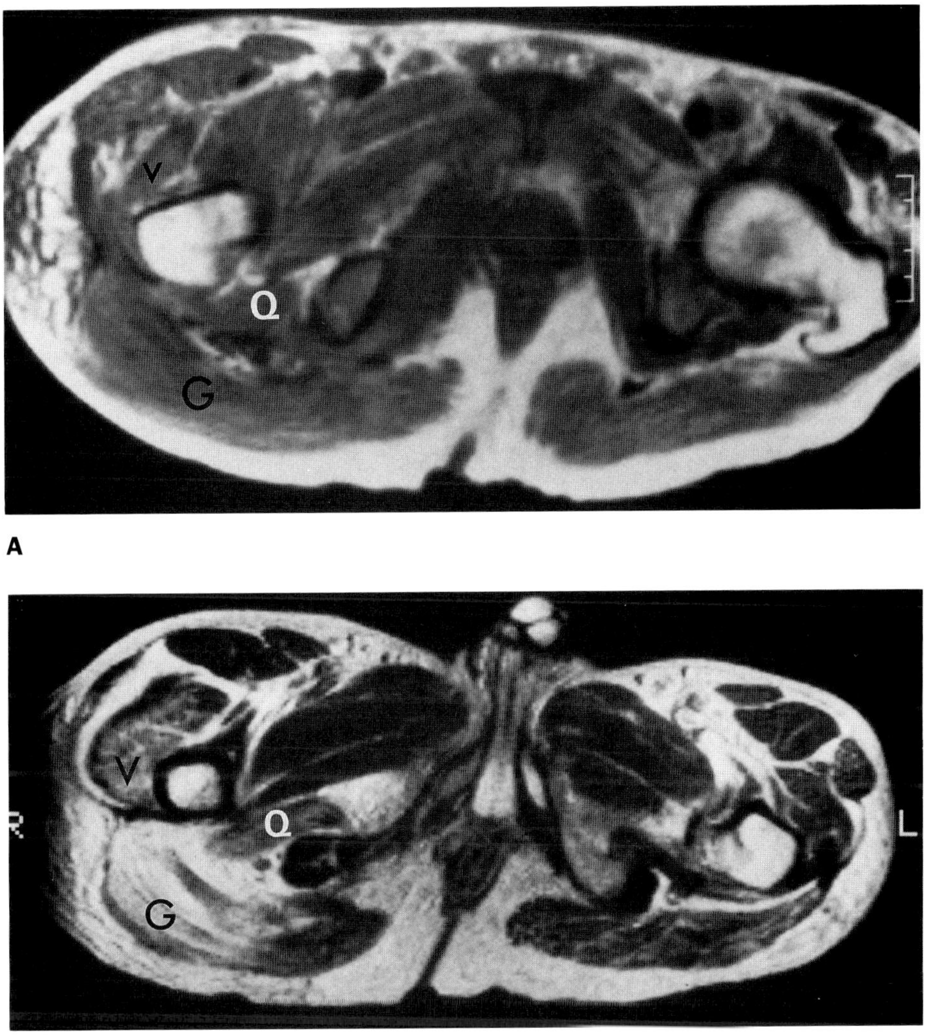

A

B

FIGURE 7.3 Pyomyositis in a 30-year-old man with AIDS. Axial (A) T1-weighted (600/15) and (B) T2-weighted (2000/60) images reveal thickening and increased signal in the right gluteus maximus (G), quadratus femoris (Q), and vastus lateralis (V) muscles.

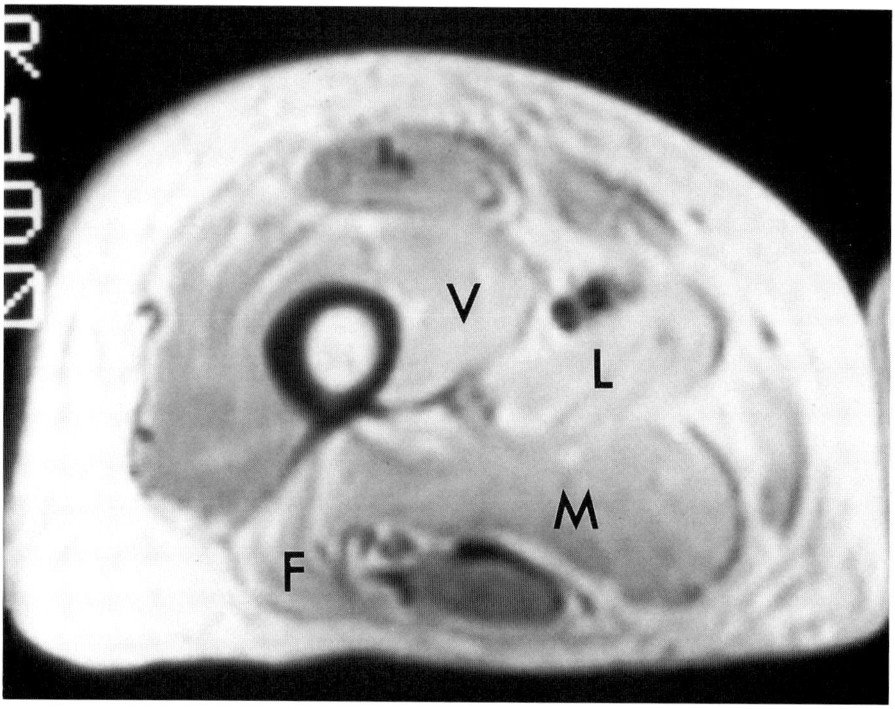

A

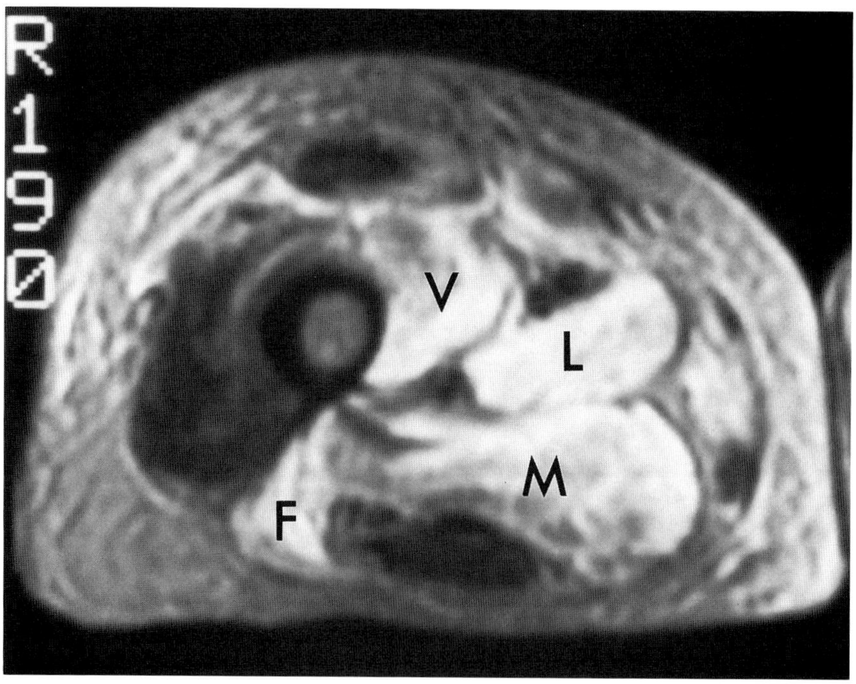

B

FIGURE 7.4 Pyomyositis in a 44-year-old diabetic woman. Axial (A) proton density (2500/20) and (B) T2-weighted (2500/80) images of the right thigh reveal prominent increased signal within the vastus medialis (V), adductor longus (L), adductor magnus (M), and biceps femoris (F) muscles. Also note subcutaneous edema versus cellulitis.

Inflammatory Myopathy (Myositis)

Definition. The inflammatory myopathies (myositides) are a group of idiopathic disorders characterized by the presence of inflammatory infiltrate within skeletal muscle.

Clinical Features. Inflammatory myopathies are relatively rare disorders which may affect adults of all ages and even children. Patients may have muscle weakness, pain, tenderness, and extremity swelling. The diagnosis is established by an elevation of serum muscle enzyme (creatine kinase) activity, electromyographic abnormalities, and typical features on muscle biopsy.

Location. There is a predilection for the proximal muscles of the upper and lower extremity, especially the shoulder girdle and thigh.

Implications. In approximately 10% of cases, muscle biopsy is nondiagnostic, presumably due to a scattered distribution of inflammatory change. Therapy for myositis includes corticosteroids and immunosuppressant medication.

MRI Findings. MRI is sensitive in the detection of myositis and is effective in depicting the extent and distribution of involvement. Acute myositis appears as a focal or diffuse increase in muscle signal intensity on T2-weighted and STIR images, due to the presence of inflammation and edema. There is preservation of normal muscle architecture and T1-weighted images may appear unremarkable. The increased signal intensity on T2-weighted and STIR images has been shown to correlate with disease activity and becomes normal following successful therapy. MRI can be used to follow a patient with myositis and assess response to therapy. In addition, MRI might be helpful in guiding muscle biopsy, which could be directed toward the most prominently inflamed and edematous regions. The findings of chronic myositis include muscle atrophy and fatty replacement. Fatty replacement of muscle is well-visualized on T1-weighted sequences, appearing as areas of high signal that are isointense to subcutaneous fat.

Differential Diagnosis. The MRI findings of myositis are typical, but not specific. Similar findings can be seen with muscle injury, infection, denervation, other types of myopathy, and rhabdomyolysis. These entities should be distinguishable based upon clinical grounds. Myositis can be differentiated from an intramuscular neoplasm by noting the preservation of normal muscle architecture.

References

Fraser D, Frank J, Dalakas M, et al. Magnetic resonance imaging in the idiopathic inflammatory myopathies. *J Rheum* 18:1693–1700, 1991.

Reimers C, Schedel H, Fleckenstein J, et al. Magnetic resonance imaging of skeletal muscles in idiopathic inflammatory myopathies of adults. *J Neurol* 241:306–314, 1994.

Stiglbauer R, Graninger W, Prayer L, et al. Polymyositis: MRI-appearance at 1.5 T and correlation to clinical findings. *Clin Radiol* 48:244–248, 1993.

Esteva-Lorenzo F, Ferreiro J, Tardagulla F, et al. Case report 866. *Skeletal Radiol* 23:572–576, 1994.

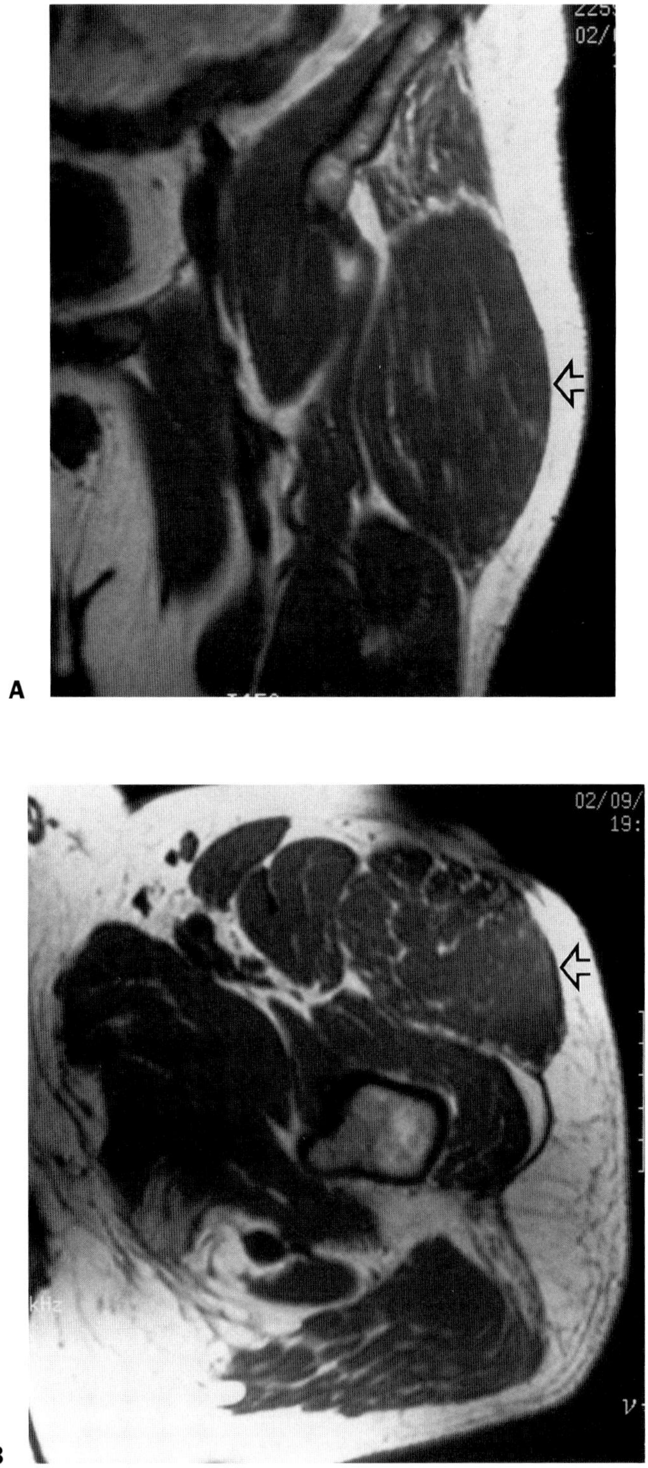

FIGURE 7.5 A 60-year-old male with biopsy-proven myositis who presented with a palpable, firm left hip region mass. T1-weighted (A) coronal (600/10) and (B) axial (533/10) images reveal marked fusiform enlargement of the tensor fasciae latae muscle (arrows). Note the preservation of normal muscle architecture. (C) Coronal FMPIR (4000/34, TI-120) and (D) axial FSE T2-weighted fat suppression (4000/102) images reveal increased signal throughout the involved muscle (arrows).

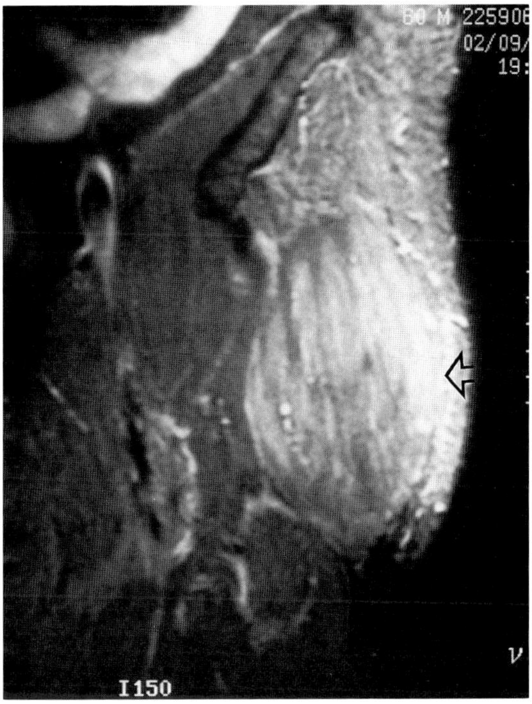

C

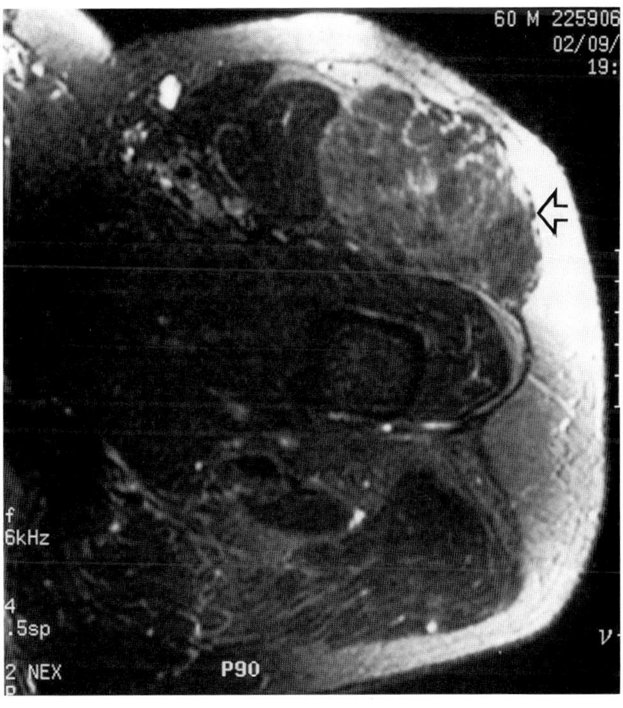

D

Post-Injection Soft Tissue Inflammation Reaction

Definition. Changes may occur in the soft tissues following intramuscular or subcutaneous injection of various medications. The associated changes may represent an inflammatory reaction or may be due to the drug itself. There may or may not be associated hemorrhage. With time, a granulomatous response may develop which can calcify.

Clinical Features. Numerous drugs are commonly injected into the soft tissues, most notably intramuscular pain medications and subcutaneous insulin.

Location. Intramuscular injections are most commonly performed in the upper-outer buttocks and anterior thigh, but may be administered in other sites, including the deltoid muscle.

Implications. These lesions should not be mistaken for neoplasms or other soft tissue processes. No treatment is necessary.

MRI Findings. On MRI, post-injection sites typically appear as stellate-shaped or ill-defined lesions which are hypointense on T1-weighted images and hyperintense on T2-weighted sequences. The signal intensity is variable when there is associated hemorrhage. The presence of hemosiderin or of calcification within a granuloma would result in areas of signal void on all pulse sequences. These lesions are often multiple and bilateral. Injected material may dissect along intramuscular fascial planes. The internal muscle architecture should be preserved and there should not be significant mass effect. A needle tract may be present.

Differential Diagnosis. The MR appearance may resemble muscle injury, infection, muscle infarction, previous biopsy site, or an infiltrating neoplasm. Multiplicity/bilaterality and a typical location are strong clues to the diagnosis, which should be readily confirmed by clinical history.

Reference

Resendes M, Helms C, Fritz R, et al. MR appearance of intramuscular injections. *AJR* 158:1293–1294, 1992.

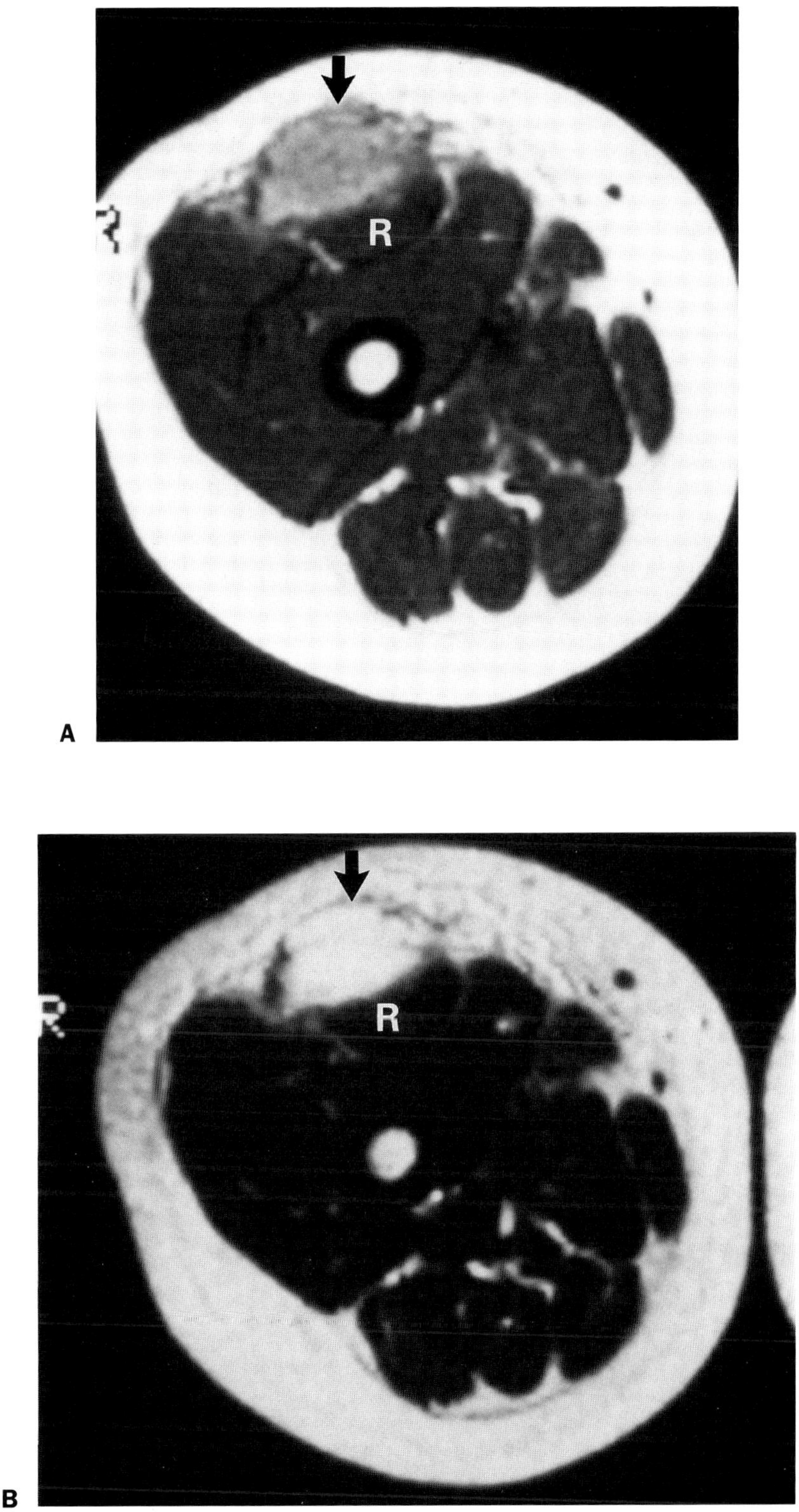

FIGURE 7.6 An 18-month-old female with post-injection inflammatory reaction within the anterior right thigh. Axial (A) T1-weighted (750/40) and (B) T2-weighted (2000/80) images reveal a focal anterior subcutaneous mass (arrows). Note the mass effect on the rectus femoris muscle (R).

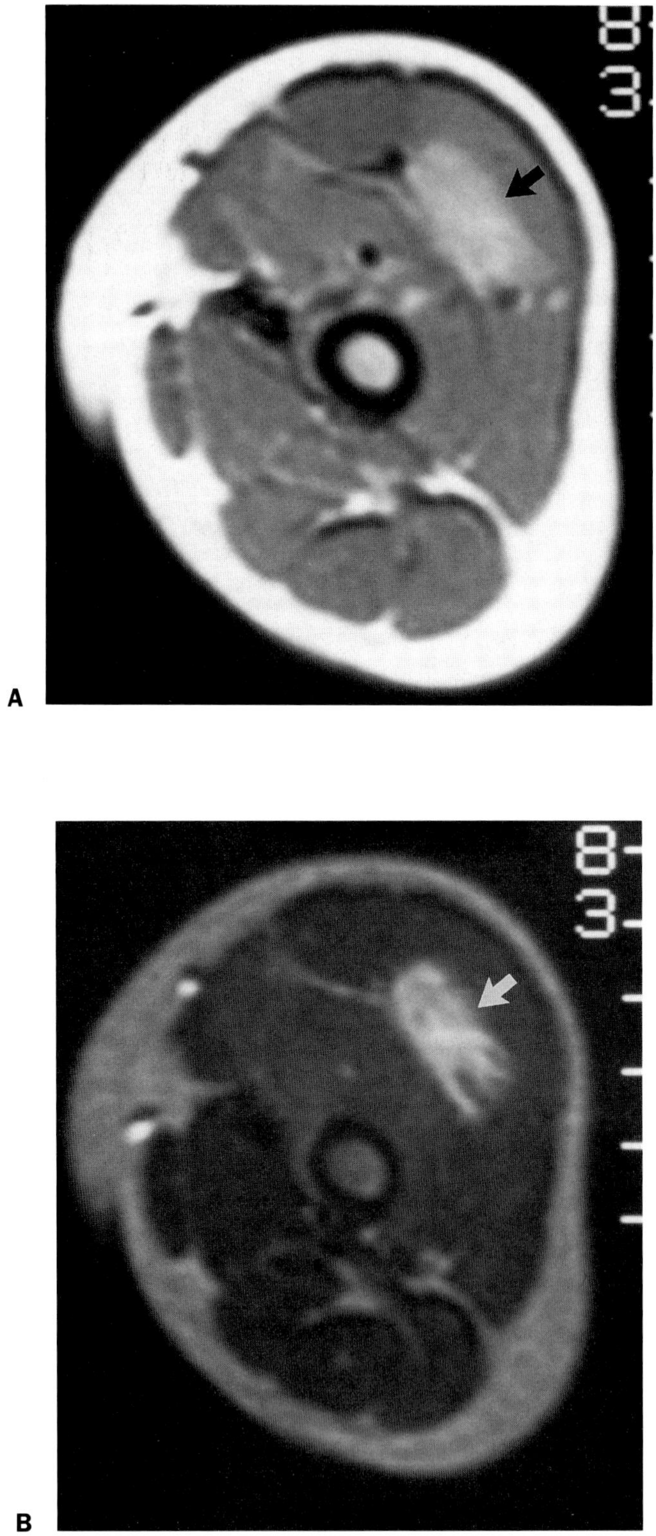

Figure 7.7 Intramuscular post-injection inflammatory reaction in a 3-year-old patient. Axial (A) proton density (2400/20) and (B) T2-weighted (2400/80) images reveal a focal lesion within the left vastus lateralis muscle (arrows).

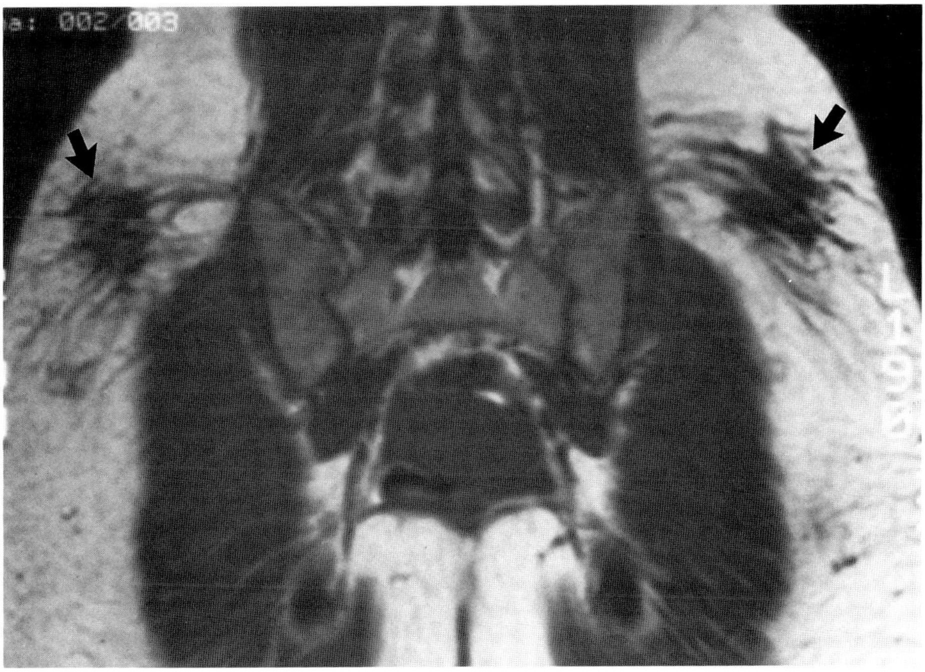

A

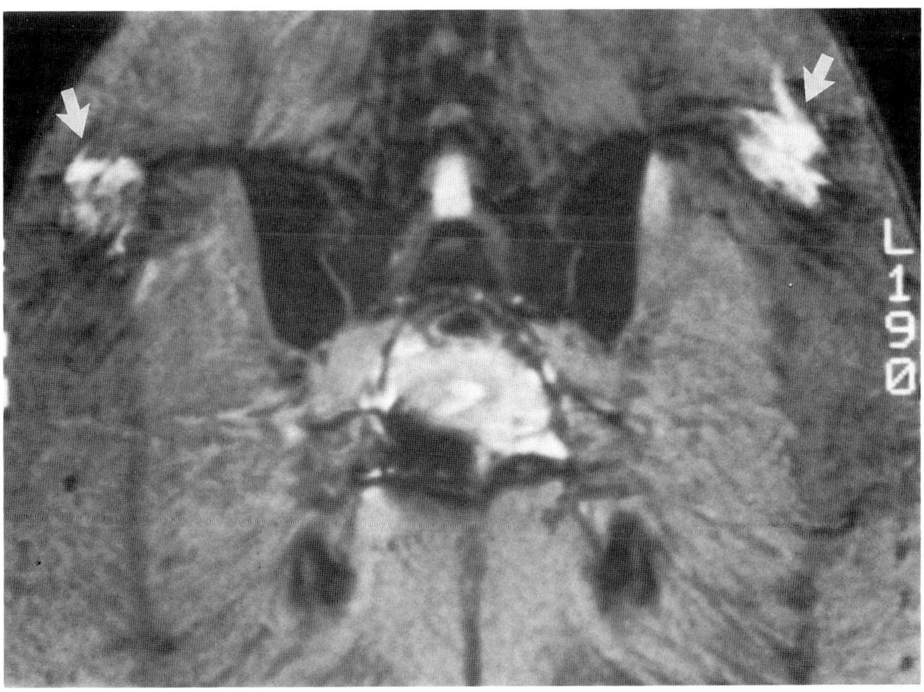

B

Figure 7.8 A 38-year-old woman with post-injection inflammatory reactions in both buttocks. Coronal (A) T1-weighted (600/20) and (B) MPGR (500/15, 15 degrees) scans demonstrate irregular, somewhat stellate-shaped areas of signal abnormality in the subcutaneous tissues (arrows).

8 Muscles Presenting as Masses

Accessory Muscle

Definition. Accessory muscles are anatomic variants. Numerous accessory muscles of the musculoskeletal system have been reported. One of the most recognized is the accessory soleus muscle, which is described separately (*see* Index for listing).

Clinical Features. Accessory muscles of the hand/wrist and foot/ankle are relatively common. Accessory muscles are often asymptomatic. However, they may present as palpable masses or can be associated with pain, swelling, and tenderness or with symptoms related to nerve entrapment, vascular compression, or muscle ischemia. Symptoms may be precipitated by exercise or manual labor.

Location. Accessory muscles may occur throughout the musculoskeletal system, but are encountered most frequently on imaging studies in the hand/wrist and foot/ankle regions. Accessory muscles are frequently bilateral.

Implications. Therapy is not required for asymptomatic lesions. Conservative treatment is preferred for symptomatic lesions, but fasciotomy or surgical excision may be required. Patients are typically symptom-free following surgical treatment.

MRI Findings. The MRI findings are characteristic and consist of a homogeneous hypointense "mass" which is isointense to the adjacent muscles on all pulse sequences. This "mass" generally demonstrates the typical marbled appearance and architecture of skeletal muscle.

Differential Diagnosis. Familiarity with these lesions should enable the correct diagnosis to be made with MRI and help prevent unnecessary surgery. Scanning of the opposite extremity may be helpful due to the frequent bilaterality of accessory muscles. Other lesions which may exhibit low signal intensity on T2-weighted sequences include giant cell tumor of tendon sheath, fibrous tumors, and scar tissue.

References

Anderson M, Benedetti P, Walter J, et al. Case report. MR appearance of the extensor digitorum manus brevis muscle: A pseudotumor of the hand. *AJR* 164:1477–1479, 1995.

Yu J, Resnick D. MR imaging of the accessory soleus muscle appearance in six patients and a review of the literature. *Skeletal Radiol* 23:525–528, 1994.

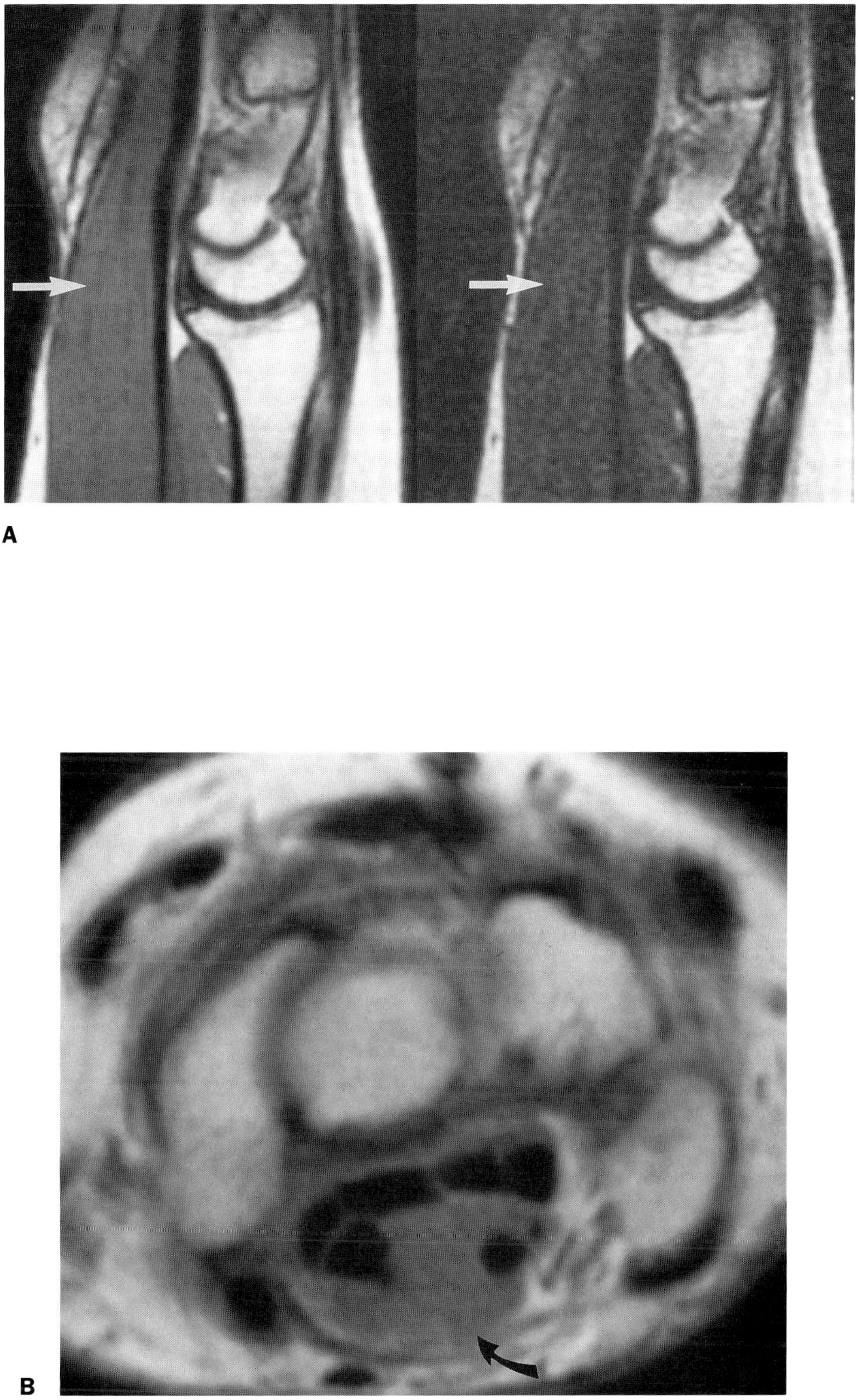

A

B

FIGURE 8.1 A 16-year-old female with exercise-induced wrist swelling, pain, and weakness. (A) Sagittal dual-echo T2-weighted (1700/30, 80) images reveal an abnormal soft tissue density (arrows) extending from the distal forearm through the carpal tunnel and into the volar soft tissues of the hand. Note that this lesion is isointense with the adjacent muscles. Axial (B) proton density (1700/30) and

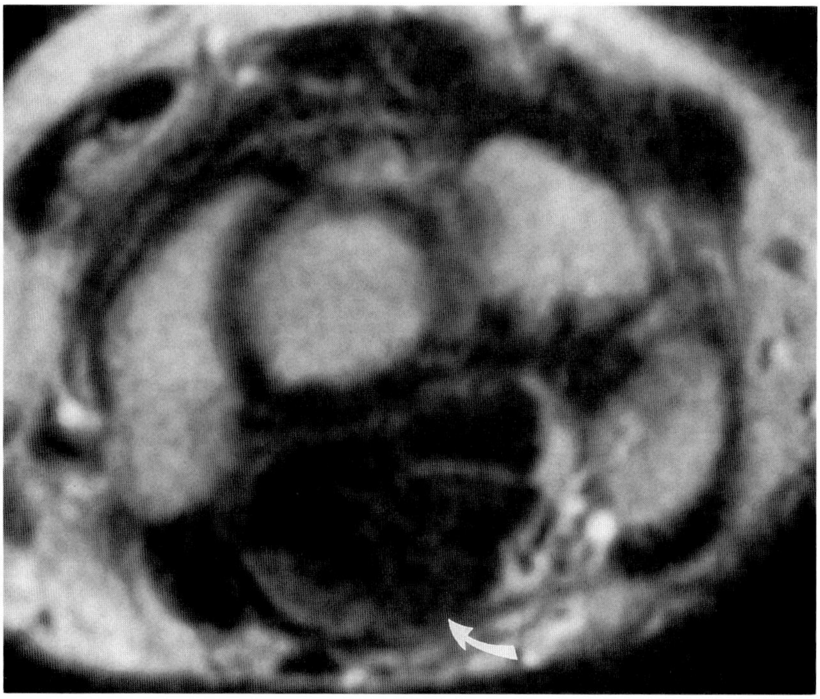

C

FIGURE 8.1 (continued) (C) T2-weighted (1700/80) images reveal that the soft tissue lesion (curved arrows) is associated with the flexor tendons. Findings are consistent with anomalous distal extension of the flexor digitorum superficialis muscle. Symptoms are presumably related to mass effect on the median nerve.

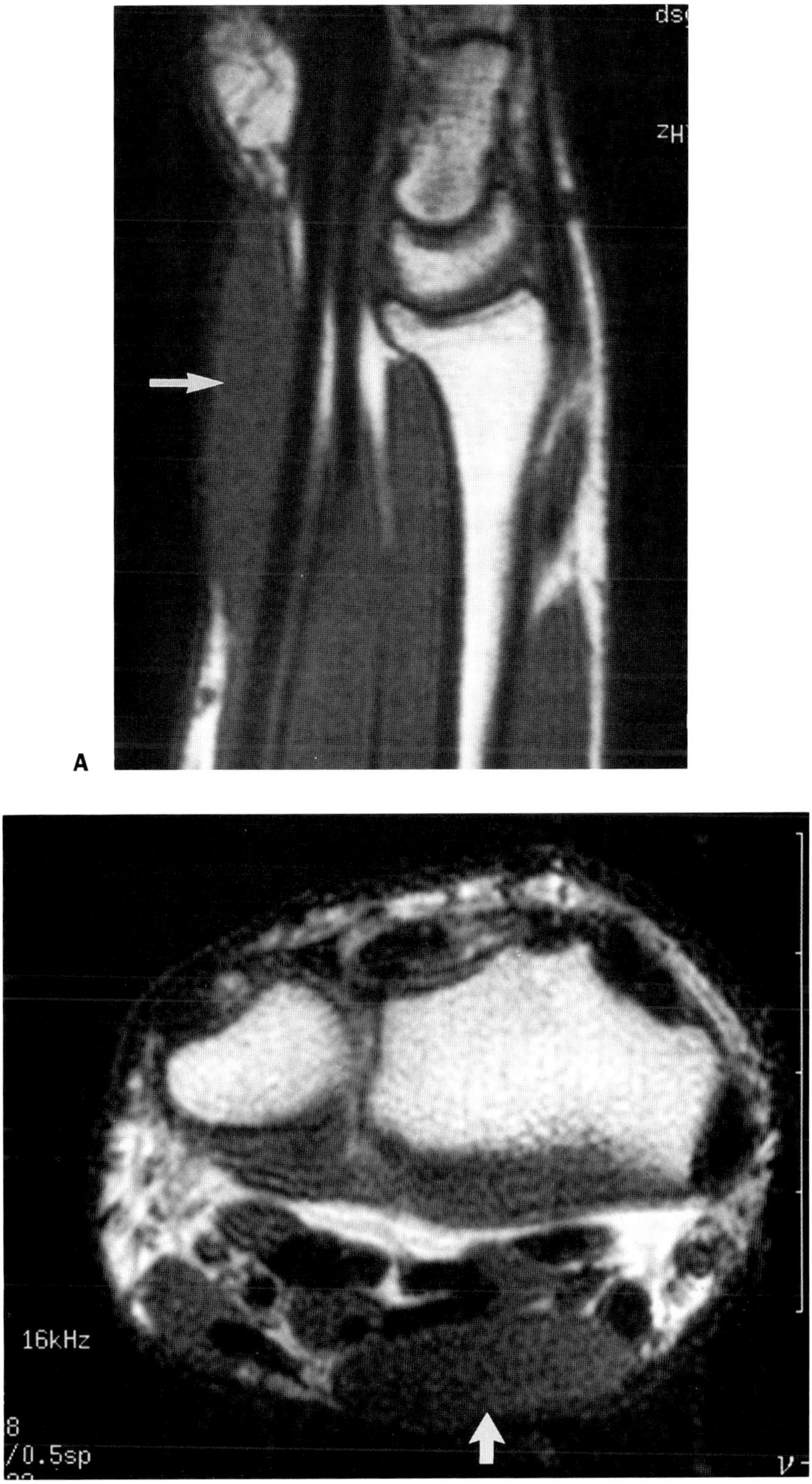

A

B

FIGURE 8.2 A 26-year-old male with palpable swelling at the volar aspect of the wrist. T1-weighted (A) sagittal (516/15) and (B) axial (550/22) images reveal an anomalous palmaris longus muscle (arrows). Note the isointensity and similar appearance to the surrounding musculature.

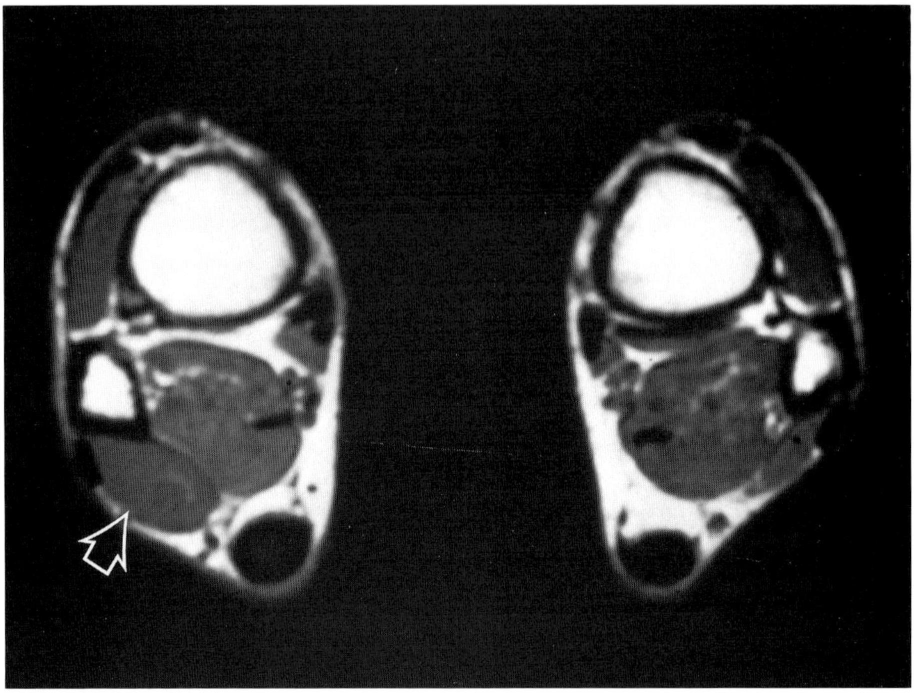

FIGURE 8.3 Anomalous leg muscle in a 49-year-old male. Axial T1-weighted image (600/20) demonstrates an anomalous muscle known as peroneus quartus (arrow). This is the second most common accessory muscle of the ankle region.

Accessory Soleus Muscle

Definition. An accessory soleus muscle is a normal variant consisting of persistence of the distal muscular portion of the soleus in the region of the pre-Achilles fat pad. It is probably the most well-recognized accessory muscle and is worthy of separate discussion (*see* Index for accessory muscle listing).

Clinical Features. Accessory muscles of the foot and ankle occur in up to 6% of individuals. The most common of these anomalous muscles is the accessory soleus. Most patients present with a fullness/soft tissue mass in the posteromedial aspect of the ankle or with exercise-induced pain and swelling, which may result from closed compartment ischemia, a tenuous blood supply, or compression of the posterior tibial nerve. Patients are typically young at presentation (age range: 9–35 years old), which likely reflects a response to increased muscle mass during adolescence or an increase in physical activity. An accessory soleus may also be asymptomatic and noted incidentally on imaging studies.

Location. An accessory soleus muscle extends into the pre-Achilles fat pad (Kager's triangle) and may insert onto the Achilles tendon, the medial aspect of the calcaneus, or the flexor retinaculum. Bilateral accessory soleus muscles may be present.

Implications. No therapy is required for asymptomatic lesions. Symptomatic lesions may be treated with fasciotomy (for compartment syndrome) or surgical excision (for compression neuropathy or claudication). Patients are generally symptom-free following surgery.

MRI Findings. At the level of the ankle, a "mass" is identified between the flexor hallicus longus muscle and the Achilles tendon. Normally, this region contains only pre-Achilles fat. This mass demonstrates the typical marbled appearance and architecture of muscle and is isointense to the adjacent muscles on all pulse sequences, appearing hypointense on both T1-weighted and T2-weighted sequences.

Differential Diagnosis. An accessory soleus muscle is readily differentiated from other masses based upon the typical location and signal characteristics described above.

References

Deutsch A, Mink J, Kerr R. *MRI of the Foot and Ankle*. New York, NY; Raven Press, Ltd: 1992: pp 255–256, 149–150.

Yu J, Resnick D. MR imaging of the accessory soleus muscle appearance in six patients and a review of the literature. *Skeletal Radiol* 23:525–528, 1994.

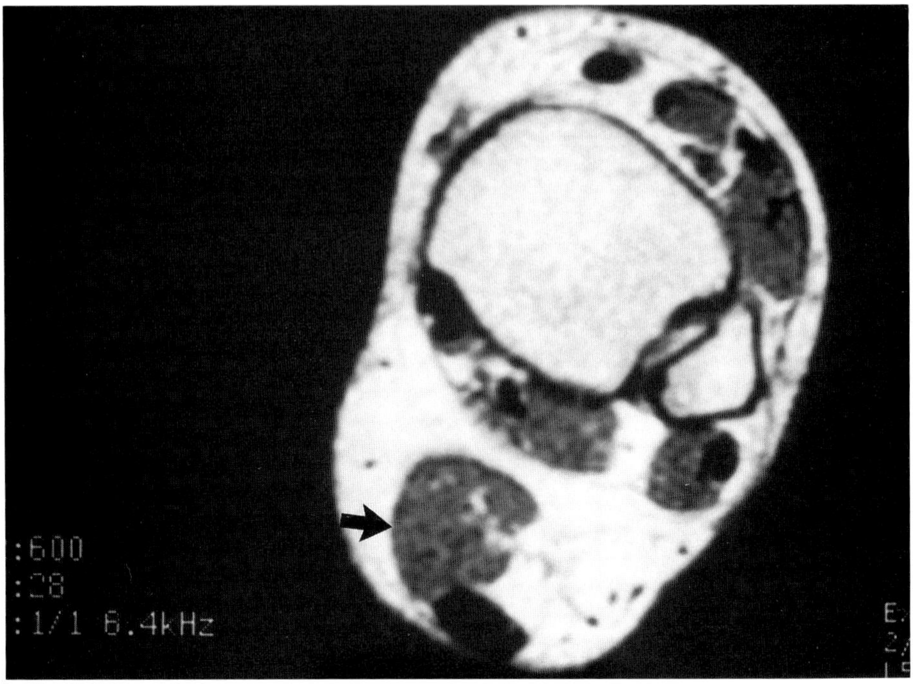

A

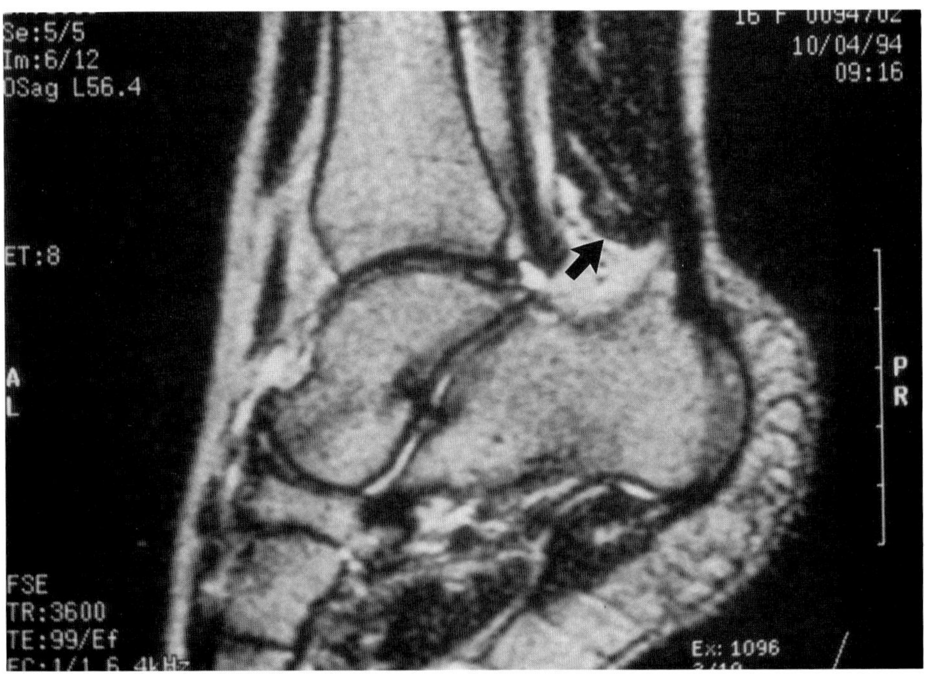

B

FIGURE 8.4 Accessory soleus in a 16-year-old female. (A) Axial T1-weighted (600/28) and (B) sagittal FSE T2-weighted (3600/99) images reveal an accessory soleus muscle (arrows) in the pre-Achilles fat pad (Kager's triangle). Note that this structure is isointense and similar in appearance to the surrounding muscles.

Retracted Muscle

Definition. If there is a complete or significant partial tear of a muscle or tendon, the muscle often retracts resulting in enlargement/mass effect of the retracted portion.

Clinical Features. In most cases, the patient can relate the swelling/mass to a specific traumatic event, thus allowing a straightforward clinical diagnosis. However, sometimes there is only a questionable history of remote injury or the traumatic insult is not recalled by the patient. Under these circumstances, patients may present with a palpable soft tissue mass, with or without persistent pain, which is worrisome clinically for a neoplasm. In other cases, atrophy of a previously torn muscle results in hypertrophy of the surrounding muscles, which may be mistaken clinically for a soft tissue tumor. The mass effect associated with a muscle tear is usually fixed and independent of the amount of muscle contraction. However, some patients present with a mass that is only palpable in certain positions (e.g., flexion).

Location. These injuries can occur throughout the musculoskeletal system depending on the specific activity and mechanism of injury.

Implications. MRI should allow confident diagnosis of a torn and retracted muscle, thereby allowing appropriate therapy. MRI also provides information about the extent of the muscle injury, degree of retraction, and amount of muscle atrophy, as well as delineating the margins of normal versus abnormal muscle and tendon. This information may be helpful in preoperative planning if surgical treatment is performed. If the patient has a position-dependent mass, it is important to image the involved muscle in both relaxed and contracted positions. This scanning technique may reveal a partial muscle tear or muscle herniation through a fascial defect. If the MR findings are not obvious, comparison with the unaffected extremity may prove useful.

MRI Findings. MRI will reveal a "mass" adjacent to a muscle or tendon tear. Depending on the age of the injury, there may be surrounding edema and hemorrhage. Edema exhibits high signal intensity on T2-weighted sequences, whereas methemoglobin demonstrates bright signal intensity on both T1- and T2-weighted images. The mass of retracted muscle will appear hypointense on all pulse sequences, paralleling that of the adjacent musculature. Internal architecture typical for that of skeletal muscle should also be identified. There may be atrophy of the injured muscle or compensatory hypertrophy of the adjacent muscles. Atrophic muscle demonstrates increased fat content (which appears bright on T1-weighted sequences) compared with the adjacent muscles. Atrophy or adjacent muscle hypertrophy is readily diagnosed upon comparison with the contralateral extremity. The size of the defect at the tear site is proportional to the severity of the muscle tear. This defect is also accentuated by the adjacent muscle retraction.

Differential Diagnosis. MRI should allow accurate diagnosis of a retracted muscle in the vast majority of cases. If prominent edema and hemorrhage are present, the retracted muscle mass may exhibit heterogeneous signal intensity similar to that of a soft tissue sarcoma or other aggressive soft tissue lesion. In these cases, careful evaluation of the muscle anatomy and possibly comparison with the contralateral extremity should confirm the diagnosis.

Reference

DeSmet A. Magnetic resonance findings in skeletal muscle tears. *Skeletal Radiol* 22:479–484, 1993.

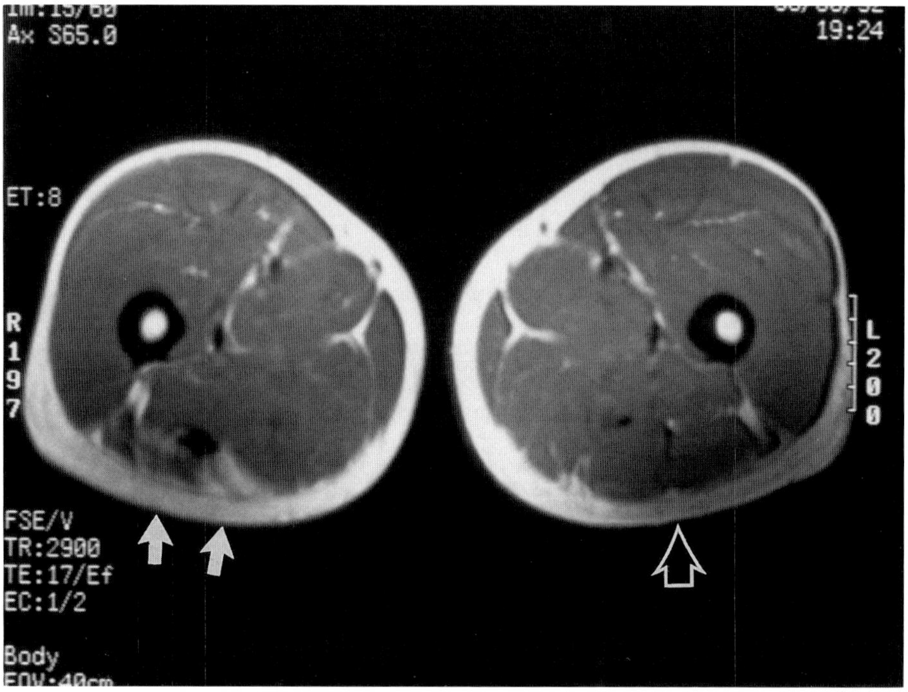

FIGURE 8.5 Hamstring avulsion in a 33-year-old male. Axial FSE proton density (2900/17) image at the mid-thigh level reveals biceps femoris, semitendinosus, and semimembranosus musculotendinous retraction (arrows) as a result of complete avulsion from the ischial tuberosity. This finding is readily apparent upon comparison with the normal left hamstring musculature (open arrow). (Case courtesy of Phillip Tirman, MD).

9 Miscellaneous Benign Masses

Giant Cell Tumor of the Tendon Sheath

Definition. Giant cell tumor of the tendon sheath (GCTTS) is an idiopathic condition which is histologically similar to pigmented villonodular synovitis (PVNS). Pathologic examination reveals masses with lipid-laden foam cells, histiocytes, giant cells, and hemosiderin. The growth pattern of GCTTS is not villous or frond-like as in PVNS. GCTTS can be localized or diffuse. The localized form is also known as nodular tenosynovitis and the diffuse form is often referred to as florid or proliferative synovitis. Localized GCTTS consists of a nodular or polypoid mass. Diffuse GCTTS is less well-defined and grows in a multinodular pattern which is more irregular than the localized form. As the name implies, this condition is associated with a tendon sheath.

Clinical Features. Localized GCTTS is one of the most common tumors involving the hands and feet. It is the second most frequent mass of the hand and wrist, behind only ganglion cyst. It typically presents as a firm, lobulated, nontender mass which is adherent to the underlying deep tissue. The diffuse form of GCTTS is more irregular and infiltrating. The size of the mass typically ranges from 5 mm to 5 cm with localized GCTTS, but tends to be larger with the diffuse form. It occurs along the distribution of a tendon and may present with symptoms of nerve compression or restricted range of motion.

Location. These masses are usually attached to tendons. Localized GCTTS most commonly involves the digits. The diffuse form typically occurs about the knee and ankle.

Implications. Distinguishing between the local and diffuse forms of GCTTS and differentiating these forms from PVNS has therapeutic and prognostic significance. Surgical excision may be tedious, requiring meticulous technique to avoid spillage and incomplete excision, which increase the chance of local recurrence. Recurrence is common, with reported rates ranging from 7 to 27% for the localized form and 40 to 50% for the diffuse form. Malignant transformation has not been reported, even following multiple recurrences.

MRI Findings. The signal intensity of GCTTS may be slightly lower, slightly higher, or isointense to that of skeletal muscle on both T1- and T2-weighted images. The signal intensity depends primarily on the amount of hemosiderin present. The diffuse form typically contains more hemosiderin and therefore its signal intensity is more frequently hypointense to that of skeletal muscle. With less hemosiderin, intermediate signal intensity is more likely. Due to magnetic susceptibility, the hypointense signal of hemosiderin becomes more prominent on gradient-echo images. The lesion may appear heterogeneous, with areas of increased and decreased signal intensity on T2-weighted sequences. The localized form appears as a well-marginated nodule or polypoid mass, whereas the diffuse form demonstrates an irregular, infiltrating appearance. If the lesion is in contact with the underlying cortex, a pressure erosion may be seen in the involved bone.

Differential Diagnosis. If located away from a joint, GCTTS is easily distinguished from PVNS, which is an intra-articular process. If located near a joint, the absence of joint effusion and hyperplastic synovium should enable differentiation of GCTTS from PVNS. The unusual signal characteristics of GCTTS (i.e., hypointense on both T1- and T2-weighted images) allows differentiation from the vast majority of soft tissue masses. Moreover, the presence of markedly hypointense signal (i.e., from hemosiderin) is distinctly unusual in soft tissue masses. Fibrous tumors, such as a desmoid, may demonstrate hypointense signal on T1- and T2-weighted images. However, most desmoid tumors demonstrate increased signal on T2-weighted sequences and are frequently characterized by linear or lace-like areas of hypointense signal throughout the lesion, which is not seen with GCTTS.

References

Jelinek J, Kransdorf M, Shmookler B, et al. Giant cell tumor of the tendon sheath: MR findings in nine cases. *AJR* 162:919–922, 1994.

Froimson A. Benign solid tumors. *Hand Clinics* 3:215–216, 1987.

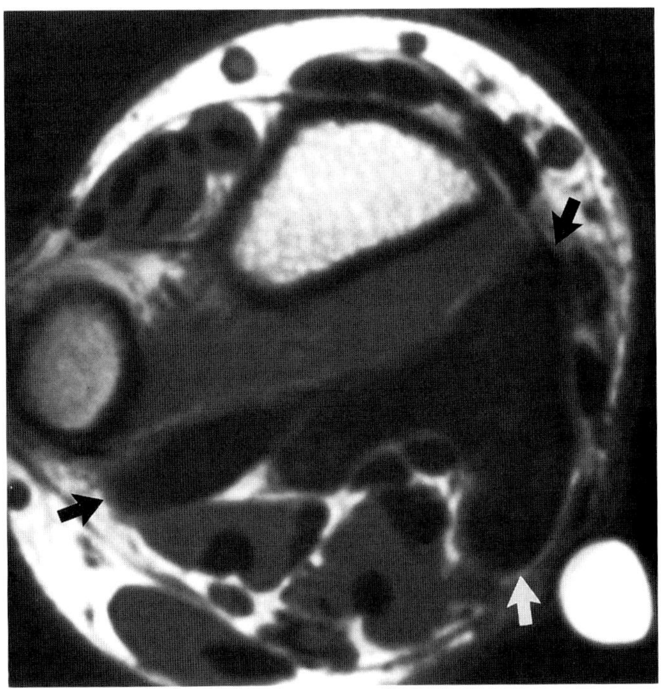

A

FIGURE 9.1 A 50-year-old male with a three-month history of a mass and mild discomfort in the distal left forearm. Axial (A) T1-weighted (800/17) and (B) T2-weighted (2000/80) images demonstrate a well-marginated, lobulated mass (arrows) around the flexor tendons of the distal forearm. Note the hypointense signal in relation to muscle on both images. (C) Coronal T1-weighted image (949/15) demonstrates portions of the hypointense mass (long arrows).

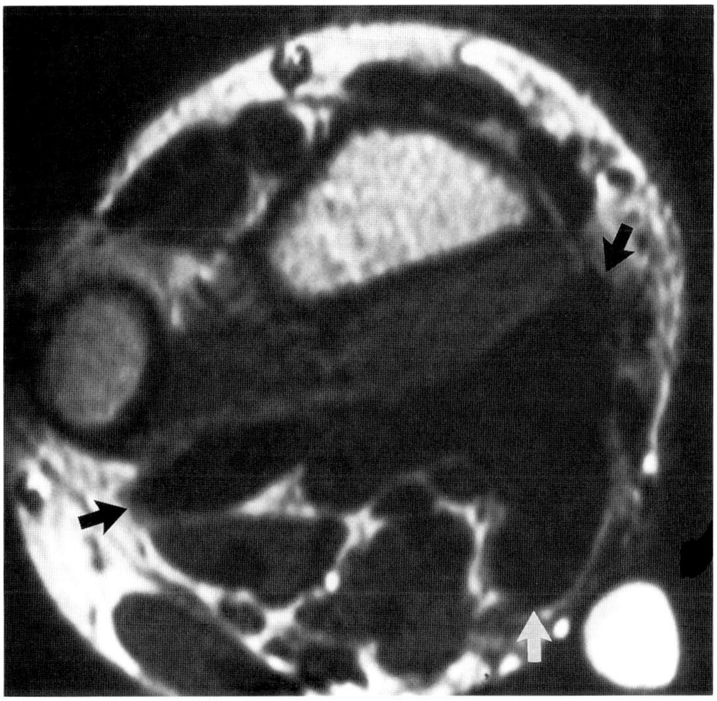

B

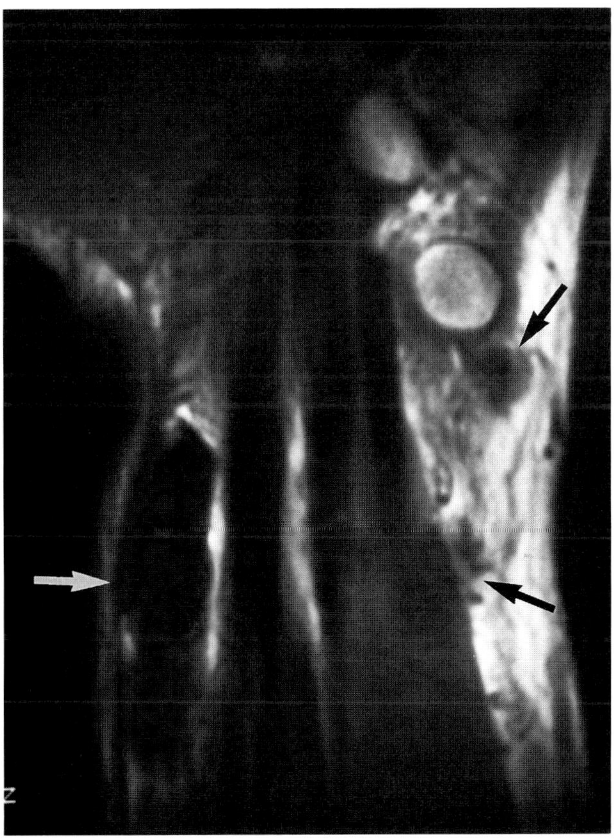

C

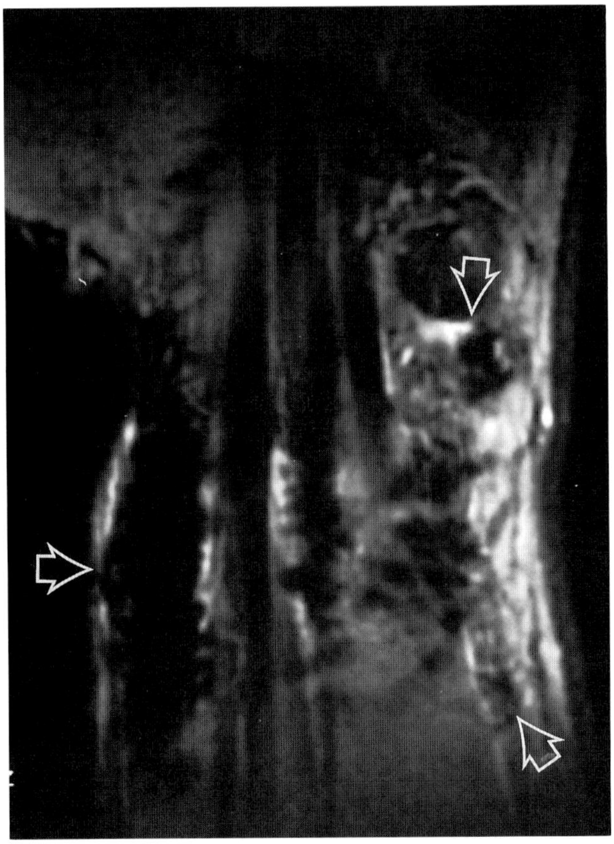

D

FIGURE 9.1 (continued) (D) Coronal MPGR image (600/20, 30 degrees) reveals "blooming" of these hypointense areas (open arrows) due to magnetic susceptibility. These findings strongly suggest the presence of hemosiderin associated with a localized giant cell tumor of the tendon sheath. The biopsy results were compatible with this diagnosis, revealing numerous iron pigment-laden cells and foamy histiocytes.

Myxoma

Definition. A myxoma is a benign mesenchymal neoplasm composed of stellate cells in a matrix of mucoid material which contains hyaluronic acid. Cyst-like spaces within the lesion are not uncommon. There is a delicate fibrous capsule, but nearly all lesions infiltrate the adjacent soft tissues on pathologic examination.

Clinical Features. Soft tissue myxomas are rare lesions which typically occur between the fourth and seventh decades of life, although they may appear at any age. They usually present as a painless mass, although approximately 20% are associated with pain and/or tenderness. There is a variable rate of tumor growth and occasionally there may be long periods of time in which the size of the lesion remains stable.

Location. The most common location of myxomas is the heart. Soft tissue myxomas may be intramuscular or less commonly juxta-articular. The majority of extracardiac soft tissue myxomas occur in the thigh, shoulder, and elsewhere in the extremities.

Implications. These lesions may recur following surgery, but metastasis has not been reported. There is an association between intramuscular myxomas and fibrous dysplasia, especially the polyostotic variety. In these cases, the myxomas are usually located near the most severely involved bones and may be multiple.

MRI Findings. On MRI, soft tissue myxomas appear as oval or round well-marginated masses. They demonstrate homogeneous hypointense signal in relation to skeletal muscle on T1-weighted images and homogeneous hyperintense signal in relation to fat on T2-weighted sequences. They typically exhibit an inhomogeneous increase in signal intensity following gadolinium administration. In atypical cases, the mass may have margins which are not sharply defined or may contain calcification, which appears as a signal void on all pulse sequences.

Differential Diagnosis. Since fluid and myxoid tissue have similar MR imaging characteristics, myxomas often resemble cystic masses or other fluid collections. Myxomas can be differentiated from ganglia or other cystic lesions by the administration of intravenous gadolinium, which results in inhomogeneous enhancement of the myxoma versus rim enhancement of most cystic masses. A hematoma would typically exhibit heterogeneous signal intensity and may contain methemoglobin which appears bright on T1-weighted images. An abscess also typically has heterogeneous signal intensity, depending on the amount of necrosis and internal debris present. Numerous additional benign and malignant lesions have similar signal characteristics, but most do not appear as homogeneous as myxomas.

References

Abdelwahab A, Kenan S, Hermann G, et al. Intramuscular myxoma: Magnetic resonance features. *Br J of Radiol* 65:485–490, 1992.

Peterson K, Renfrew D, Feddersen R, et al. Magnetic resonance imaging of myxoid containing tumors. *Skeletal Radiol* 20:245–250, 1991.

King D, Saifuddin A, Preston H, et al. Magnetic resonance imaging of juxta-articular myxoma. *Skeletal Radiol* 24:145–147, 1995.

Gober G, Nicholas R. Case report 800. *Skeletal Radiol* 22:452–455, 1993.

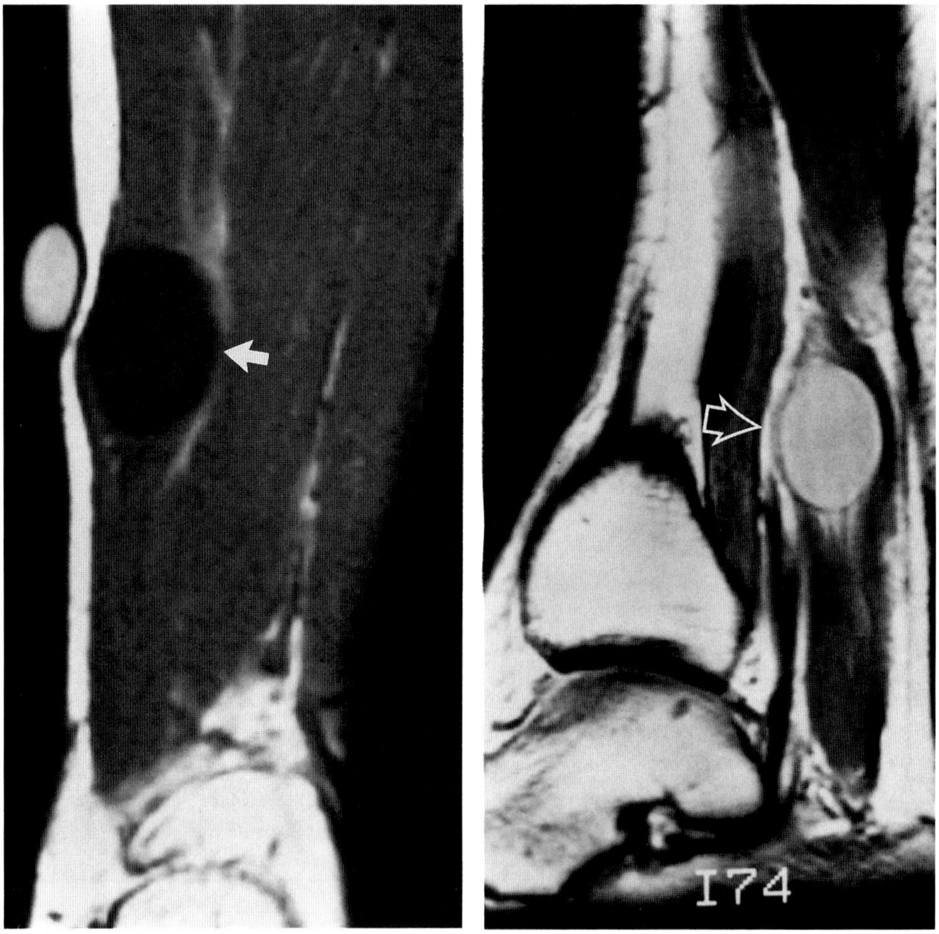

A B

FIGURE 9.2 Intramuscular myxoma of the distal calf in a 38-year-old woman. (A) Coronal T1-weighted image reveals a mass with homogeneously low signal intensity (arrow). (B) Sagittal proton density image demonstrates uniformly high signal intensity within the oval-shaped, well-marginated lesion (open arrow). (Courtesy of James O. Johnston, MD).

Lymphangioma

Definition. Lymphangiomas arise from sequestered lymphatic sacs which fail to communicate with peripheral draining channels due to congenital obstruction. Based upon the size of the lymphatic channels, lymphangiomas can be classified histologically into three types: simple (capillary-sized), cavernous, and cystic (also known as hygroma). However, since all three varieties often coexist and pathologic distinction may be difficult, many prefer to use the term lymphangioma for all of these lesions. The lymphatic spaces may contain variable amounts of fat, blood, and necrotic debris, and can be separated by fibrofatty septations.

Clinical Features. Lymphangiomas are fairly rare lesions which typically occur in childhood. Cosmetic concern is the most common complaint, but these lesions are usually otherwise asymptomatic. There is an increased incidence of lymphangiomas with Turner syndrome and Trisomies.

Location. The majority of lesions occur in the neck (75%) and axilla (20%). Less common locations include the mediastinum, retroperitoneum, and bones.

Implications. Lymphangiomas may exhibit aggressive growth and result in significant cosmetic deformity. Surgical resection is the only effective treatment. Incomplete resection will result in tumor recurrence, thus emphasizing the importance of preoperative delineation of tumor location and extent.

MRI Findings. Lymphangiomas typically appear as round or oval heterogeneous masses exhibiting slightly hypointense or isointense signal in relation to muscle on T1-weighted images and very bright signal on T2-weighted sequences. This appearance reflects the usual histologic composition of lymphatic spaces filled with fluid. Less commonly, the cystic spaces contain blood or fat and appear bright on T1-weighted sequences. Fluid-fluid levels may be present. Nearly all lesions contain internal low signal intensity linear structures representing fibrous septations. Most lesions appear well-marginated, although ill-defined borders may be present.

Differential Diagnosis. Although the MRI findings are variable and not specific, the presence of a multiloculated fluid-filled mass in the neck or axilla of an asymptomatic child is strongly suggestive of the diagnosis. Other fluid-filled masses should also be considered.

References

Siegel M, Glazer H, St. Amour T, et al. Lymphangiomas in children: MR imaging. *Radiol* 170:467–470, 1989.

Castillo M, Dominguez R. Case Report. Congenital lymphangiectatic elephantiasis. *Magn Reson Imaging* 10:321–324, 1992.

Smith R, Sherk H, Kollmer C, et al. Case report. Cystic lymphangioma in the adult: An unusual axillary mass. *Magn Reson Imaging* 7:561–563, 1989.

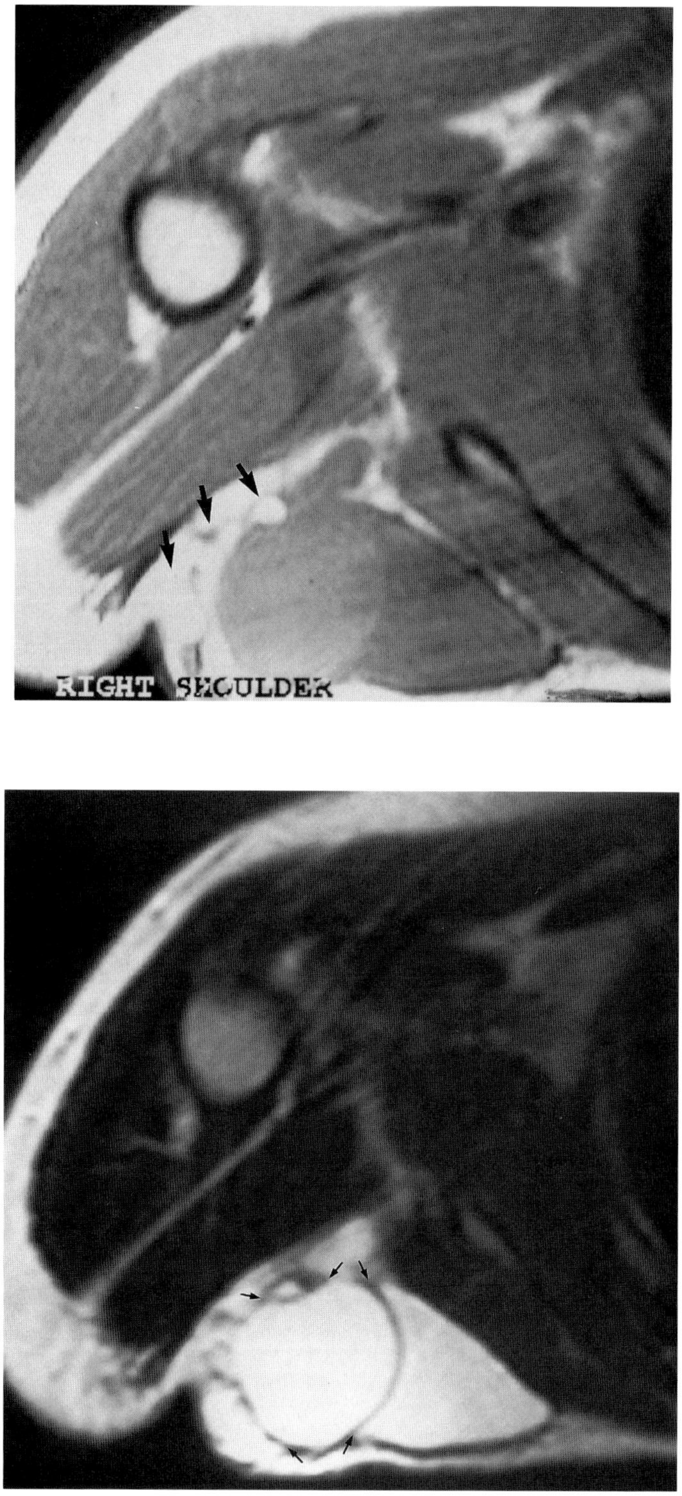

A

B

FIGURE 9.3 A 4-year-old girl with a right posterior axillary mass. Axial (A) T1-weighted (800/20) and (B) FSE T2-weighted (2620/85) images reveal a multiloculated, well-marginated mass in the posterior axillary subcutaneous tissues. Portions of the lesion are isointense, slightly hyperintense, and very hyperintense in relation to muscle with T1-weighting. The very high signal areas (arrows) may represent blood or fat within the lesion. The lesion appears very bright with T2-weighting. Note the thin internal septations (small arrows). These findings strongly suggest the diagnosis of a cystic lymphangioma.

Soft Tissue Hematoma

Definition. A soft tissue hematoma is a focal collection of blood that is distinguished from simple hemorrhage (not mass-like) within the soft tissues.

Clinical Features. Patients of all ages may be affected. Clinical settings include patients with trauma, bleeding diathesis, or anticoagulation therapy. Individuals who are otherwise healthy may not recall the traumatic event. Patients typically present with a mass, with or without associated pain. An intramuscular hematoma or hematoma of the deep soft tissues may be clinically mistaken for a neoplastic process, especially if there is no history of trauma or bleeding tendency. A hematoma may become secondarily infected.

Location. Those soft tissue hematomas requiring imaging are most commonly intramuscular, but they may occur in any location.

Implications. Percutaneous drainage or surgery may be required if the hematoma becomes secondarily infected or causes symptoms related to compression of adjacent structures. Old hematomas may calcify.

MRI Findings. The MR appearance of soft tissue hematomas is extremely variable depending on the age of the lesion and blood product composition. In contrast to soft tissue hemorrhage, the signal characteristics of soft tissue/intramuscular hematomas are similar to those of intracranial hemorrhage. This presumably results from loculation of the blood preserving the blood cell integrity. Many soft tissue hematomas exhibit intermediate signal intensity on T1-weighted images and low signal intensity on T2-weighted sequences due to the presence of intracellular deoxyhemoglobin. Subacute hematomas typically demonstrate bright signal intensity on both T1- and T2-weighted sequences due to the presence of methemoglobin. With time, the central fluid becomes serous and exhibits signal intensity similar to that of simple fluid (i.e., hypointense with T1-weighting, markedly hyperintense with T2-weighting). Fluid-fluid levels and internal debris may be seen. Surrounding edema may be present and appears as low signal intensity on T1-weighted images and bright signal intensity on T2-weighted sequences.

Differential Diagnosis. Unless there is a clear-cut history of significant trauma or bleeding tendency, it may be difficult to differentiate a soft tissue hematoma from a hemorrhagic neoplasm. Many malignant soft tissue tumors can contain significant amounts of hemorrhage. Fluid-fluid levels are a nonspecific finding and have been reported in numerous benign and malignant soft tissue lesions. Intravenous gadolinium may be helpful in selective cases because a hematoma would typically demonstrate only peripheral rim enhancement.

References

DeSmet A. Magnetic resonance findings in skeletal muscle tears. *Skeletal Radiol* 22:479–484, 1993.

Hermann G, Gilbert M, Abdelwahab I. Hemophilia: evaluation of musculoskeletal involvement with CT, sonography, and MR imaging. *AJR* 158:119–123, 1992.

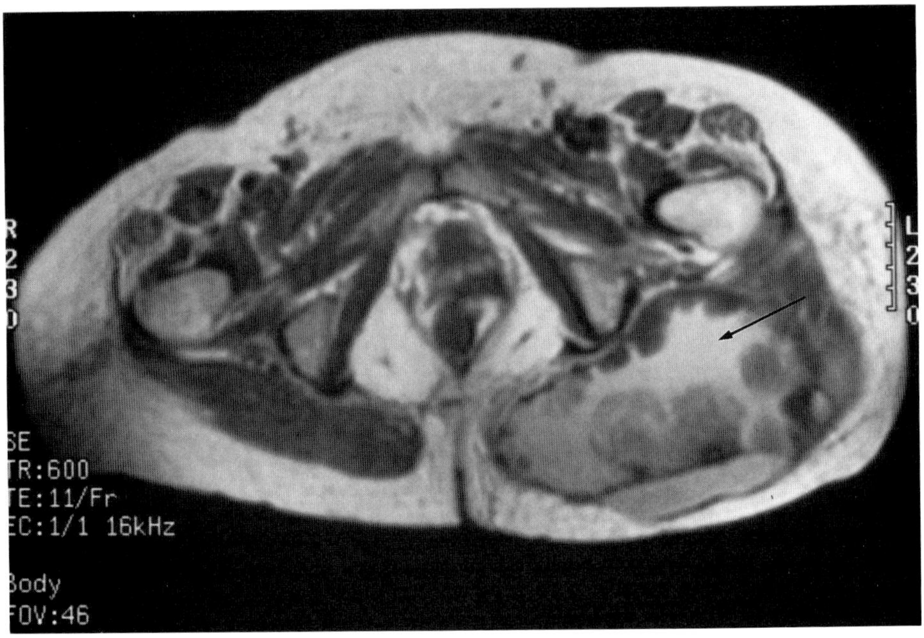

A

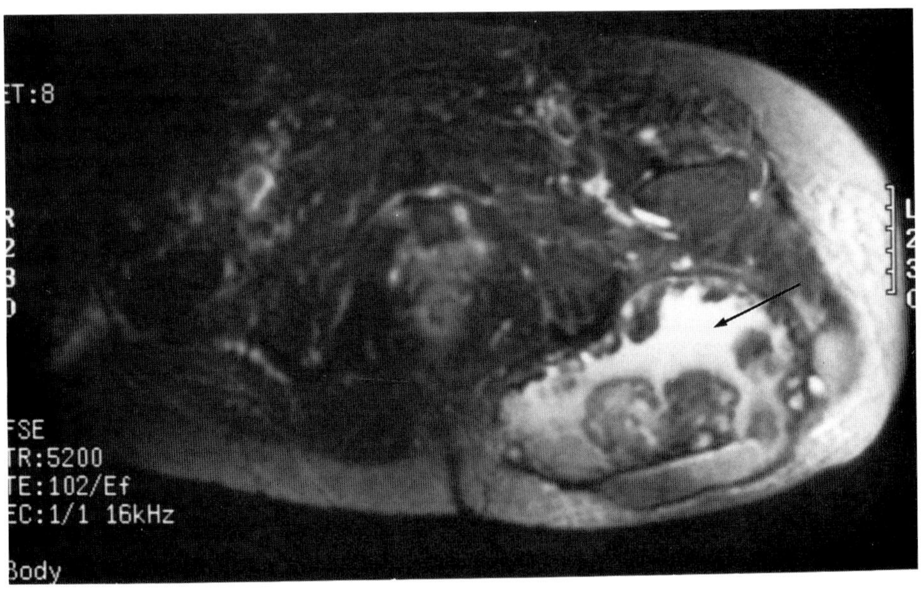

B

FIGURE 9.4 Buttock hematoma in a 78-year-old woman. Axial (A) T1-weighted (600/11) and (B) FSE T2-weighted fat suppression (5200/102) images reveal a large heterogeneous mass in the region of the left gluteus maximus muscle. The center of the lesion (arrows) exhibits hyperintense signal on both sequences indicating the presence of methemoglobin. The peripheral rim is of very low signal intensity, which likely corresponds to hemosiderin. Note the variability of signal intensity within the prominent mural nodular projections due to multiple blood products.

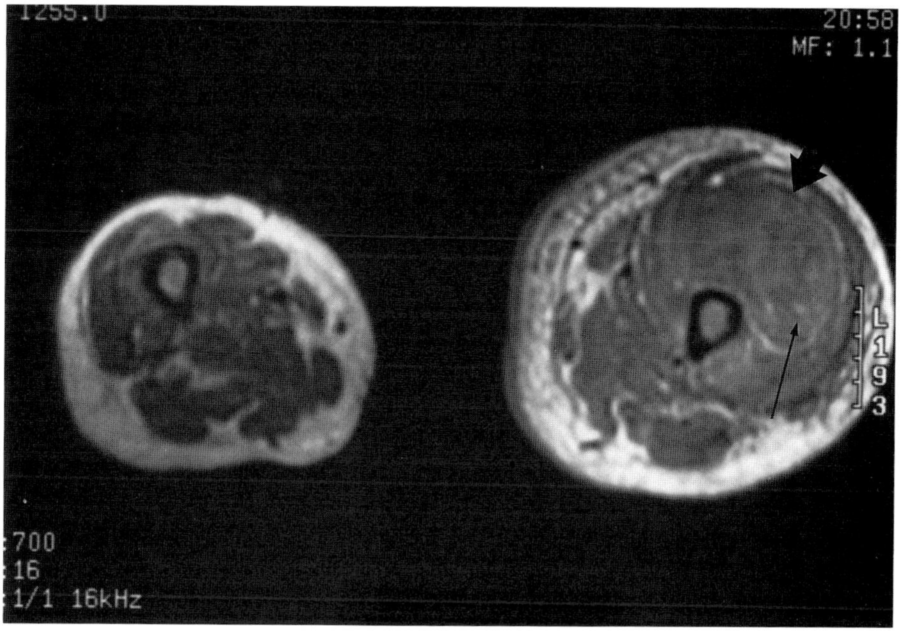

A

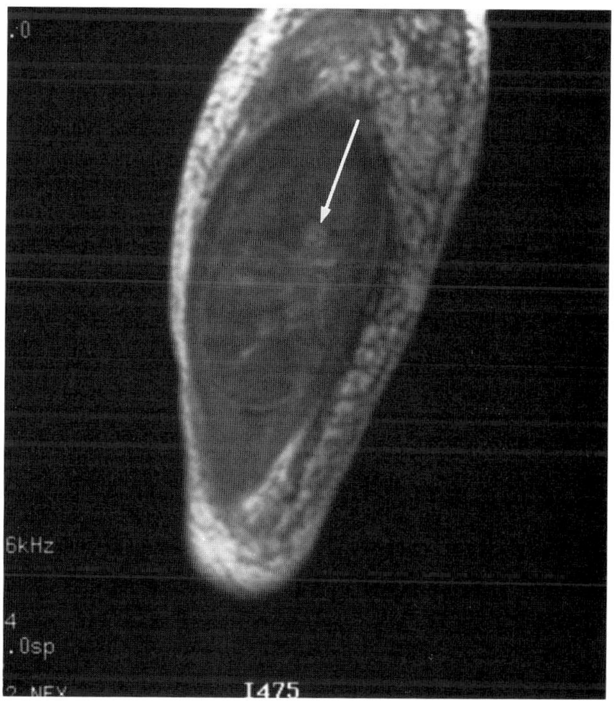

B

FIGURE 9.5 A 38-year-old woman with an intramuscular hematoma of the left thigh. T1-weighted (A) axial (700/16) and (B) sagittal (733/16) images reveal a prominent hematoma involving the vastus lateralis, vastus intermedius, and rectus femoris muscles (arrow). Note the internal component of high signal intensity consistent with methemoglobin (thin arrows).

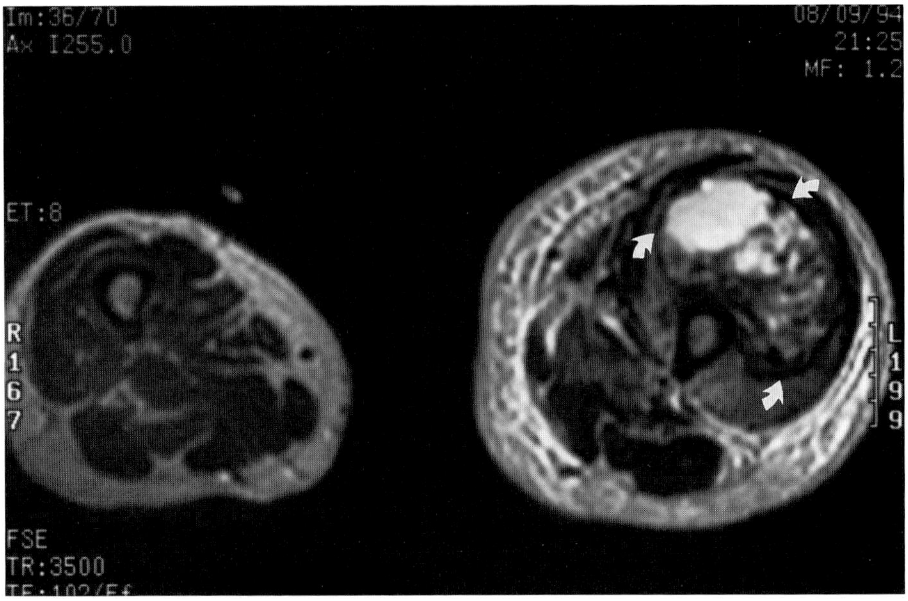

C

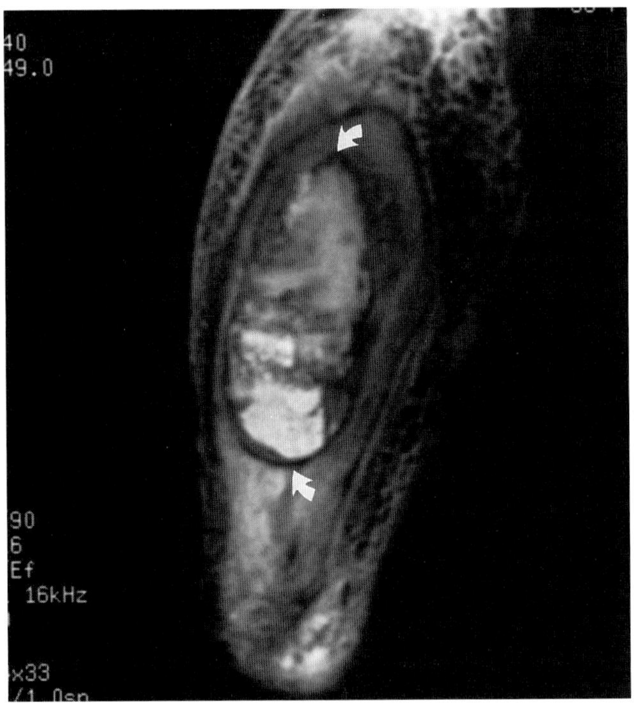

D

FIGURE 9.5 (continued) (C) Axial FSE T2-weighted (3500/102) and (D) sagittal FMPIR (3016/51, TI-150) images reveal heterogeneous signal intensity within the lesion indicating variable blood product composition. Note the peripheral rim of very low signal intensity (curved arrows), which likely represents hemosiderin.

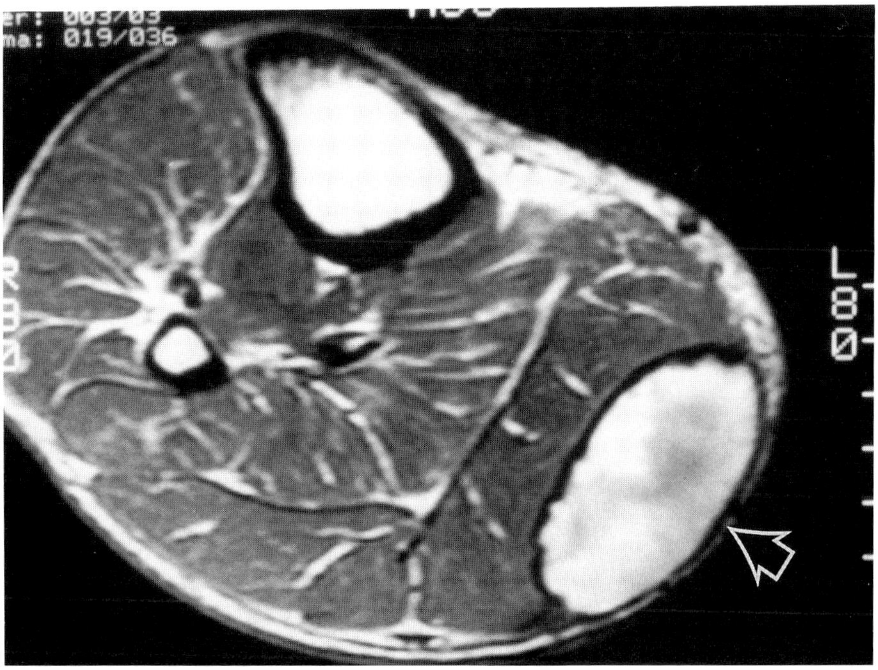

A

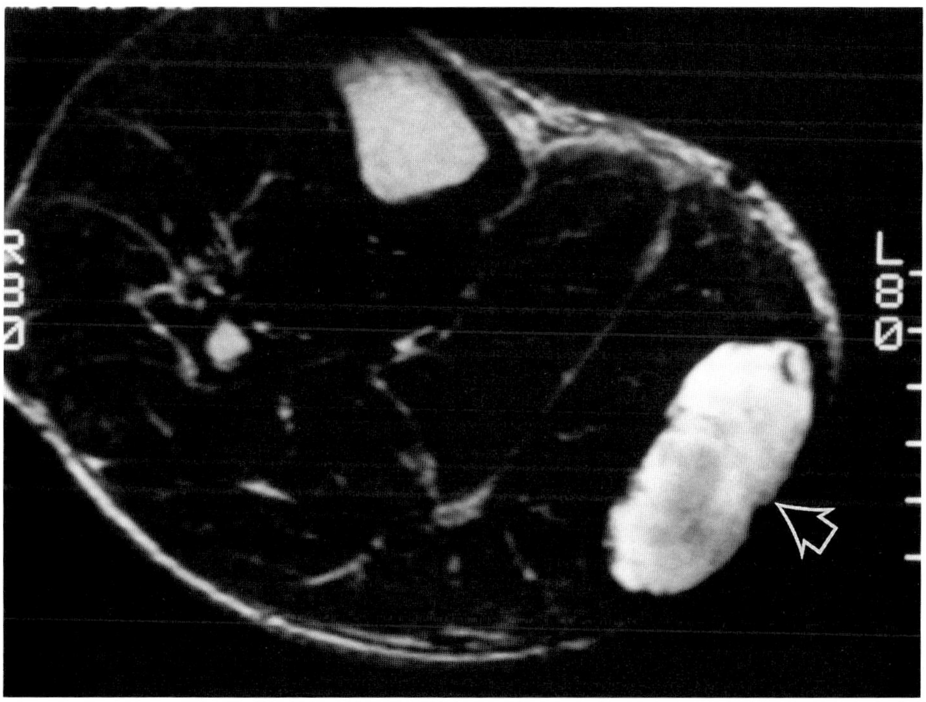

B

FIGURE 9.6 A 57-year-old male with an intramuscular hematoma of the calf. (A) Axial proton density (2000/20), (B) axial T2-weighted (2000/80), and

(*continued*)

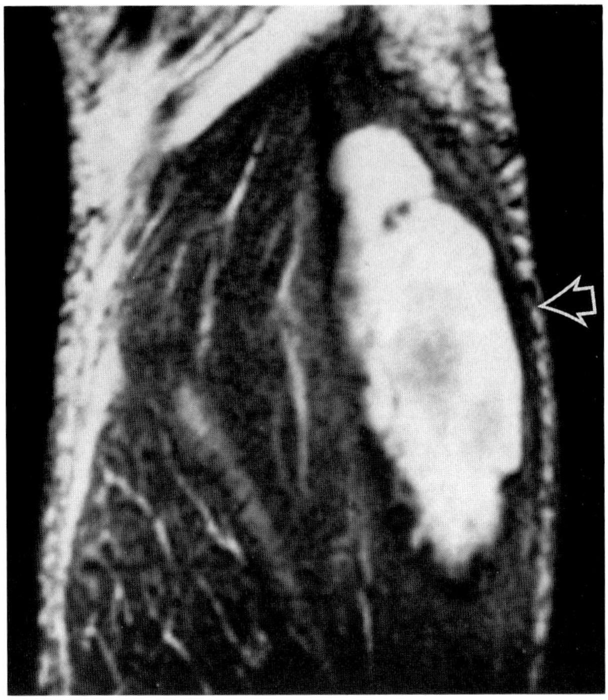

C

FIGURE 9.6 (continued) (C) sagittal T1-weighted (600/20) images demonstrate a hematoma within the medial head of the gastrocnemius muscle (arrows). Note the predominantly high signal intensity internally consistent with methemoglobin as well as the peripheral rim of signal void consistent with hemosiderin.

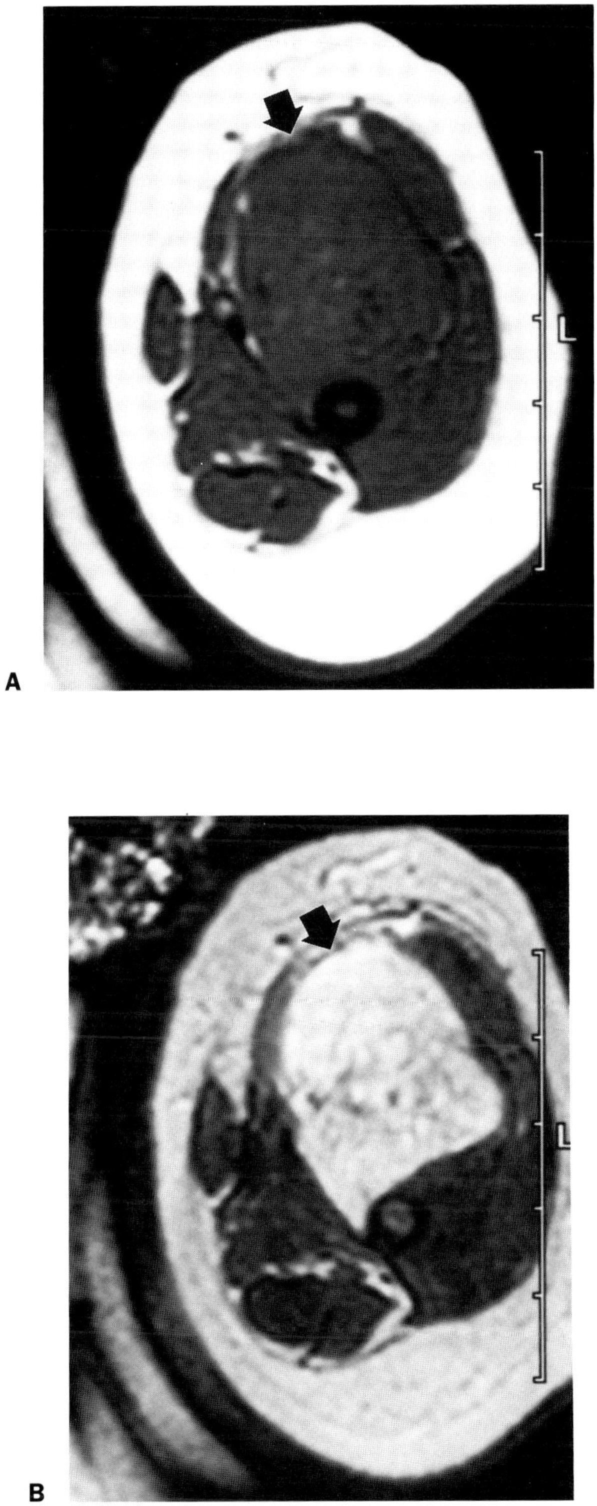

FIGURE 9.7 Intramuscular hematoma of the left thigh in a 2-year-old boy. Axial (A) T1-weighted (700/15) and (B) FSE T2-weighted (4000/92) images reveal a prominent hematoma in the region of the vastus intermedius muscle (arrows). The lesion is predominantly isointense to muscle with T1-weighting and hyperintense with T2-weighting.

Myositis Ossificans

Definition. Myositis ossificans is a benign, ossifying soft tissue mass within skeletal muscle. It occurs most commonly in association with trauma, burns, and recent immobilization/paralysis. The exact pathogenesis is unknown, although proposed etiologies include metaplasia of connective tissue cells and ossification of a hematoma. Over time, a process of bony maturation occurs within the mass creating different histologic appearances. Within the first month, there is a central fibroblastic reaction which becomes organized peripherally. As the process progresses, there is peripheral new bone formation by 6–8 weeks. Continued maturation of this new bone results in a dense zone of compact bone surrounding a central zone of lamellar bone by 6 months. Various terms have been used to describe this entity including myositis ossificans circumscripta, heterotopic ossification, pseudomalignant osseous tumor of soft tissue, pseudomalignant myositis ossificans, and extraosseous localized non-neoplastic bone and cartilage formation.

Clinical Features. Myositis ossificans may occur at any age. A history of trauma is present in only half of the cases. In the early stages, patients may present with pain, swelling, and limited range of motion. These symptoms may be mistaken clinically for infection or tumor, especially if there is no history of antecedent trauma or other predisposing factor. In the later stages, myositis ossificans may present as a firm, palpable mass which is worrisome for malignancy.

Location. This process may occur throughout the musculoskeletal system. The quadriceps muscle is a classic location.

Implications. Myositis ossificans is a self-limiting process. In the clinical setting of previous trauma, burns, or recent immobilization/paralysis, the diagnosis is readily established by observing the development of peripheral, mature ossification ("zonal phenomenon") on plain radiographs. Serial radiographs can be used to observe the progressive maturation of this process and confirm the diagnosis. In general, these lesions should not be biopsied because they can be mistaken pathologically for malignancy, especially in the earlier stages.

MRI Findings. Like the plain film findings, the MRI findings depend on the stage of maturation. In the early (acute) phase, myositis ossificans typically appears as a relatively well-defined mass with inhomogeneous signal intensity that is low (isointense to muscle) on T1-weighted images and bright on T2-weighted sequences. There is diffuse surrounding soft tissue edema (appearing as low signal with T1-weighting and high signal with T2-weighting) and possibly adjacent bone marrow edema. There may or may not be a low signal intensity rim. With subacute lesions, the central zone appears hypointense (isointense or slightly hyperintense to muscle) on T1-weighted images and markedly hyperintense on T2-weighted sequences. On both T1- and T2-weighted images, an incomplete or complete low signal intensity rim is present which corresponds to early peripheral ossification. T2-weighted images demonstrate extensive peripheral edema and there may be adjacent bone marrow edema as well. Occasionally, fluid-fluid levels may be seen within the lesion. In chronic myositis ossificans, the central zone consists of fatty marrow infiltration between bone trabeculae. The fat appears bright on T1-weighted sequences and parallels subcutaneous fat on additional pulse sequences. The bone trabeculae appear as low signal intensity on all pulse sequences. Fibrosis within the central zone also contributes to the low signal intensity areas observed on all pulse sequences. Chronic lesions typically have a low signal intensity peripheral zone on all pulse sequences corresponding to mature ossification.

Differential Diagnosis. Although there are typical MR patterns for the various phases of myositis ossificans, the findings are not pathognomonic and MR images must be interpreted with corresponding radiographs or CT images. Similar signal characteristics have been reported in hematomas, abscesses, and various benign and malignant neoplasms.

References

DeSmet A, Norris M, Fisher D. Magnetic resonance imaging of myositis ossificans: Analysis of seven cases. *Skeletal Radiol* 21:503–507.

Kransdorf M, Meis J, Jelinek J. Myositis ossificans: MR appearance with radiologic-pathologic correlation. *AJR* 157:1243–1248, 1991.

Cvitanic O, Sedlak J. Acute myositis ossificans. *Skeletal Radiol* 24:139–141, 1995.

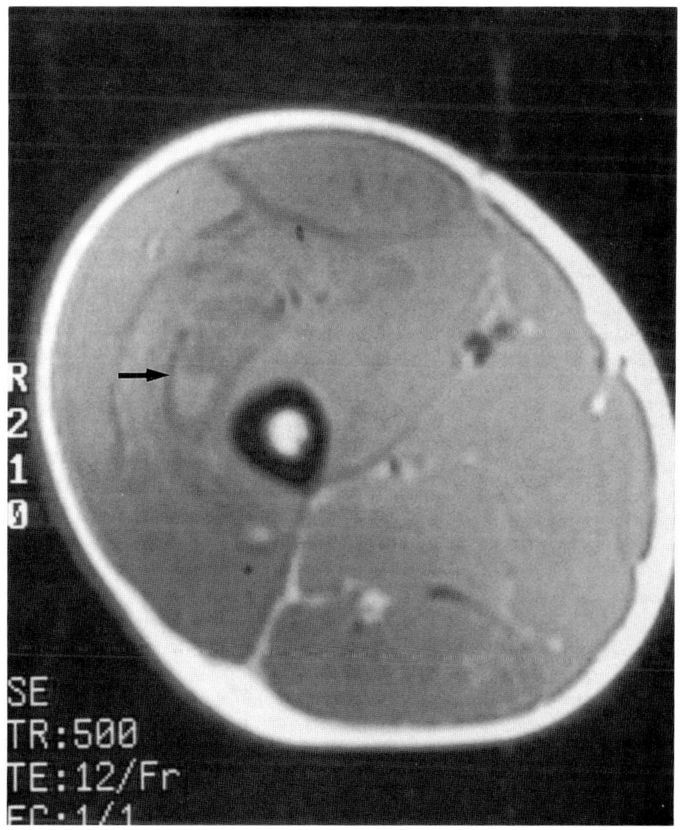

A

FIGURE 9.8 Myositis ossificans of the right thigh in a 17-year-old male with a history of trauma. Axial (A) T1-weighted (500/12) and

(*continued*)

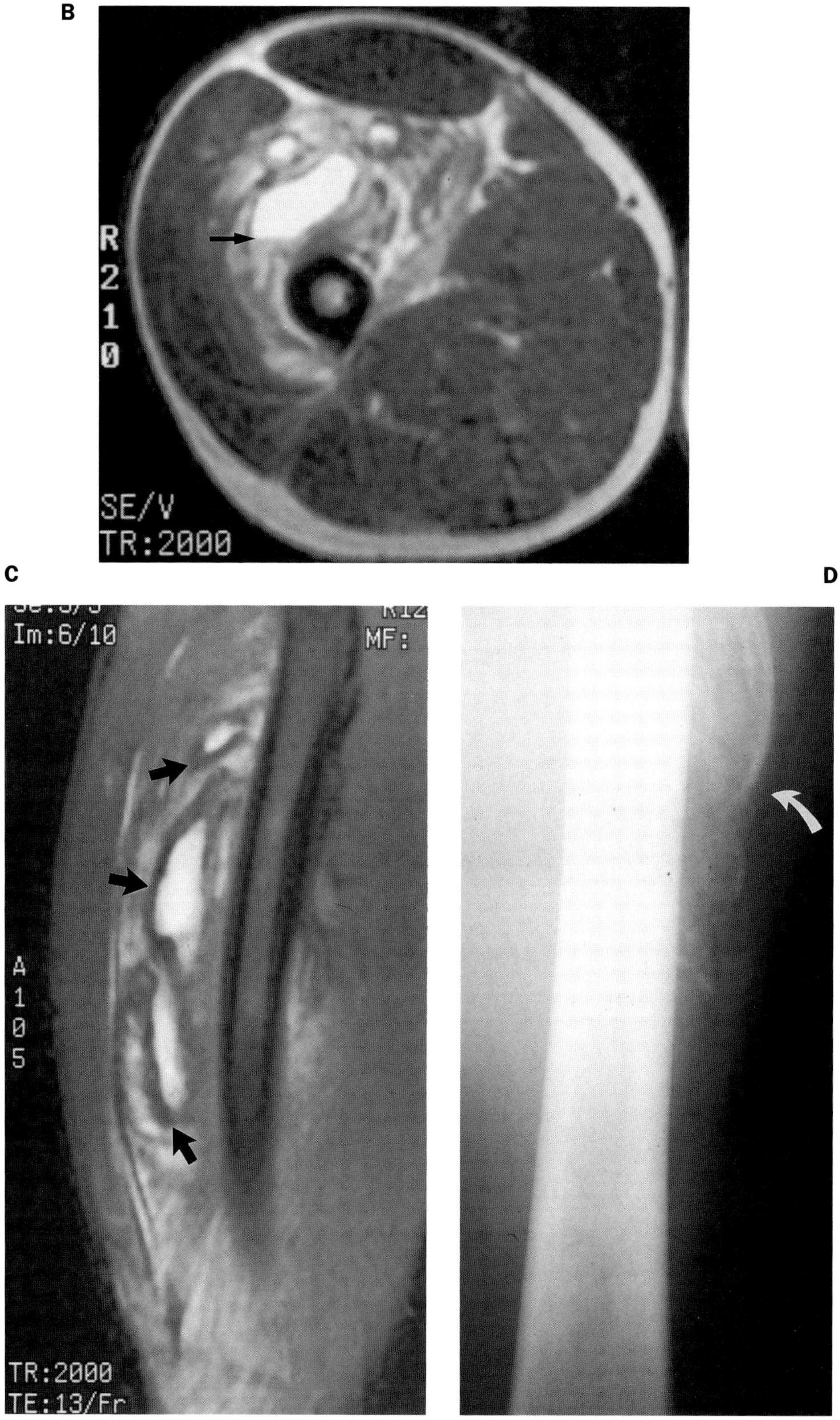

FIGURE 9.8 (continued) (B) T2-weighted (2000/80) images reveal a mass within the vastus intermedius muscle. Note the fluid-fluid level (thin arrows) and surrounding edema. (C) Sagittal proton density image (2000/13) demonstrates margins of low signal intensity (arrows) corresponding to peripheral ossification (curved arrow) noted on corresponding lateral radiograph (D). Findings are consistent with subacute myositis ossificans.

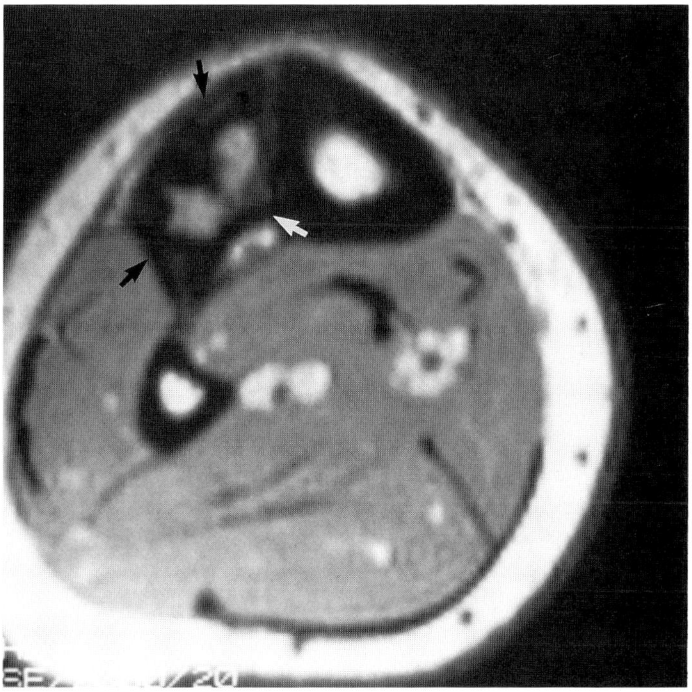

A

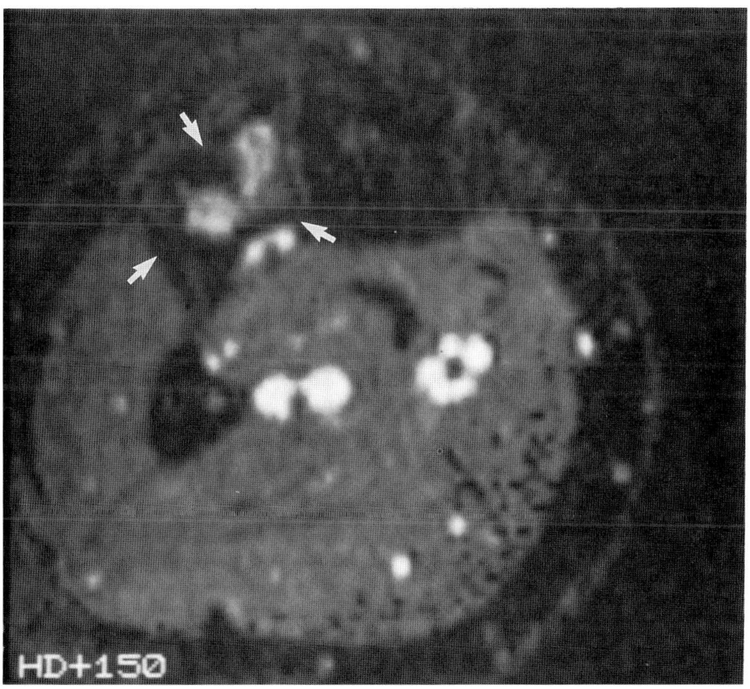

B

FIGURE 9.9 A 27-year-old male with myositis ossificans involving the tibialis anterior, extensor pollicis longus, and extensor digitorum longus muscles. (A), (B) Axial proton density (2000/20) and T2-weighted (2000/100) scans demonstrate a central zone of high signal intensity surrounded by a rim of very low signal intensity (arrows), which corresponds to peripheral ossification. Findings are consistent with a more mature stage of myositis ossificans than in Figure 9.8.

Achilles Tendon Xanthoma

Definition. Xanthomas are composed of connective tissue and foam cells which contain cholesterol, cholesterol esters, triglycerides, and phospholipids. Histologic examination reveals infiltration of the Achilles tendon with foam cells, which spread apart the collagen fibers. An inflammatory response to the lipid may occur within the tendon as well.

Clinical Features. These lesions are asymptomatic and do not predispose to Achilles tendon tear. Achilles tendon xanthomas are present in the vast majority of patients with familial hyperlipidemia. Approximately half of the lesions can be palpated as thickening, nodularity, or a mass on physical examination.

Location. Xanthomas involve the Achilles tendon diffusely, although the greatest thickening occurs in the middle third of the tendon, followed by the proximal third.

Implications. Establishing a clinical diagnosis of familial hyperlipidemia depends on the detection of xanthomas, which are not detectable on physical examination until they become large. MRI is more sensitive than physical examination and plain films for detecting Achilles tendon xanthomas. With early diagnosis, therapy can be administered in hopes of preventing or controlling atherosclerotic disease.

MRI Findings. Achilles tendon xanthomas demonstrate abnormal signal characteristics prior to enlarging or distorting the shape of the Achilles tendon. The abnormal signal is diffuse rather than focal and discrete nodules are not identified. The tendon has a uniform stippled appearance composed of numerous low signal round structures of equal size surrounded by high signal material on both T1-weighted and gradient-echo images. The uniformly sized, round low signal intensity structures most likely represent collagen fibers with the surrounding high signal intensity between these fibers representing infiltrating foam cells and associated inflammation. On sagittal images, the appearance consists of parallel vertical striations. With disease progression, there is enlargement of the Achilles tendon in the anteroposterior dimension (7–14 mm compared to 5–6 mm in normal tendons) as well as a convex anterior tendon margin on axial images. The greatest tendon thickening occurs in the middle third of the tendon. Full thickness tears are not identified in these patients. Kager's (pre-Achilles) fat triangle appears normal. The changes are bilateral and symmetrical.

Differential Diagnosis. The main differential diagnosis consists of Achilles tendinopathy, namely tendon degeneration, partial tear, and tendonitis. Typically with Achilles tendinopathy, the tendon appears thickened and has abnormally increased signal, which is nonuniform and may be focal or diffuse. In these instances, Achilles tendinopathy is easily distinguishable from a xanthoma. However, in approximately 30% of cases, Achilles tendinopathy is associated with a diffuse, uniform stippled pattern which is indistinguishable from a xanthoma. Differentiation in these cases must be made on clinical and laboratory grounds.

Reference

Dussault R, Kaplan P, Roederer G. MR imaging of Achilles tendon in patients with familial hyperlipidemia: Comparison with plain films, physical examination, and patients with traumatic tendon lesions. *AJR* 164:403–407, 1995.

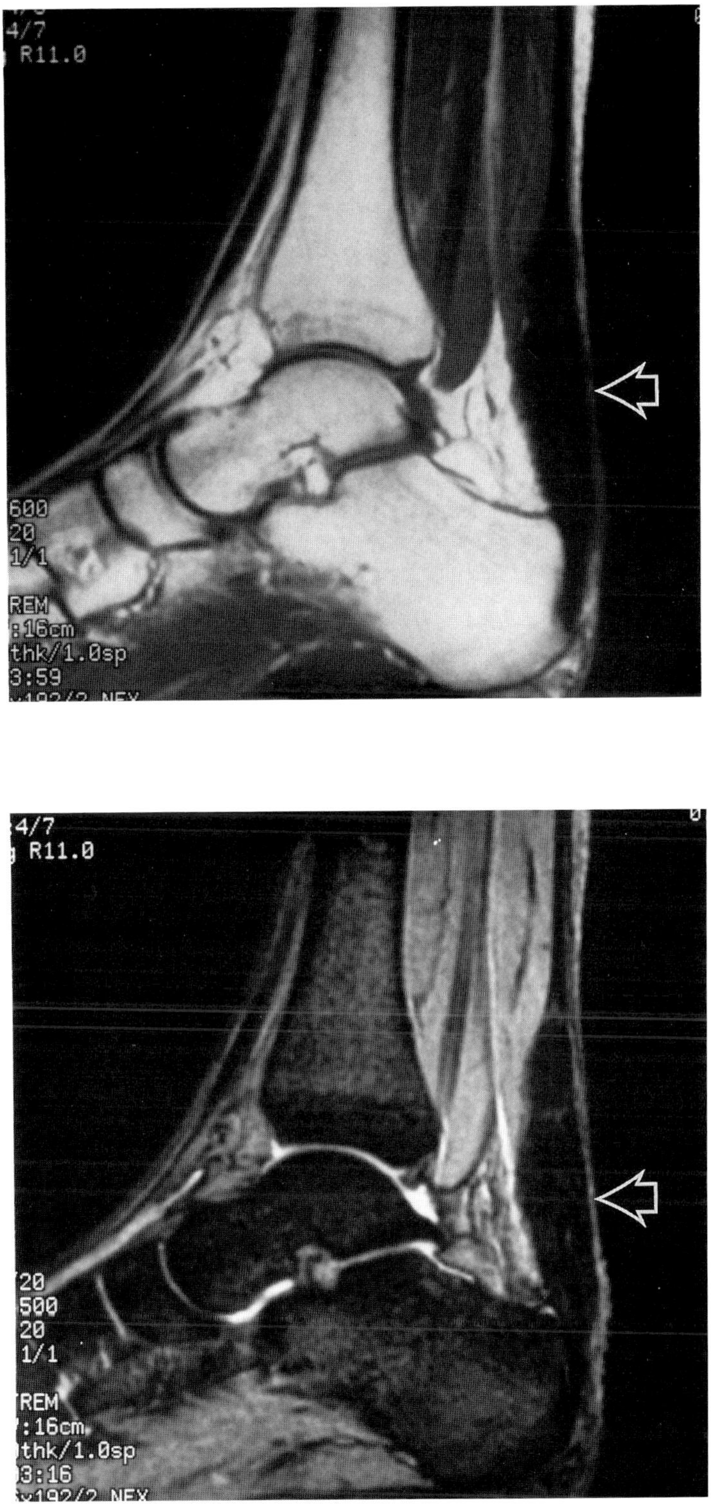

A

B

FIGURE 9.10 Achilles tendon xanthoma in a 30-year-old woman with familial hyperlipidemia. Sagittal (A) T1-weighted (600/20) and (B) GRE (500/20, 20 degrees) images reveal fusiform Achilles tendon thickening, which is greatest in the mid portion of the tendon (arrows). Note the very thin vertical striations.

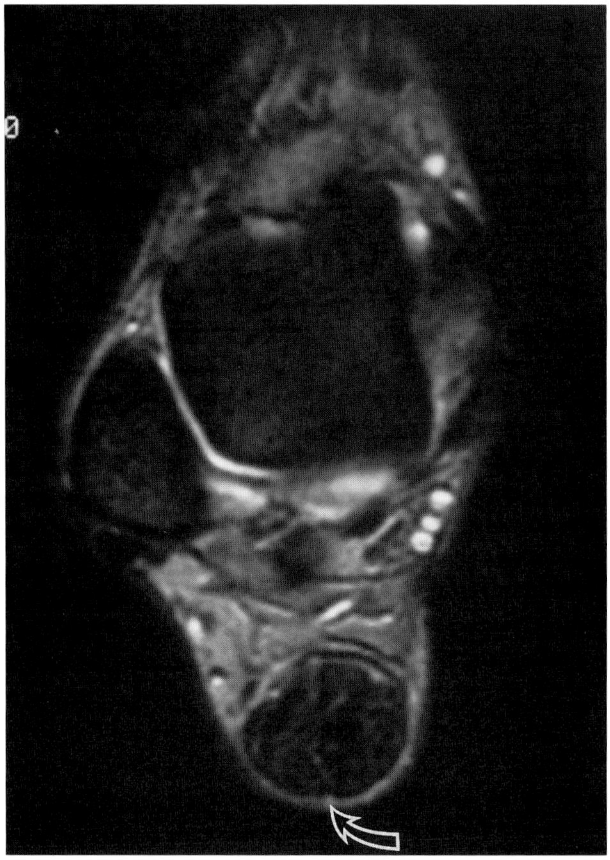

C

FIGURE 9.10 (continued) (C) Axial GRE image (500/20, 20 degrees) demonstrates the characteristic uniform stippled appearance (curved arrow). (Courtesy of Phoebe Kaplan, MD).

10 Miscellaneous Malignant Tumors

Synovial Sarcoma

Definition. Synovial sarcoma is a malignant mesenchymal neoplasm arising in the soft tissues. The name is derived from an appearance resembling synovium on histologic examination and not because it arises from synovium. Pathologic examination classically demonstrates both epithelial and spindle cell components.

Clinical Features. Synovial sarcoma is the fourth most common soft tissue malignancy. It typically affects young adults between the ages of 15 and 35 years, although all ages may be affected. It usually presents as a slowly growing soft tissue mass. Symptoms depend on size, location, and neurovascular involvement. Males are more frequently affected than females.

Location. This lesion is most frequently encountered in the extremities, more often in the lower extremities than the upper. It typically occurs in a periarticular location or adjacent to a bursa or tendon sheath. An intra-articular location is rare, accounting for 1 to 10% of cases.

Implications. Approximately 25% have metastasis at presentation, most frequently to the lungs. Local recurrence following surgery is very common and associated with a poor prognosis.

MRI Findings. This lesion appears as a soft tissue mass, with or without invasion of the adjacent structures, which demonstrates nonspecific signal characteristics. On T1-weighted images, this lesion demonstrates homogeneous or heterogeneous hypointense signal. Hyperintense signal is seen on T2-weighted sequences which may be similar to or less than that of the adjacent subcutaneous fat. Approximately 1/3 of these lesions contain calcification, which appears as hypointense foci on all pulse sequences. Involvement of the adjacent bone may be seen (5–25% of cases). The lesion may contain fluid-fluid levels due to hemorrhage or have a multilocular appearance with internal septations.

Differential Diagnosis. Although possessing a nonspecific MR appearance, this lesion typically occurs in a younger age group than malignant fibrous histiocytoma or liposarcoma. Also, synovial sarcoma is the most common soft tissue sarcoma to contain calcification.

References

Resnick D. *Bone and Joint Imaging.* Philadelphia, PA, W.B. Saunders Company, 1989, pp 1188, 1271.

Kransdorf M, Jelinek J, Moser R, et al. Soft-tissue masses: Diagnosis using MR imaging. *AJR* 153:541–547, 1989.

Tsai J, Dalinka M, Fallon M, et al. Fluid-fluid level: A nonspecific finding in tumors of bone and soft tissue. *Radiology* 175:779–782, 1990.

Blacksin M, Adesokan A, Benevenia J. Case report 871. *Skeletal Radiol* 23:589–591, 1994.

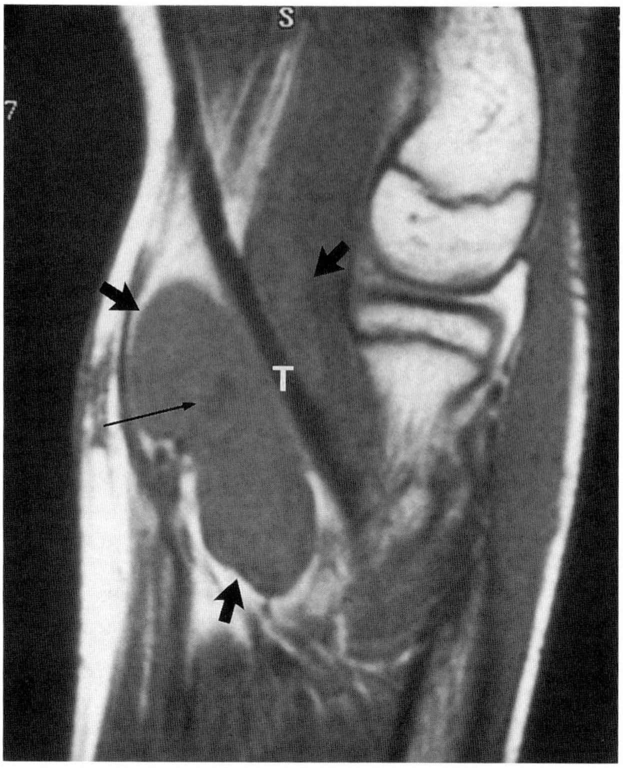

A

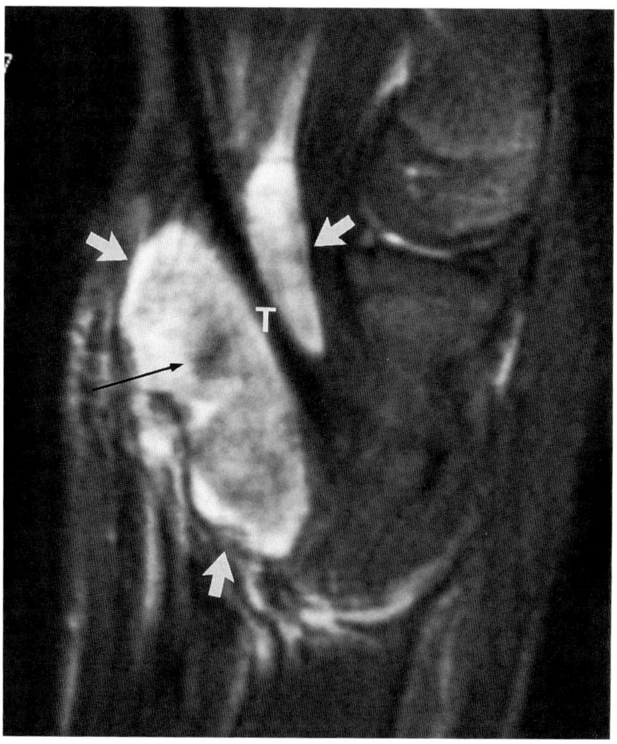

B

FIGURE 10.1 Synovial sarcoma of the antecubital fossa in a 13-year-old patient. Sagittal (A) T1-weighted and (B) FSE T2-weighted fat suppression images demonstrate a well-marginated mass (arrows) surrounding the biceps tendon (T). The predominant signal is approximately isointense to muscle with T1-weighting and heterogeneous with T2-weighting. The central focus of hypointense signal on both images (thin arrows) may represent calcification.

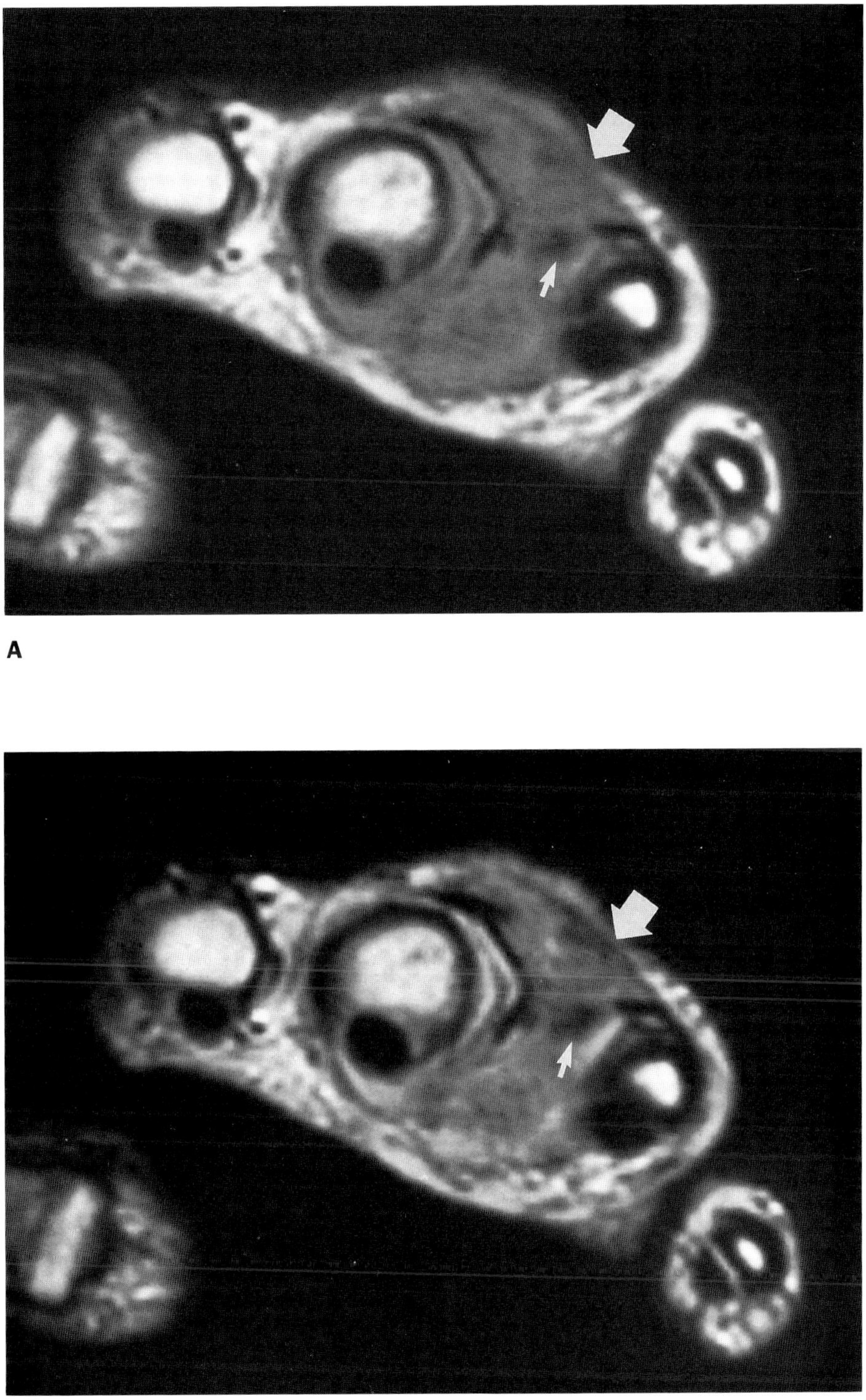

A

B

FIGURE 10.2 A 15-year-old female with synovial sarcoma of the hand. (A), (B) Axial proton density (2000/20) and T2-weighted (2000/60) images demonstrate an infiltrative mass in the 3rd-4th web space (arrows). Interestingly, the signal is predominantly hypointense on the T2-weighted image. A central focus of very low signal (thin arrows) could represent calcification.

Rhabdomyosarcoma

Definition. Rhabdomyosarcoma is a malignant mesenchymal neoplasm of the soft tissues. The name is derived from its histologic appearance resembling striated muscle. The three histologic subtypes are embryonic, alveolar, and pleomorphic. The alveolar and pleomorphic types are those typically encountered in the musculoskeletal system.

Clinical Features. Musculoskeletal involvement accounts for approximately 30% of all rhabdomyosarcomas. These lesions more frequently occur in the head and neck, orbit, and bladder of pediatric patients. Musculoskeletal lesions typically occur from late childhood to middle age, presenting as soft tissue masses. Symptoms depend on size, location, and neurovascular involvement.

Location. These lesions tend to occur in the deep soft tissues of the extremities and torso.

Implications. The prognosis is poor. Infiltration of the adjacent tissues is common and probably accounts for the frequent recurrence rate following surgery. Pulmonary metastasis is common.

MRI Findings. MRI demonstrates a soft tissue mass with nonspecific signal characteristics. The lesion may appear homogeneous or heterogeneous on MR images. Hypointense signal is seen on T1-weighted images with corresponding hyperintense signal on T2-weighted sequences. Infiltration of the adjacent structures is common. The adjacent bone may be involved. Calcification within the mass may occur, appearing as hypointense foci on all pulse sequences.

Differential Diagnosis. The MRI appearance is nonspecific and the differential diagnosis includes other soft tissue sarcomas such as malignant fibrous histiocytoma, fibrosarcoma, liposarcoma, synovial sarcoma, and leiomyosarcoma.

References

Resnick D. *Bone and Joint Imaging*. Philadelphia, PA, W.B. Saunders Company, 1989, pp 1173, 1188–1189, 1266.

Kransdorf M, Jelinek J, Moser R, et al. Soft-tissue masses: Diagnosis using MR imaging. *AJR* 153:541–547, 1989.

Shapeero L, Couanet D, Vanel D, et al. Bone metastases as the presenting manifestation of rhabdomyosarcoma in childhood. *Skeletal Radiol* 22:433–438, 1993.

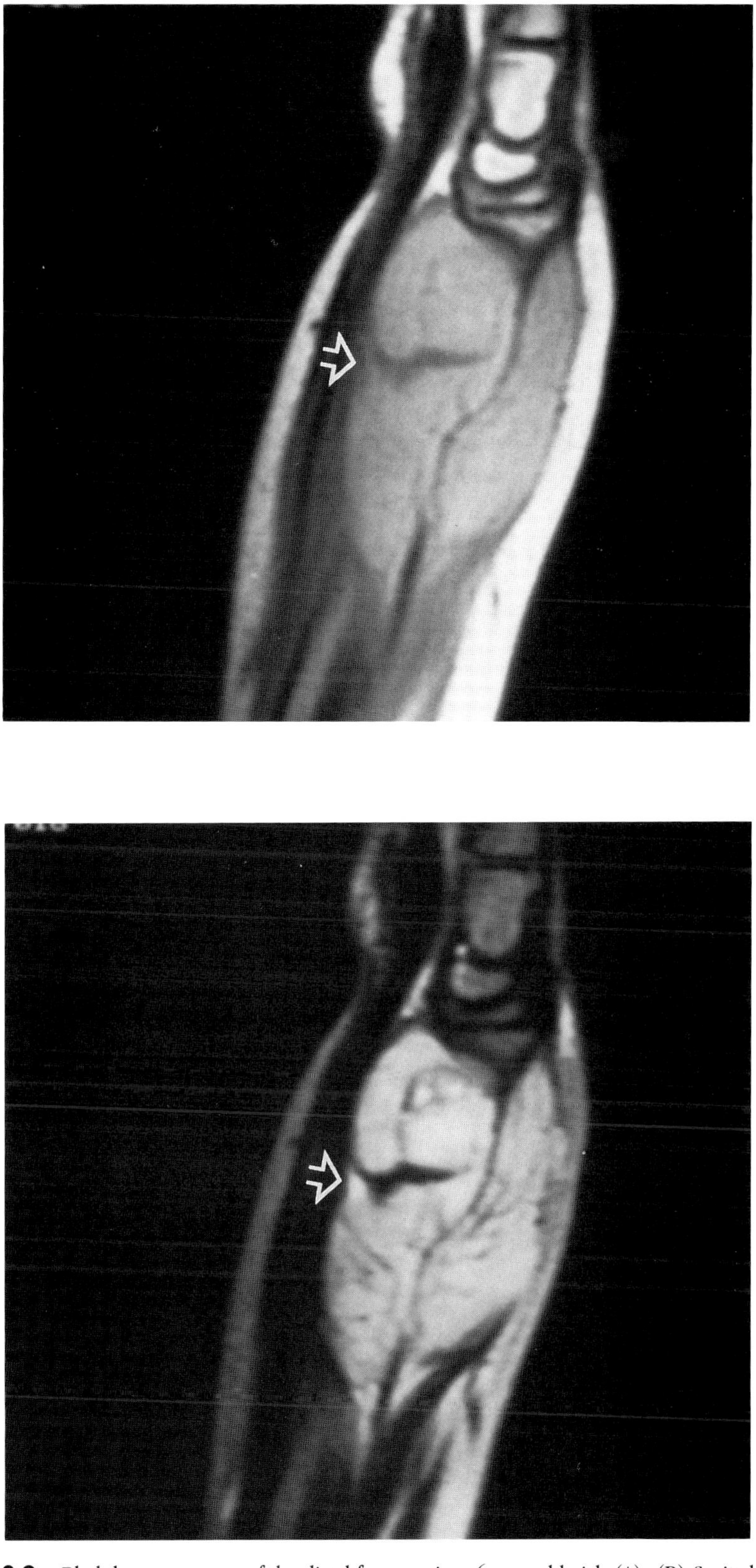

A

B

FIGURE 10.3 Rhabdomyosarcoma of the distal forearm in a 6-year-old girl. (A), (B) Sagittal dual-echo T2-weighted images (2000/20, 100) demonstrate a fairly well-marginated mass (arrows) adjacent to the distal radius. The mass contains internal septations and exhibits predominantly bright signal intensity with T2-weighting. The MR appearance is nonspecific, but rhabdomyosarcoma should be considered in a patient of this age.

Leiomyosarcoma

Definition. Leiomyosarcoma is a malignant neoplasm of smooth muscle cells which may occur in the soft tissues. Hemorrhage, necrosis, and cystic change are frequently present. Calcification is not typically identified.

Clinical Features. This uncommon tumor primarily affects adults. It typically presents as a soft tissue mass. Symptoms depend on size, location, and neurovascular involvement.

Location. Lesions of the musculoskeletal system are less common than those occurring in the alimentary tract, retroperitoneum, and genitourinary system. Musculoskeletal lesions may arise in any soft tissue location. These lesions may also arise from blood vessels.

Implications. Treatment depends on size, location, neurovascular involvement, and invasion of adjacent structures. Metastasis is common.

MRI Findings. MRI demonstrates a soft tissue mass which may be homogeneous or heterogeneous in appearance. Signal characteristics depend on the amount of hemorrhage, necrosis, and cystic change present. In general, the signal intensity is low to intermediate on T1-weighted sequences and increased on T2-weighted images.

Differential Diagnosis. The MR imaging appearance is nonspecific with the differential diagnosis including other soft tissue sarcomas such as malignant fibrous histiocytoma, fibrosarcoma, liposarcoma, synovial sarcoma, and rhabdomyosarcoma.

References

McLeod A, Zornoza J, Shirkhoda A. Leiomyosarcoma: Computed tomographic findings. *Radiology* 152:133–136, 1984.

Sundaram M, McGuire M, Herbold D. Magnetic resonance imaging of soft tissue masses: An evaluation of fifty-three histologically proven tumors. *Magn Reson Imaging* 6:237–248, 1988.

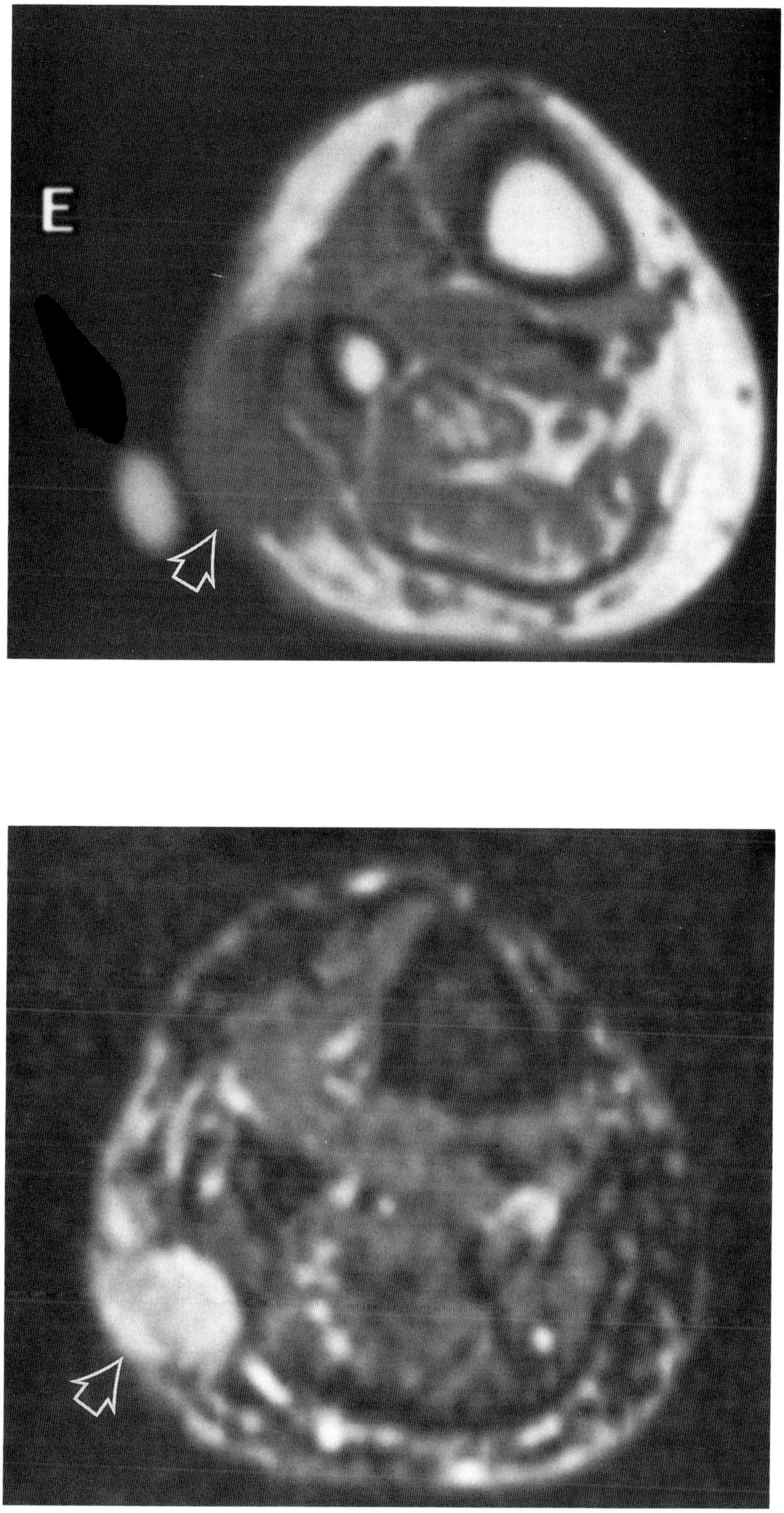

A

B

FIGURE 10.4 Leiomyosarcoma of the calf in an 87-year-old woman. (A), (B) Axial T1-weighted (600/17) and FMPIR (5000/36, TI-160) images demonstrate a mass in the lateral subcutaneous tissues (arrows). The signal characteristics are nonspecific.

Alveolar Soft Part Sarcoma

Definition. Alveolar soft part sarcoma (ASPS) is a hypervascular malignant soft tissue tumor of unknown cellular origin. It was named for its appearance histologically, in which there are large granular cells dispersed in alveolar-like arrangements separated by vascular channels. Gross pathologic examination typically reveals a partially or completely encapsulated well-circumscribed mass. There may be infiltration of the surrounding tissues. The lesion contains multiple large, tortuous vessels as well as arteriovenous shunting. Marked hemorrhage and necrosis are usually present centrally within the tumor.

Clinical Features. ASPS is one of the least common malignant soft tissue neoplasms, accounting for less than 1% of all soft tissue sarcomas. This lesion most frequently occurs between the second and fourth decades of life, with a female predominance. It usually presents as a slow-growing, firm, immobile mass which may or may not be painful. The mass may be pulsatile and associated with an audible bruit, and can be clinically misdiagnosed as an arteriovenous malformation.

Location. ASPS most commonly involves the lower extremity (particularly the thigh, buttock, and popliteal region), followed by the head and neck, upper extremity, and trunk, in order of decreasing frequency. It tends to be located deep within the soft tissues.

Implications. At the time of presentation, there is a high incidence (23–67%) of distant metastasis, most frequently to the lung, as well as to the brain and skeleton. Metastasis may occur many years (more than 25 years) after the primary tumor has been excised. Lymph node involvement occurs in about 10% of cases. Reported five-year survival rates range from 50–67%. Surgery is the treatment of choice in the management of ASPS, with limited roles for both chemotherapy and irradiation. Aggressive treatment of metastatic disease is often recommended, including resection of pulmonary metastases. Due to the hypervascular nature of this lesion, surgery may be complicated by significant hemorrhage. It is important to note that ASPS can be mistaken histologically for metastatic renal, adrenal, or hepatocellular carcinoma.

MRI Findings. ASPS typically exhibits moderately high signal intensity (greater than muscle, but less than fat) on T1-weighted sequences and very high signal intensity (greater than fat) on T2-weighted images. The relatively high signal on T1-weighted images is most likely related to the presence of slow blood flow within some tumor vessels. This lesion is also characterized by the presence of tubular areas of signal void (on both T1- and T2-weighted sequences) centrally and near the tumor margin, corresponding to rapid blood flow within other tumor vessels. These lesions may also contain small calcifications, appearing as areas of signal void on T1- and T2-weighted sequences that become more prominent on gradient-echo sequences due to magnetic susceptibility. Central necrosis is commonly present and appears as very bright signal on T2-weighted images. These tumors may cause destruction of the adjacent bone.

Differential Diagnosis. A soft tissue mass with relatively high signal intensity with T1-weighting as well as central and marginal flow voids is characteristic of ASPS. The majority of soft tissue sarcomas exhibit hypointense or isointense signal in relation to muscle on T1-weighted images. Liposarcomas may contain significant amounts of fat, but these areas would appear brighter (isointense to subcutaneous fat, yellow marrow) on T1-weighted images than ASPS. ASPS also affects a younger age distribution than liposarcoma. Like ASPS, hemangioma typically exhibits signal which is hyperintense to muscle on T1-weighted images and may also have areas of signal void due to calcification or phleboliths. However, the shape and distribution of the signal voids should allow differentiation. In ASPS, the signal voids are tubular in shape and occur within and at the periphery of the mass. The identification of phleboliths on radiographs would confirm the diagnosis of hemangioma.

References

Iwamoto Y, Morimoto N, Chuman H, et al. The role of MR imaging in the diagnosis of alveolar soft part sarcoma: A report of 10 cases. *Skeletal Radiol* 24:267–270, 1995.

Lorigan J, O'Keefe F, Evans H, et al. The radiologic manifestations of alveolar soft-part sarcoma. *AJR* 153:335–339, 1989.

Nakashima Y, Kotoura Y, Kasakura K, et al. Alveolar soft-part sarcoma. A report of ten cases. *Clin Orthop* 294:259–266, 1993.

Hermann G, Abdelwahab I, Klein M, et al. Case report 796. *Skeletal Radiol* 22:386–389, 1993.

Daly B, Cheung H, Gaines P, et al. Imaging of alveolar soft part sarcoma. *Clin Radiol* 46:253–256, 1992.

Temple H, Scully S, O'Keefe R, et al. Clinical presentation of alveolar soft-part sarcoma. *Clin Orthop* 300:213–218, 1994.

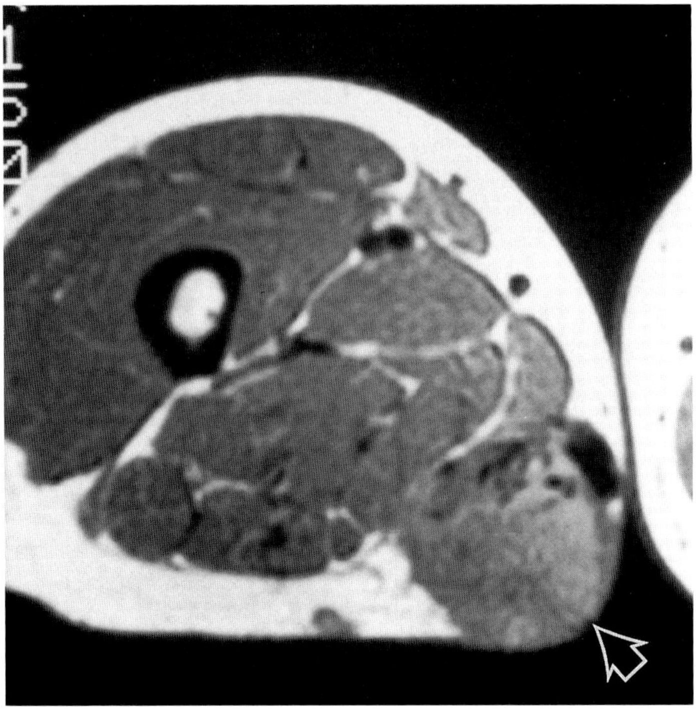

A

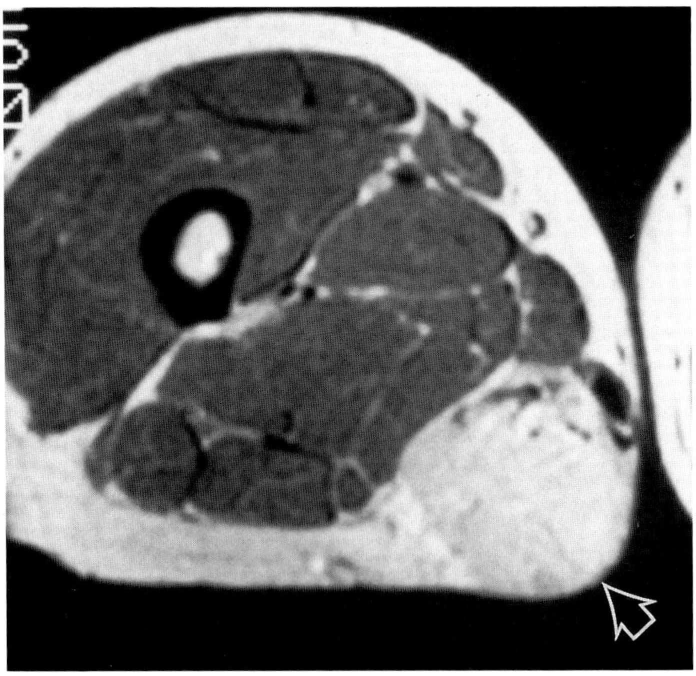

B

FIGURE 10.5 Alveolar soft part sarcoma of the right thigh in a 27-year-old woman. Axial (A) T1-weighted (600/11) and (B) proton density (2200/30) images reveal a well-marginated mass within the posteromedial subcutaneous tissues of the upper thigh (open arrows).

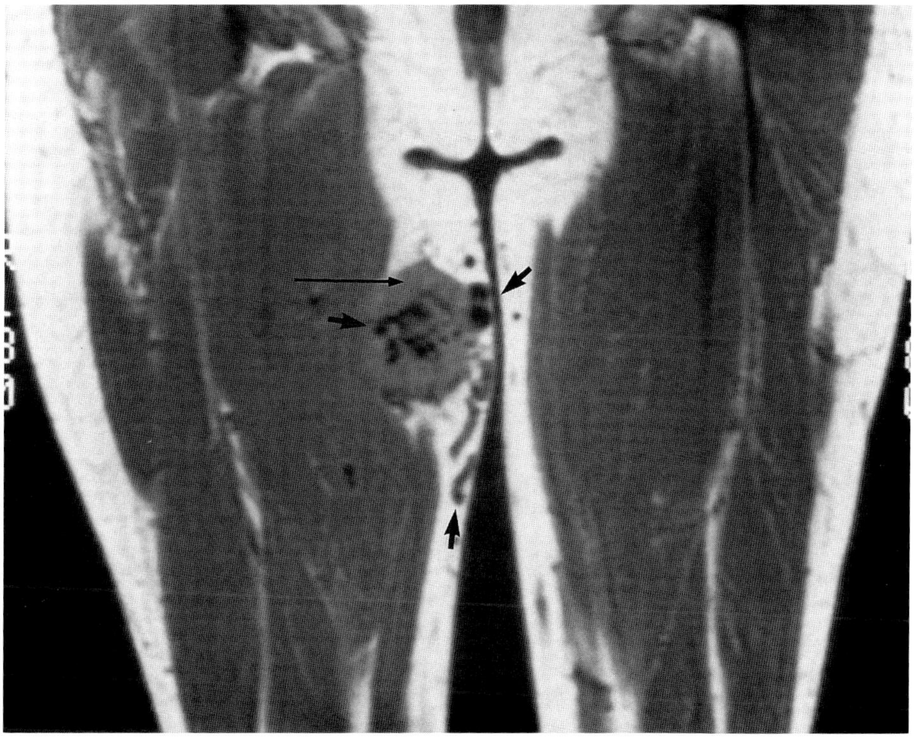

C

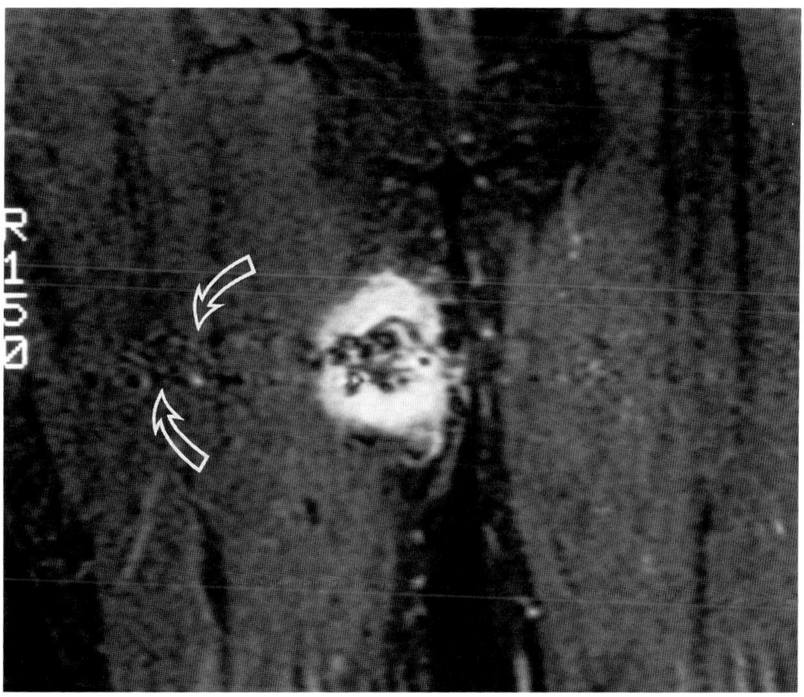

D

FIGURE 10.5 (continued) Coronal (C) T1-weighted (600/10) and (D) inversion recovery (2000/30, TI-150) images reveal numerous peripheral and central tubular areas of signal void (arrows). Note the associated pulsation artifact (curved arrows). In addition, note that the signal is hyperintense to muscle on the T1-weighted image (thin arrow), which is not typical for the majority of musculoskeletal mass lesions. The combination of these findings is characteristic for alveolar soft part sarcoma.

Lymphoma

Definition. Lymphoma is categorized as Hodgkin's disease or non-Hodgkin's lymphoma. Hodgkin's disease is histologically heterogeneous, consisting of prominent inflammatory cells, malignant (Reed-Sternberg) cells, and variable fibrosis. Non-Hodgkin's lymphoma is relatively homogeneous on histologic examination, consisting predominantly of malignant lymphocytes.

Clinical Features. Lymphoma may occur at any age. Patients may present with one or more palpable masses and often have constitutional symptoms such as weight loss, night sweats, fever, fatigue, and weakness.

Location. Lymphoma arises from lymphoid tissue and may disseminate throughout the body via hematogenous spread, lymphagenous spread, or direct extension.

Implications. Therapy and prognosis depend on the disease extent at the time of diagnosis and the histologic type. If the musculoskeletal system is involved, the disease is typically widespread.

MRI Findings. In general, lymphoma appears intermediate in signal intensity (slightly hyperintense to muscle) on T1-weighted images and intermediate in signal intensity (hypointense or isointense to fat) on T2-weighted sequences. Areas of bright signal on T2-weighted images may be seen in the presence of intratumoral necrosis. The signal intensity tends to be fairly homogeneous unless there is significant necrosis present.

Differential Diagnosis. In most cases of lymphoma, the diagnosis is established prior to the performance of a musculoskeletal MR examination, which is used to assess the disease extent. Although lymphoma is not typically as bright as most neoplasms on T2-weighted sequences, areas of very high signal intensity can be seen if necrosis is present. In addition, numerous lesions have been reported to exhibit hypointense signal with T2-weighting including fibrous lesions, peripheral nerve sheath tumors, and lesions containing calcification or ossification.

References

Negendank W, Al-Katib A, Karanes C, et al. Lymphomas: MR imaging contrast characteristics with clinical-pathologic correlations. *Radiology* 177:209–216, 1990.

Metzler J, Fleckenstein J, Vuitch F, et al. Skeletal muscle lymphoma: MRI evaluation. *Magn Reson Imaging* 10:491–494, 1992.

A

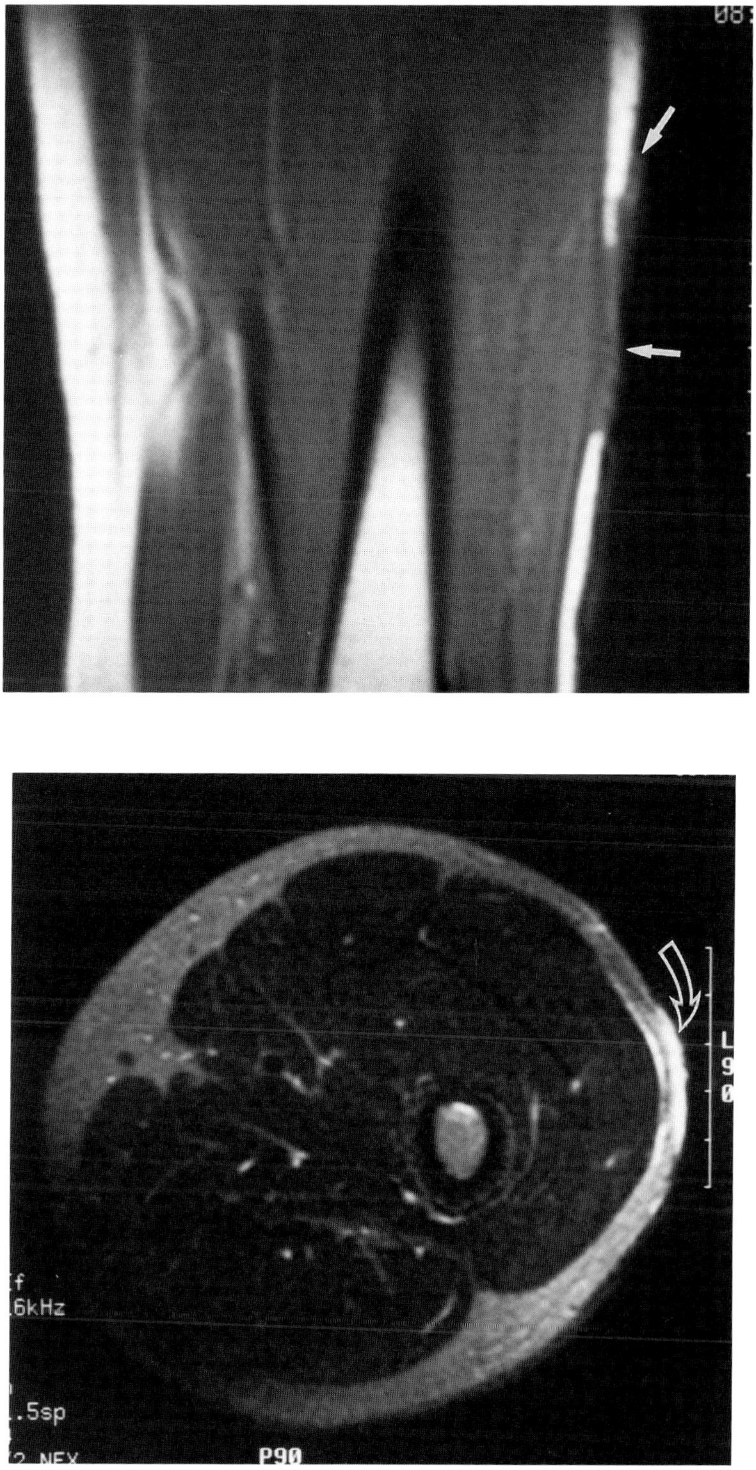

B

FIGURE 10.6 Cutaneous T-cell lymphoma of the thigh in a 15-year-old male. (A) Coronal T1-weighted image (400/16) demonstrates an elongated lesion which is isointense to muscle involving the cutaneous and subcutaneous tissues (arrows). (B) Axial FSE T2-weighted fat suppression image (4000/102) demonstrates hyperintense signal of the lesion (curved arrow). The signal characteristics are nonspecific.

SECTION II

BONE

11 Bone-Forming Masses

Bone Island (Enostosis)

Definition. A bone island (enostosis) consists of a focus of normal-appearing compact (cortical) bone within cancellous bone. It represents the mildest form of failure in resorption of the secondary spongiosa during endochondral ossification.

Clinical Features. Bone islands are asymptomatic and usually solitary. They are detected as incidental findings during radiographic examination. These lesions are frequent in all age groups. It is probably a noninherited entity. In the spine, there is a 1–14% incidence of bone islands. In this location, they have also been termed endosteomas. In most cases, bone islands measure 1 mm to 2 cm, however, "giant" bone islands (over 2 cm) may be as large as 5 cm in diameter.

Location. Any bone may be affected, although there is a predilection for the pelvis, proximal femur, and ribs.

Implications. Most bone islands are metabolically inactive. However, these lesions may increase in size or demonstrate increased activity on bone scintigraphy, thereby creating concern for an aggressive lesion. These lesions demonstrate increased scintigraphic activity in approximately 5% of cases, with the vast majority of lesions showing normal uptake. These lesions may decrease in size or completely disappear as well. When detected incidentally on MRI, these lesions require no additional workup. However, plain radiographs should be obtained for confirmation if there is a clinical possibility of sclerotic metastasis.

MRI Findings. The MR imaging features parallel the radiographic findings, which are usually diagnostic. Bone islands may be round, oval, or oblong and are usually oriented parallel to the long axis of the bone. These lesions demonstrate markedly hypointense signal on all pulse sequences, paralleling the adjacent cortical bone. If the lesion is large enough, MRI may show the classic radiographic feature of thorny, radiating bony spicules ("pseudopods") arising from the lesion and blending in with the surrounding trabeculae. Usually, bone islands are not connected with the adjacent cortical bone, but occasionally they are connected with the endocortex of the host bone.

Differential Diagnosis. In most clinical settings, the typical MRI findings may be considered diagnostic of a bone island. However, other densely sclerotic processes could demonstrate a similar appearance. Such processes include dense osteoblastic metastasis and sclerosing osteomyelitis. In the appropriate clinical setting, plain radiographs should be obtained to exclude these entities.

References

Greenspan A. Bone island (enostosis): Current concept—a review. *Skeletal Radiol* 24:111–115, 1995.

Greenspan A. Sclerosing bone dysplasias—a target-site approach. *Skeletal Radiol* 20:561–583, 1991.

Resnick D, Niwayama G. Enostosis, hyperostosis, and periostitis. In: Resnick D. *Bone and Joint Imaging*. Philadelphia, PA, W.B. Saunders Company; 1989; p 1233.

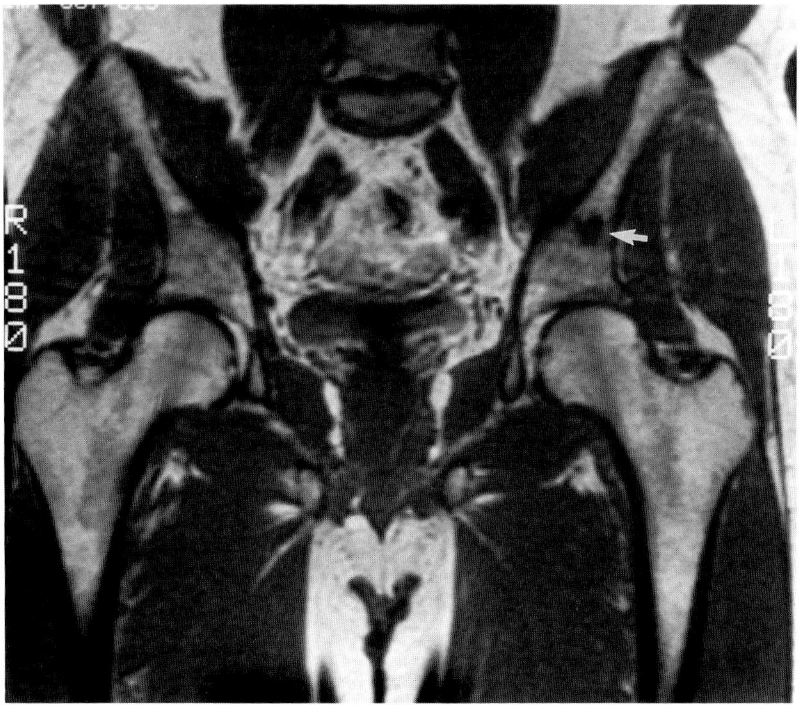

A

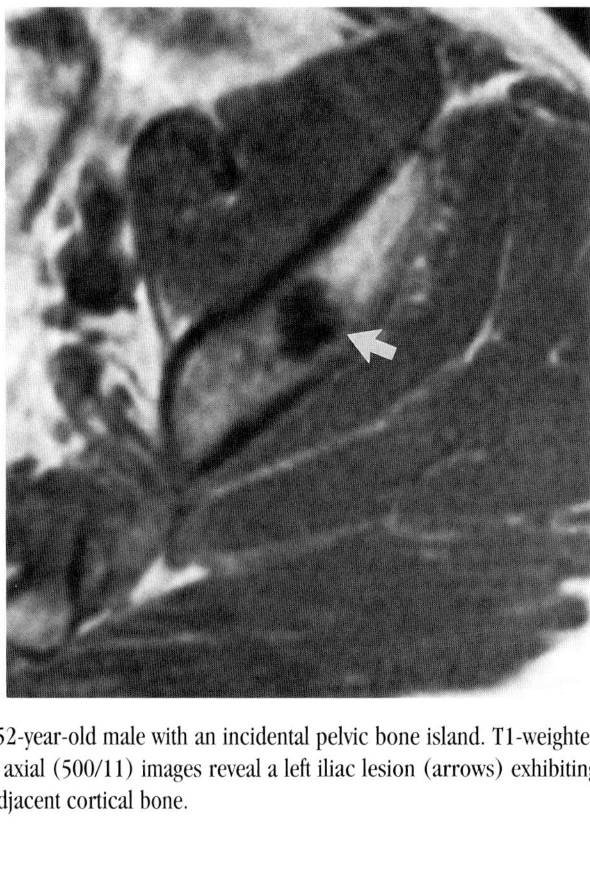

B

FIGURE 11.1 A 52-year-old male with an incidental pelvic bone island. T1-weighted (A) coronal (600/10) and (B) axial (500/11) images reveal a left iliac lesion (arrows) exhibiting signal which is isointense to the adjacent cortical bone.

C

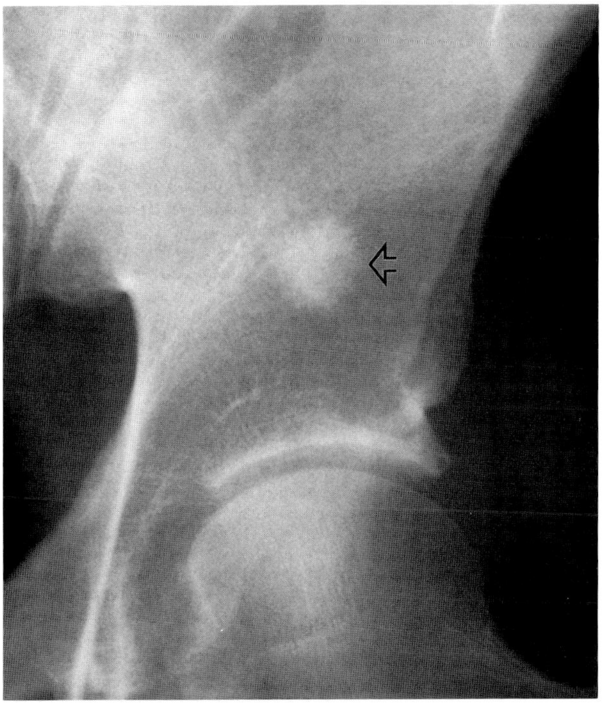

FIGURE 11.1 (continued) (C) Corresponding radiograph demonstrates small radiating spicules blending into the surrounding trabeculae, which is characteristic for a bone island (open arrow).

Osteoma

Definition. An osteoma is a juxtacortical mass composed of dense mature bone. It is a benign, slow-growing tumor.

Clinical Features. Symptoms associated with osteoma depend on the size and location of the lesion. Small osteomas are usually asymptomatic and incidental. They may be seen at any age, but predominate in the third through fifth decades of life. There is a 2:1 male predominance. Multiple lesions are nearly always associated with Gardner's syndrome, which is a familial autosomal dominant disease consisting of intestinal polyposis, multiple osteomas, soft tissue desmoid tumors, and other benign soft tissue lesions. Osteomas of the sinuses are not infrequent, but tubular bone lesions are rare.

Location. The vast majority of osteomas occur in the sinuses (about 75%, especially frontal and ethmoid), cranial vault, mandible, and maxilla. Other sites are much less commonly involved. These lesions are juxtacortical in location, arising from the periosteum.

Implications. Asymptomatic lesions do not require therapy. The presence of multiple osteomas strongly suggests Gardner's syndrome and one should be aware that osteomas frequently precede clinical and radiographic evidence of intestinal polyposis. Osteomas are usually stable on serial radiographs, but may slowly enlarge.

MRI Findings. Osteomas appear as smooth or lobular well-defined masses arising from the surface of the host bone (sinus lesions may protrude inward). The signal intensity is homogeneous and markedly hypointense (signal void) on all pulse sequences, paralleling that of the adjacent cortical bone.

Differential Diagnosis. The MR findings of an osteoma are characteristic, although plain radiographs should be obtained for confirmation. Other entities which may result in focal periosteal hyperostosis, such as osteoid osteoma or Brodie's abscess, would not remain isointense to cortical bone on all pulse sequences and should also be distinguishable based upon clinical grounds.

References

Greenspan A. Benign bone-forming lesions: Osteoma, osteoid osteoma, and osteoblastoma. Clinical, imaging, pathologic, and differential considerations. *Skeletal Radiol* 22:485–500, 1993.

Resnick D. *Bone and Joint Imaging*. Philadelphia, PA, W.B. Saunders Company; 1989; pp 1233–1234.

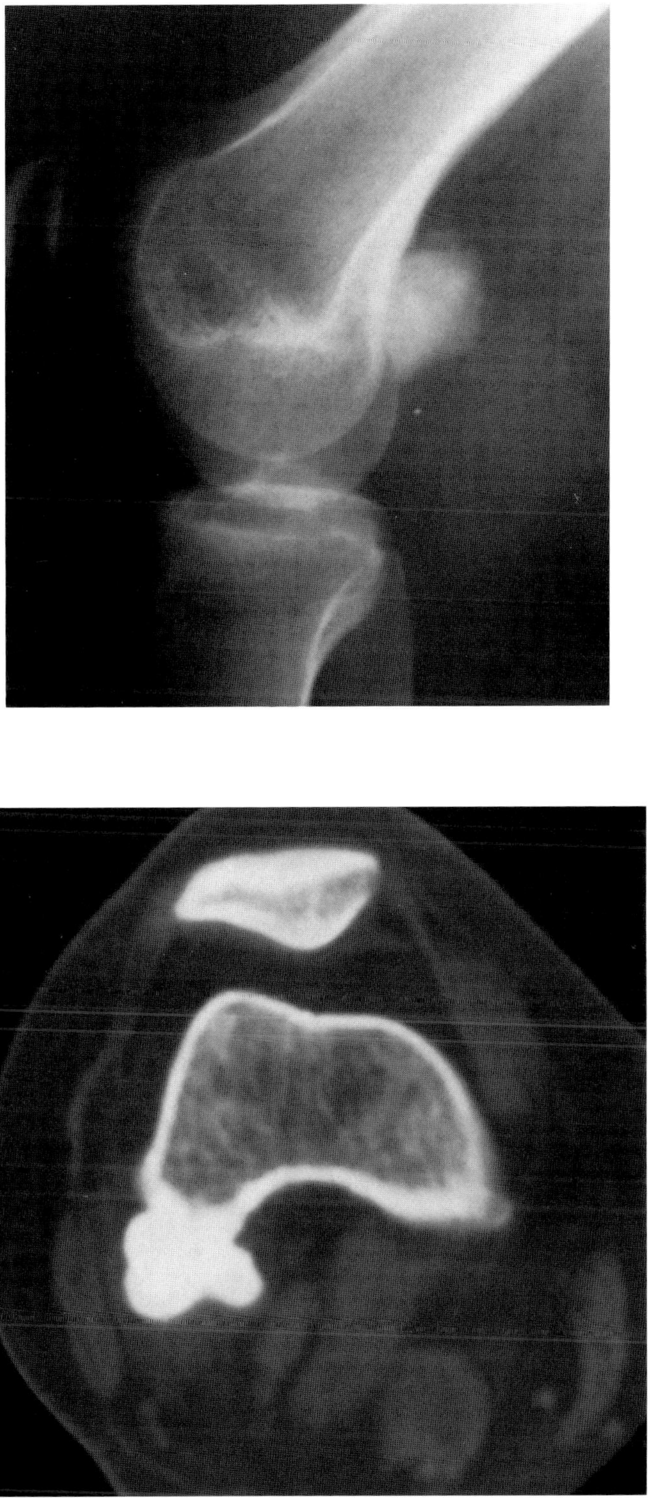

A

B

FIGURE 11.2 Biopsy-proven parosteal osteoma in a 31-year-old woman who presented with a palpable posterior knee mass. (A) Lateral radiograph and (B) axial CT image show a dense, well-marginated, lobulated, juxtacortical mass arising from the posterolateral aspect of the distal femoral metaphysis. This appearance resembles a parosteal osteosarcoma.

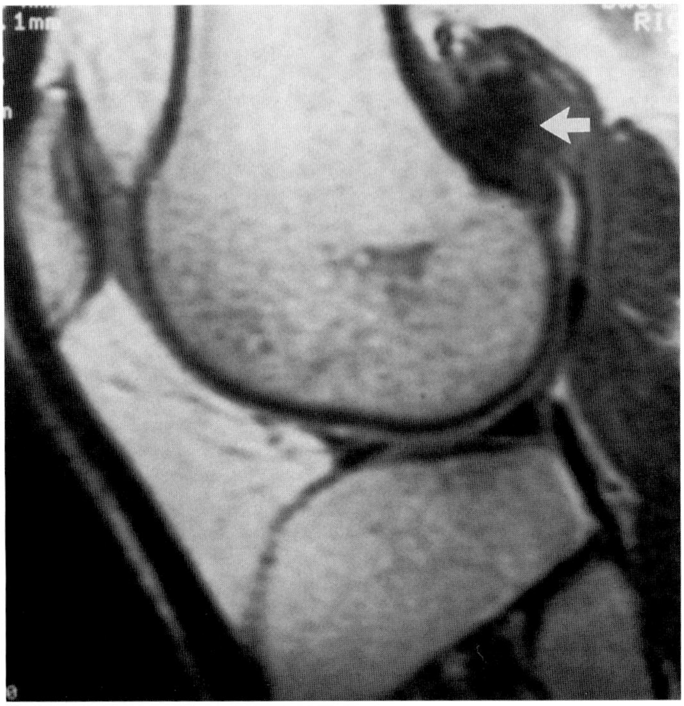

C

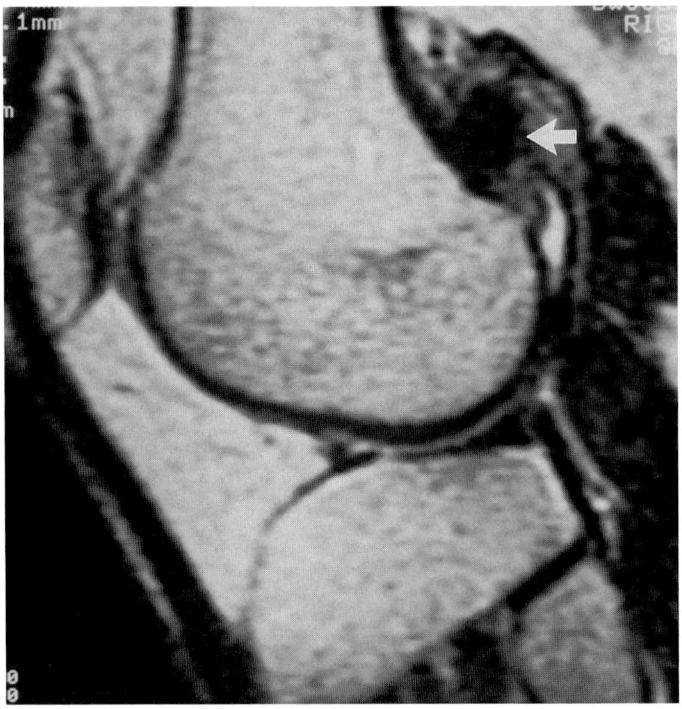

D

Figure 11.2 (continued) (C), (D) Sagittal dual-echo T2-weighted images (2000/30,80) reveal that the parosteal lesion (arrows) exhibits markedly hypointense, homogeneous signal intensity, which is equal to that of the adjacent cortex. (Courtesy of Alan Massengill, MD).

Osteoid Osteoma

Definition. Osteoid osteoma is a benign osteoblastic tumor of unknown etiology. It has very limited growth potential and is defined as being less than 1.5 cm in diameter. Histologically, osteoid osteoma strongly resembles and may be indistinguishable from osteoblastoma, which is defined as larger than 1.5 cm. The lesion consists of a nidus, which is composed of osteoid substance, woven bone, and a fibrovascular stroma. There is a variable amount of reactive sclerosis surrounding the lesion. The tumor produces prostaglandins, which induce an adjacent inflammatory response.

Clinical Features. Osteoid osteoma accounts for 11% of benign bone tumors and usually occurs between the ages of 5 and 30 years. Males are 2 to 3 times more frequently affected than females. Pain is almost invariably present and has been attributed to prostaglandin production by the lesion. The pain is classically worse at night and relieved by salicylates. This typical history has been reported in up to 75% of cases. Lesions in skeletally immature patients may result in growth disturbance, muscle atrophy, and significant deformity. Spine lesions commonly present with scoliosis. Intracapsular (intra-articular) osteoid osteomas often present with synovitis and joint effusion and are commonly misdiagnosed clinically. The synovitis is classically lymphoproliferative, mimicking rheumatoid arthritis on histologic examination.

Location. Osteoid osteomas are classified by location into cortical, medullary, subperiosteal, and intracapsular (intra-articular, periarticular) types. Cortical lesions are most common. Intracapsular lesions are least frequent, accounting for 5% of cases. 70% of lesions occur in long bones, especially the femur and tibia. 20% of cases occur in the bones of the hands and feet and 10% occur in the spine. In the long tubular bones, osteoid osteomas are usually diaphyseal, but may extend into the metaphysis. The vast majority of vertebral osteoid osteomas arise in the posterior elements.

Implications. CT is more accurate than MRI in detecting the nidus and remains the diagnostic modality of choice. Complete surgical excision of the nidus is curative and results in a dramatic relief of symptoms. Recurrence is likely if the nidus is incompletely resected. Rarely, there may be more than one nidus present (multicentric or multifocal osteoid osteoma). Osteoid osteomas may rarely (case reports) heal spontaneously. They have also been effectively treated with long-term salicylate or nonsteroidal anti-inflammatory drug administration, which may accelerate healing of the lesion. Intracapsular lesions may lead to premature osteoarthritis.

MRI Findings. MR images should not be interpreted without correlation with plain radiographs and possibly CT. The osteoid osteoma nidus, which is not visualized on MR as consistently as with CT, typically appears as a round, well-circumscribed lesion measuring 1 cm or less. The signal intensity of the nidus is low to intermediate on T1-weighted images. The signal intensity is variable (low, intermediate, or high) on enhanced T1-weighted images and on T2-weighted sequences and the intensity of the increased signal correlates with the vascularity of the nidus and the amount of osteoid substance within the nidus. Central calcification may be present within the nidus, which produces a signal void (signal isointense to cortex) on all pulse sequences. Surrounding reactive sclerosis, cortical thickening, and periosteal reaction are present in variable amounts and appear as areas of markedly hypointense signal paralleling that of cortical bone on all pulse sequences. The reactive sclerosis and periosteal reaction are prominent in cortical osteoid osteomas, but tend to be minimal with medullary, subperiosteal, and intracapsular lesions. MR commonly demonstrates adjacent areas of bone marrow and soft tissue edema and inflammation, which appear hypointense on T1-weighted images and of high signal intensity on T2-weighted sequences and gadolinium-enhanced T1-weighted images. The amount of surrounding edema and inflammation tends to be less in patients who have been treated with salicylates or nonsteroidal anti-inflammatory agents. Intracapsular osteoid osteomas are associated with synovitis and joint effusion.

Differential Diagnosis. MR images should be interpreted in the presence of plain films and/or CT images. The differential diagnosis for cortically-based lesions includes stress fracture and Brodie's abscess. A stress fracture should be distinguishable on MRI by the identification of the fracture line. A Brodie's abscess can be differentiated clinically in most cases. An osteoblastoma may have the appearance of a "giant osteoid osteoma", but the nidus is greater than 1.5 cm in size. The associated bone marrow and soft tissue changes may mimic infection, trauma, eosinophilic granuloma, or malignant lesions. Intracapsular lesions may resemble an infectious or inflammatory arthritis.

References

Assoun J, Richardi G, Railhac J, et al. Osteoid osteoma: MR imaging versus CT. *Radiology* 191:217–223, 1994.

Goldman M, Schneider R, Pavlov H. Osteoid osteomas of the femoral neck: Report of four cases evaluated with isotopic bone scanning, CT and MR imaging. *Radiology* 186:227–232, 1993.

Greenspan A. Benign bone-forming lesions: Osteoma, osteoid osteoma, and osteoblastoma. Clinical, imaging, pathologic, and differential considerations. *Skeletal Radiol* 22:485–500, 1993.

Woods E, Martel W, Mandell S, et al. Reactive soft-tissue mass associated with osteoid osteoma: Correlation of MR imaging features with pathologic findings. *Radiology* 186:221–225, 1993.

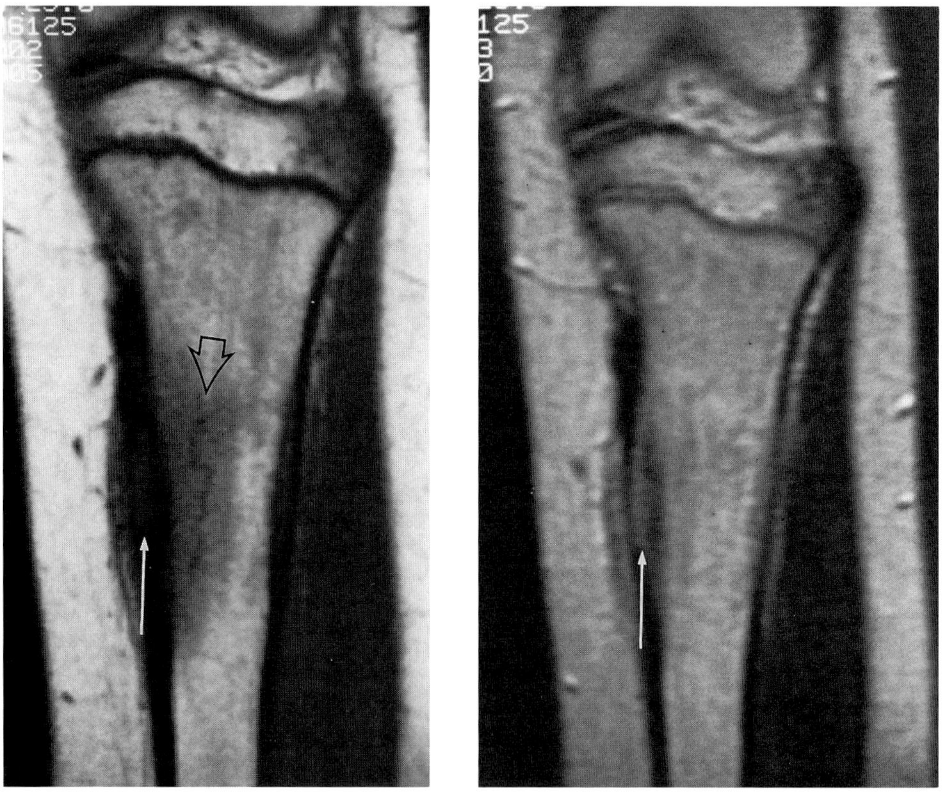

A B

FIGURE 11.3 An 8-year-old girl with a cortical osteoid osteoma in the proximal diaphysis of the left tibia. (A), (B) Coronal T1-weighted (600/20) and T2-weighted (2000/80) images demonstrate an elongated nidus of intermediate signal intensity (thin arrows) with associated cortical thickening and periosteal reaction. Note that the associated bone marrow edema is better seen on the T1-weighted image (open arrow). (C), (D) Axial T1-weighted (500/20) and T2-weighted (2200/80) scans optimize delineation of the nidus (curved open arrows), which may have a small central calcification (small arrow).

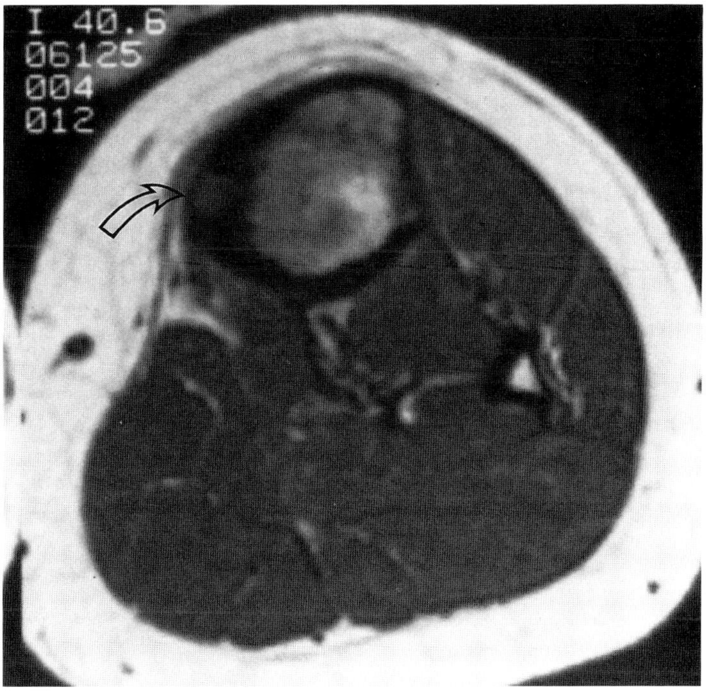

C

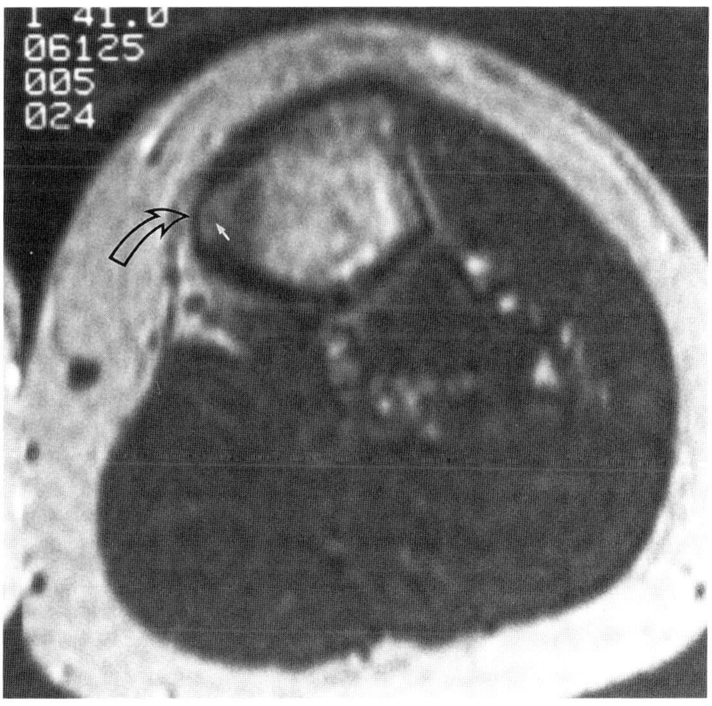

D

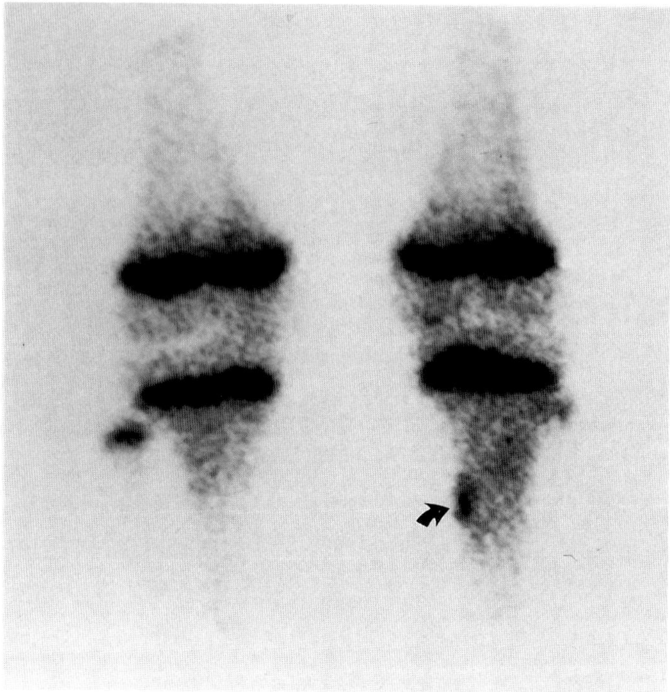

E

Figure 11.3 (continued) (E) Corresponding scintigram demonstrates the characteristic "target" appearance (curved arrow) of an osteoid osteoma with moderate increased activity surrounding a central focus of markedly increased uptake representing the hypervascular nidus.

Osteoblastoma

Definition. Osteoblastoma is a benign primary bone tumor characterized by osteoid and woven bone production. It resembles osteoid osteoma histologically and is sometimes indistinguishable based upon pathologic examination alone. In these instances, lesions larger than 1.5 cm are diagnosed as osteoblastoma, whereas smaller lesions are classified as osteoid osteoma.

Clinical Features. Osteoblastomas are rare, accounting for approximately 1% of all primary bone tumors and 3% of all benign bone tumors. Although all ages may be affected, about 90% of lesions occur between 6 and 30 years of age. Males are affected twice as commonly as females. Nearly all patients present with localized, dull, gradually increasing pain. As a general rule, the pain is not worse at night and not relieved by salicylates (which are classic features of osteoid osteoma). Localized swelling or muscle wasting may be identified and limited range of motion is frequently present. Scoliosis and neurologic deficits occur commonly with osteoblastomas of the spine.

Location. One-third of osteoblastomas occur in the spine. The vast majority of spine lesions arise in the posterior vertebral elements, with frequent extension into the vertebral body. Only rarely does the tumor arise in the vertebral body itself. The second most common site of osteoblastoma is in the long tubular bones (especially the femur and tibia), accounting for 25–30% of cases. These lesions occur in the diaphysis or metaphysis and may be eccentric, intracortical, or central. Additional sites include the bones of the hands and feet (especially the talus), craniofacial bones, and pelvis.

Implications. The treatment of choice is en bloc resection. Curettage also has a high success rate. The recurrence rate of osteoblastoma is 10 to 15% and the presence of recurrence raises the possibility of the variant known as aggressive (malignant) osteoblastoma. Secondary aneurysmal bone cyst formation may occur.

MRI Findings. The signal characteristics of osteoblastomas are nonspecific and plain films must be obtained for correlation. These lesions demonstrate low to intermediate signal intensity on T1-weighted images and hyperintense signal with T2-weighting. Areas of calcification or ossification, which appear hypointense on all pulse sequences, are often present within the lesion. Surrounding edema, which appears as hypointense signal on T1-weighted images and bright signal on T2-weighted sequences, may be seen in the marrow or soft tissues. In the spine, osteoblastomas typically appear as well-marginated, expansile masses arising in the posterior vertebral elements and may extend into the vertebral body. In long tubular bones, osteoblastomas typically appear as well-marginated round or oval expansile lesions which may be associated with cortical thinning or destruction and may have a prominent soft tissue component. The lesion may have the appearance of a "giant osteoid osteoma" with surrounding sclerosis (typically less sclerosis than that of osteoid osteoma) and periosteal reaction. The surrounding sclerosis and cortical thickening appear as hypointense signal on all pulse sequences.

Differential Diagnosis. The MR appearance of osteoblastoma is nonspecific. Plain films should be obtained for correlation. On both plain radiographs and MRI, an osteoblastoma may resemble an osteoid osteoma. In these cases, the lesion is arbitrarily classified as an osteoblastoma if it is greater than 1.5 cm in diameter. In the posterior vertebral elements, the expansile ("blown-out") appearance of an osteoblastoma resembles that of an aneurysmal bone cyst. In addition, an osteoblastoma may give rise to secondary aneurysmal bone cyst formation. In those lesions associated with soft tissue extension, the appearance may resemble malignant tumors such as osteosarcoma and Ewing's sarcoma.

References

Kroon H, Schurmans J. Osteoblastoma: Clinical and radiologic findings in 98 new cases. *Radiology* 175:783–790, 1990.

Greenspan A. Benign bone-forming lesions: Osteoma, osteoid osteoma, and osteoblastoma. Clinical, imaging, pathologic, and differential considerations. *Skeletal Radiol* 22:485–500, 1993.

Resnick D. *Bone and Joint Imaging*. Philadelphia, PA, W.B. Saunders Company; 1989; pp 1114–1116.

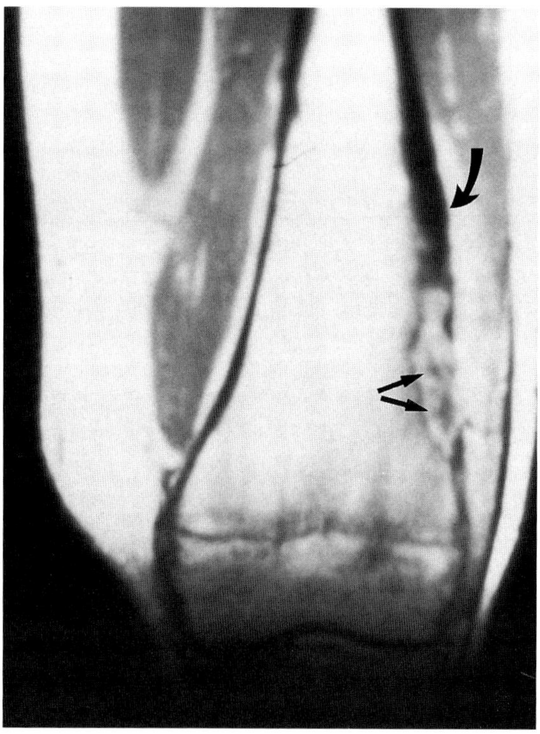

A

FIGURE 11.4 Osteoblastoma in a 16-year-old patient. (A) Contrast-enhanced coronal T1-weighted image (750/30) demonstrates an elongated intracortical lesion in the lateral metadiaphyseal region of the distal left femur. Note the nonenhancing foci of calcification within the lesion (arrows) as well as associated cortical thickening (curved arrow). Axial (B) contrast-enhanced T1-weighted (600/30) image demonstrates central hypointense foci (thin white arrow) corresponding to foci of calcification (thin black arrow) seen on CT scan (C). Adjacent reactive sclerosis is present.

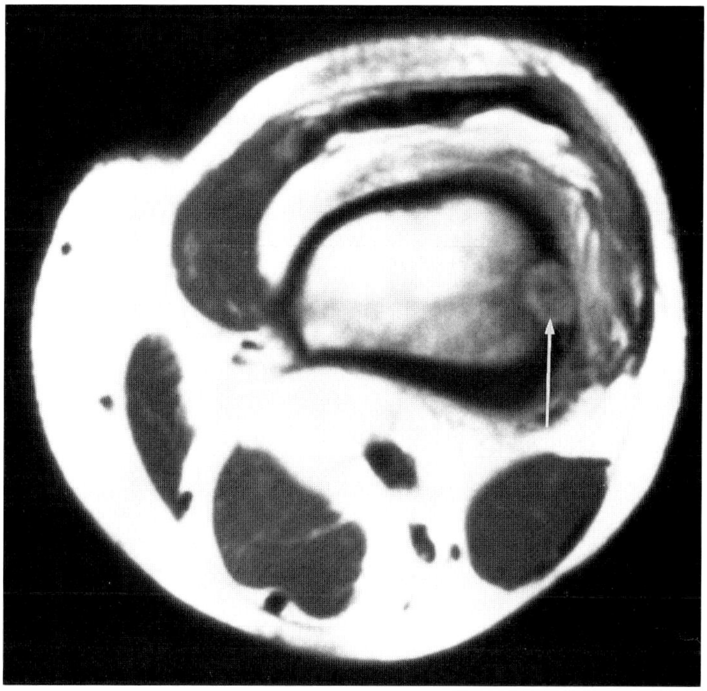

B

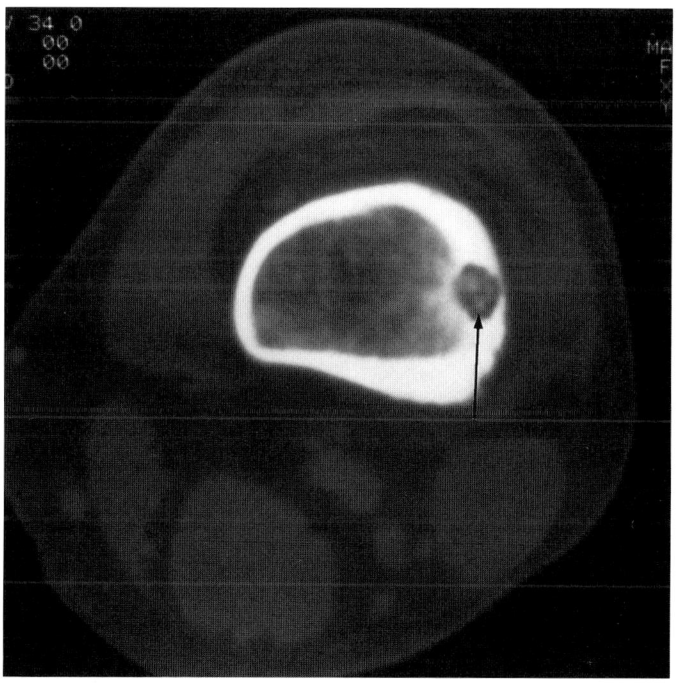

C

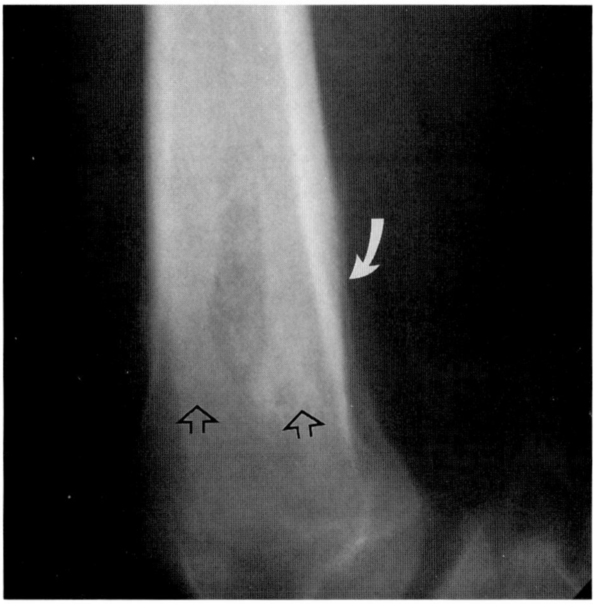

D

FIGURE 11.4 (continued) (D) Lateral radiograph demonstrates adjacent reactive sclerosis (open arrows) and periosteal reaction (curved white arrow). This osteoblastoma has a "giant osteoid osteoma" appearance. (Courtesy of Rusty Fritz, MD).

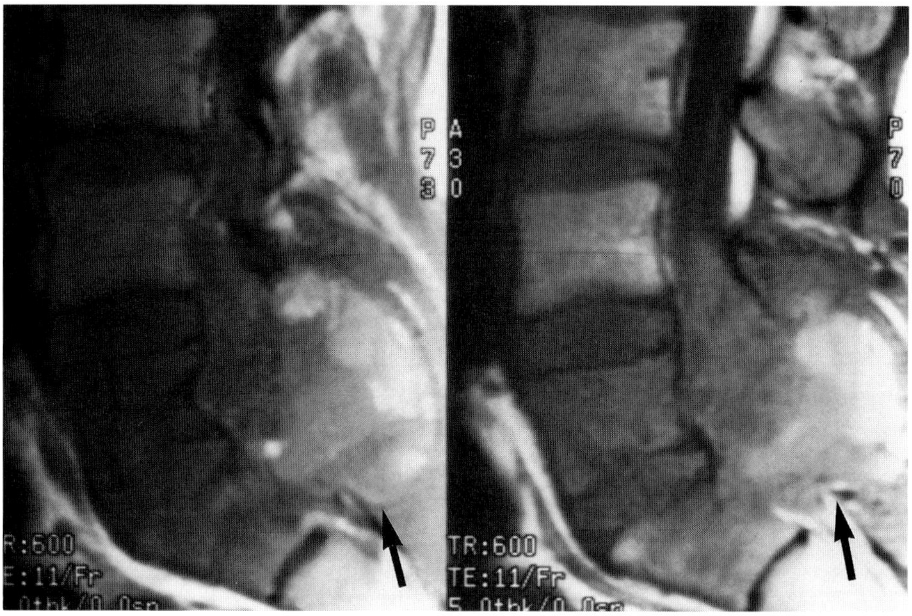

A

FIGURE 11.5 A 23-year-old male with a spinal osteoblastoma which has secondary aneurysmal bone cyst formation. (A), (B) Sagittal T1-weighted (600/11) and FSE T2-weighted (3000/102) images reveal an expansile mass involving the L5 posterior elements (arrows). Note extension into the L5 and S1 vertebral bodies (curved open arrows). Heterogeneous signal intensity and numerous fluid-fluid levels are present within the lesion consistent with extensive hemorrhage and various blood products. (C) Axial FSE T2-weighted image (3500/102) again demonstrates numerous fluid-fluid levels throughout the lesion. The mass results in very severe stenosis of the spinal canal (small arrows) and extends well into the vertebral body (curved arrow). In light of the location and patient's age, the MR findings are highly suggestive of an aneurysmal bone cyst. Surgery confirmed the diagnosis of osteoblastoma with secondary aneurysmal bone cyst formation.

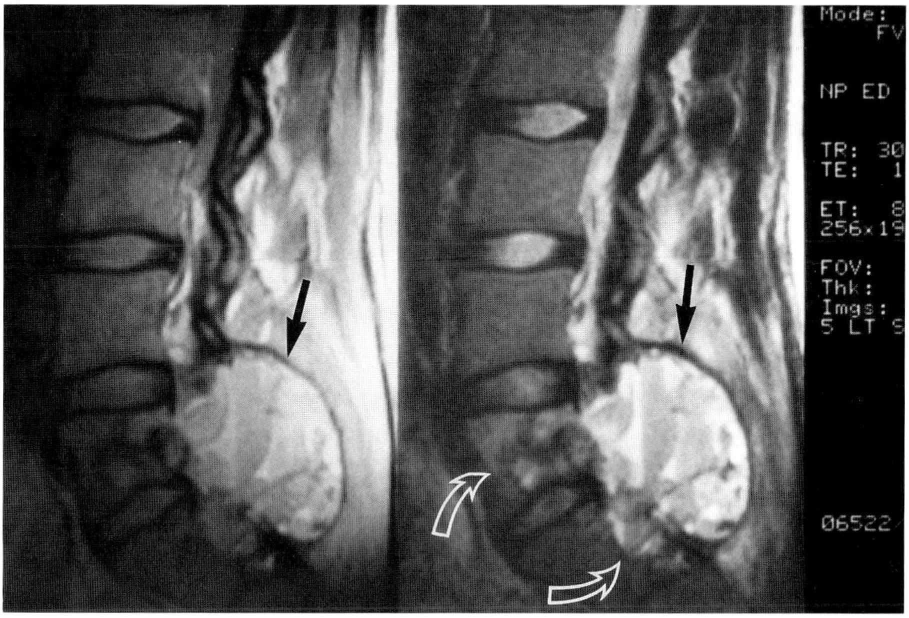
Mode:
FV
NP ED
TR: 30
TE: 1
ET: 8
256x19
FOV:
Thk:
Imgs:
5 LT S
06522

B

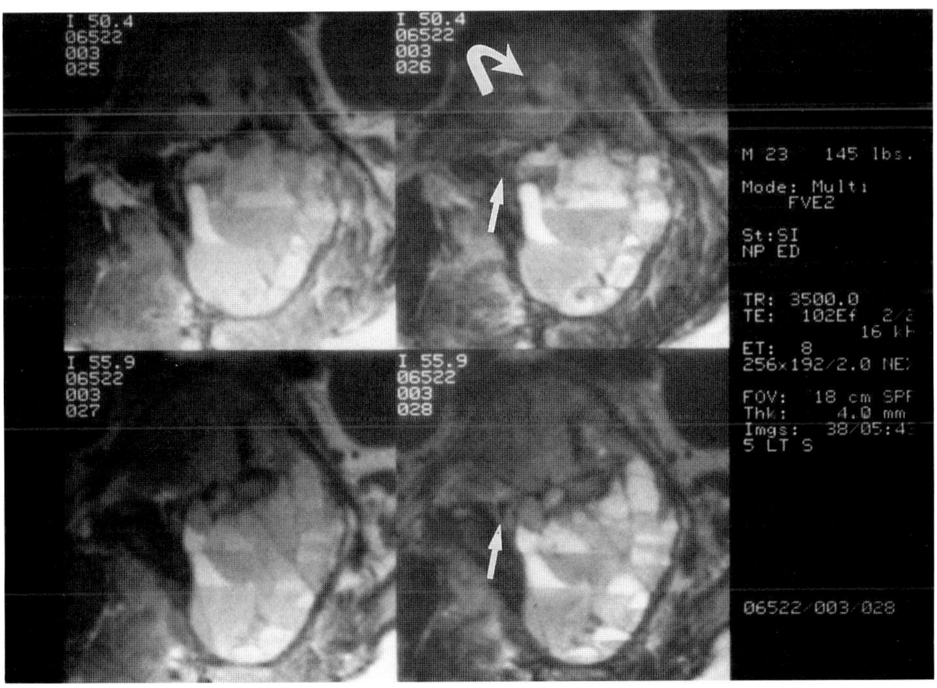
I 50.4
06522
003
025
I 50.4
06522
003
026
M 23 145 lbs.
Mode: Multi
FVE2
St:SI
NP ED
TR: 3500.0
TE: 102Ef
16 kH
ET: 8
256x192/2.0 NE
FOV: 18 cm SPF
Thk: 4.0 mm
Imgs: 38/05:4
5 LT S
I 55.9
06522
003
027
I 55.9
06522
003
028
06522/003/028

C

Osteosarcoma (Osteogenic Sarcoma)

Definition. Osteosarcoma is a malignant mesenchymal neoplasm characterized by the production of osteoid or immature bone. Osteosarcomas may be classified according to their location within the bone into central/intramedullary, intracortical, surface, periosteal, and parosteal types. Conventional (intramedullary) osteosarcoma accounts for approximately 75% of all osteosarcomas. They are also classified according to histologic grade and composition. One histologic subtype is telangiectactic osteosarcoma which is a very vascular and hemorrhagic lesion with only scant osteoid production. Secondary osteosarcomas may occur and Paget's disease is by far the most common precursor for these lesions. Osteosarcoma may very rarely be multicentric.

Clinical Features. Conventional osteosarcoma typically affects patients in the second and third decades of life. Older patients are only rarely affected and more than half of all osteosarcomas occurring beyond the age of 50 are secondary (arising most commonly from Paget's disease, irradiated bone). Except for multiple myeloma, osteosarcoma is the most common primary malignant bone tumor. Patients typically present with pain and swelling, but may also have restricted range of motion, warmth, or pathologic fracture.

Location. Most osteosarcomas involve the metaphysis of long bones, especially around the knee and the proximal humerus. Any bone may be affected.

Implications. Treatment of osteosarcomas consists of chemotherapy and surgery. Surgical alternatives include limb-sparing procedures, amputation, and disarticulation. The choice of surgical procedure depends upon the intraosseous and extraosseous extent of the tumor, including intra-articular and neurovascular involvement. Extension of tumor into an adjacent joint requires en bloc resection of the involved joint, resulting in poorer postoperative function. MR is the imaging modality of choice for staging musculoskeletal neoplasms. Advances in chemotherapy have allowed increased limb-sparing procedures, which result in improved function and survival rates of approximately 55–70%. "Skip" lesions (tumor foci which are separate from the main neoplasm) are present in a minority of cases and are associated with a poor prognosis.

MRI Findings. Most osteosarcomas are associated with a soft tissue mass. On T1-weighted images, both the intraosseous and soft tissue components typically have hypointense signal (hypointense or isointense to muscle) that tends to be homogeneous. On T2-weighted sequences, the intraosseous component generally exhibits heterogeneous signal intensity ranging from hypointense to hyperintense. Lesions containing more tumor mineralization will demonstrate lower signal on T2-weighted images and lesions containing significant necrosis will demonstrate areas of very high signal intensity. The associated extraosseous component tends to exhibit heterogeneous hyperintense signal with T2-weighting. On both T1- and T2-weighted images, the soft tissue mass is generally sharply delineated by a low signal intensity capsule or pseudocapsule. Increased peritumoral signal on T2-weighted and gadolinium-enhanced T1-weighted images is a nonspecific finding, which may represent peritumoral edema or tumor infiltration. Intra-articular tumor extension is present in about 20% of cases. MRI is very sensitive in detecting joint involvement, but false-positive cases may occur due to tumor bowing the joint capsule and peritumoral or synovial inflammatory changes. A joint effusion adjacent to the tumor is a common finding in patients with and without intra-articular involvement and is not a useful sign for staging. However, the absence of a joint effusion is a reliable indicator that the joint space is not involved. MRI is highly accurate in depicting the presence or absence of tumor spread across the physis. In our experience, intravenous gadolinium has not been helpful in further defining tumor extent.

Differential Diagnosis. Plain radiographs remain the standard for diagnosing osteosarcoma. The MR images should be interpreted in the presence of the corresponding plain films. In a younger age group, a symptomatic lesion with both intraosseous and extraosseous components on MRI could represent various entities including osteosarcoma, Ewing's sarcoma, infection, and eosinophilic granuloma.

References

Seeger L, Widoff B, Bassett L, et al. Preoperative evaluation of osteosarcoma: Value of gadopentetate dimeglumine-enhanced MR imaging. *AJR* 157:347–351, 1991.

Schima W, Amann G, Stiglbauer R, et al. Preoperative staging of osteosarcoma: Efficacy of MR imaging in detecting joint involvement. *AJR* 163:1171–1175, 1994.

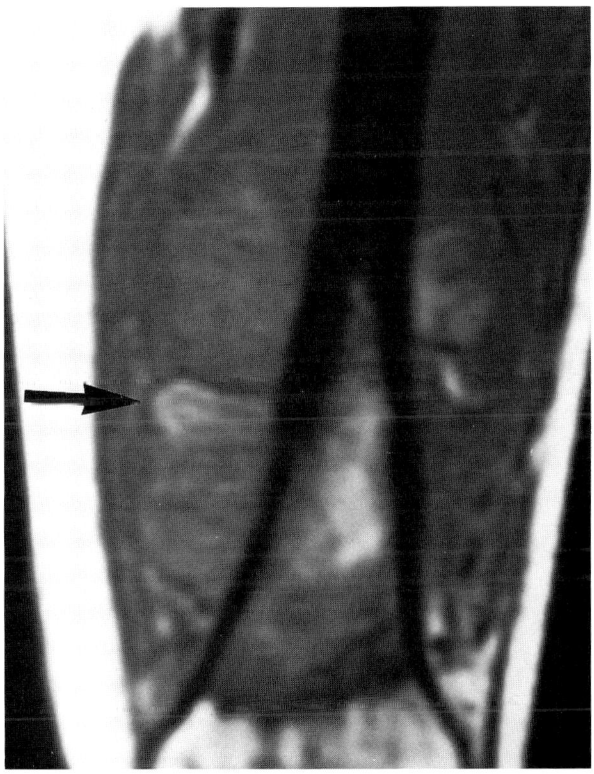

A

FIGURE 11.6 Conventional osteosarcoma of the distal left femur in a 20-year-old male. (A), (B) Coronal T1-weighted (750/16) and FMPIR (4500/18, TI-150) images demonstrate a metadiaphyseal lesion with large intraosseous and extraosseous components (arrows). Note the heterogeneous signal intensity throughout the lesion on both sequences.

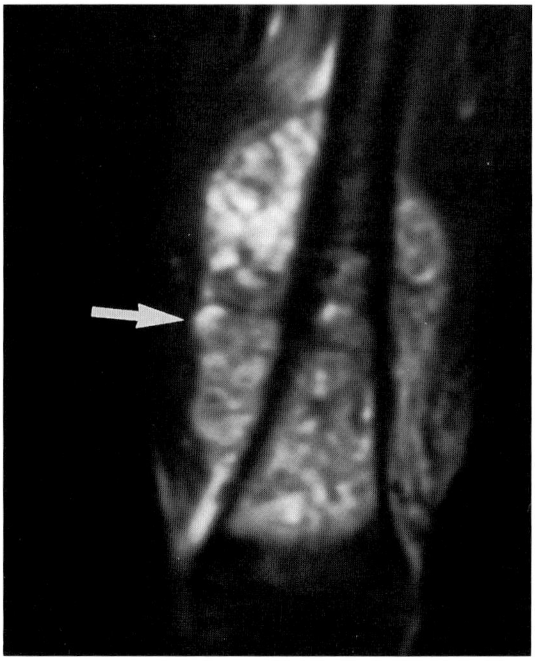

B

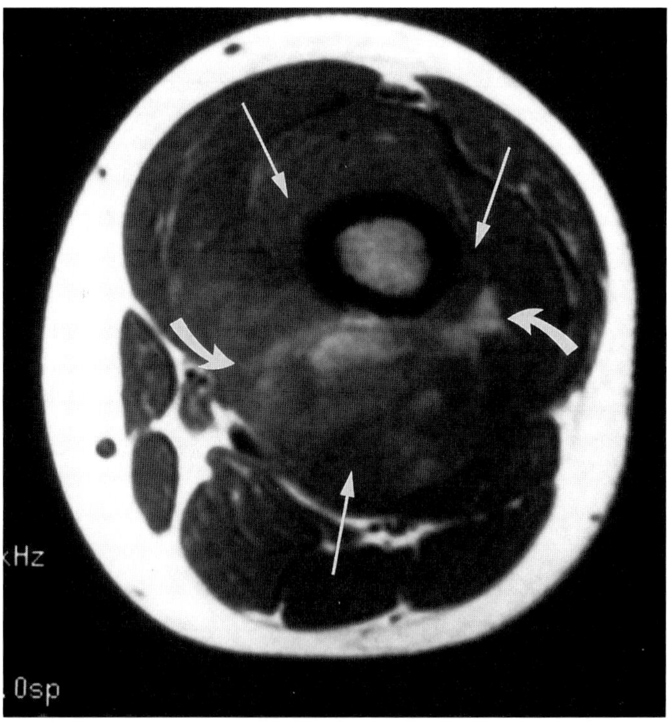

C

Figure 11.6 (continued) (C) Axial T1-weighted image (500/17) reveals that much of the soft tissue component (thin arrows) is isointense with surrounding muscle. The areas of increased signal indicate the presence of methemoglobin (curved arrows).

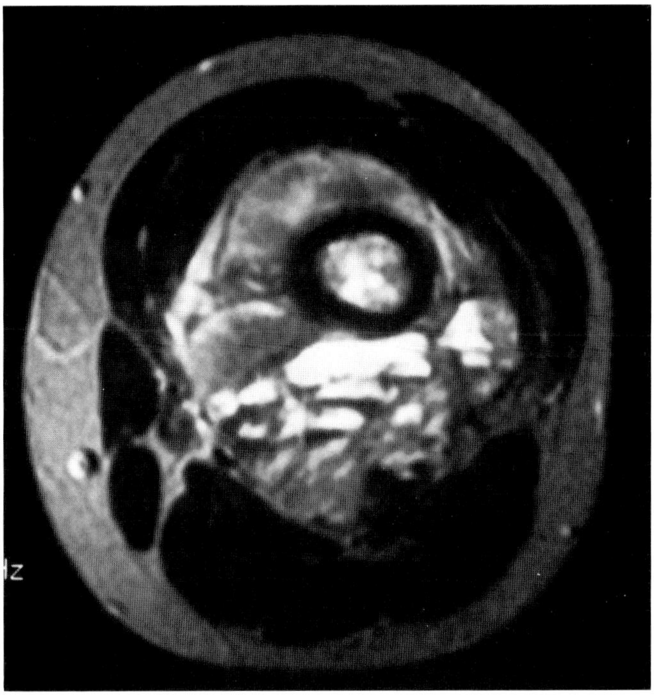

D

Figure 11.6 (continued) (D) Axial FSE T2-weighted fat suppression image (3000/90) demonstrates numerous fluid-fluid levels within the soft tissue mass consistent with hemorrhage.

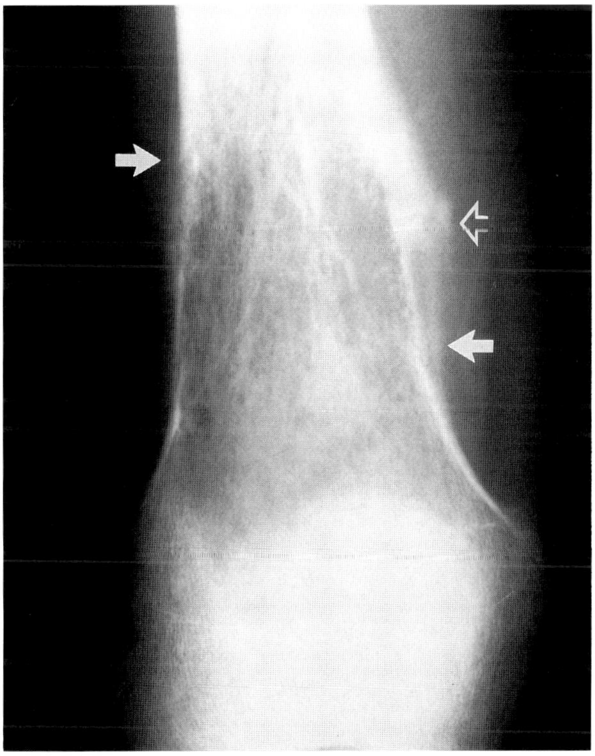

A

Figure 11.7 Telangiectactic osteosarcoma of the distal femur. (A) AP radiograph demonstrates a lytic, destructive mass in the metadiaphyseal region of the distal right femur. Note the aggressive periosteal reaction (arrows) and Codman's triangle (open arrow).

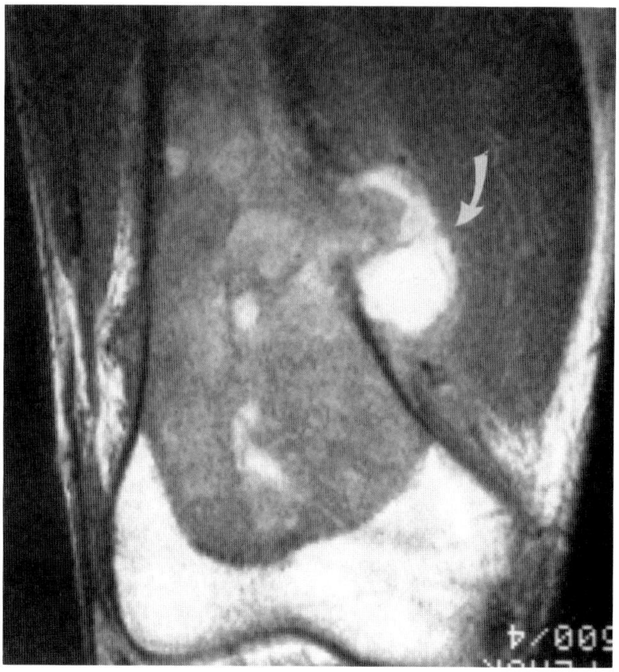

B

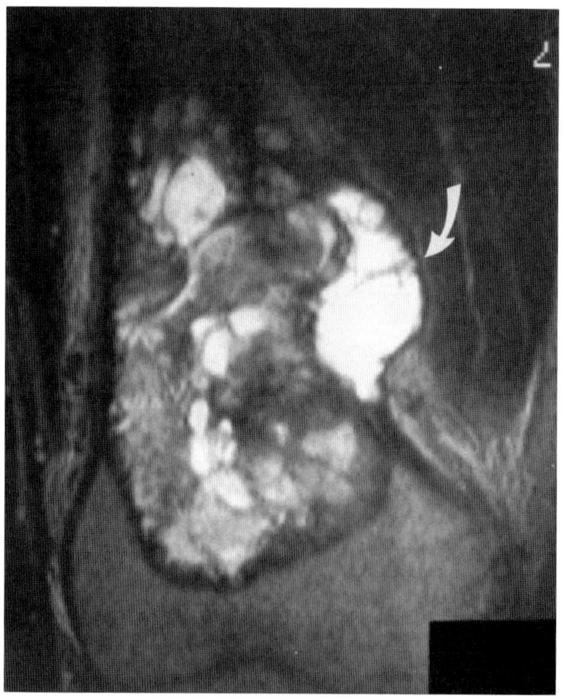

C

FIGURE 11.7 (continued) (B), (C) Coronal T1-weighted (500/30) and T2-weighted (2000/120) images demonstrate an associated soft tissue mass (curved arrows). Heterogeneous signal intensity is seen on both sequences. Areas of bright signal are seen on the T1-weighted image in both intraosseous and extraosseous components consistent with methemoglobin.

Parosteal Osteosarcoma

Definition. Parosteal osteosarcoma is typically a well-differentiated (low-grade) malignancy which arises from the surface of a bone. Histologically, it consists of well-formed osteoid and trabeculae within a spindle-cell stroma. If medullary involvement is present, there must be less than 25% of the medullary cavity affected.

Clinical Features. Parosteal osteosarcoma is an uncommon tumor which comprises about 5% of all primary osteosarcomas. It typically appears between the ages of 15 and 55 years and most commonly presents as painless swelling of relatively long duration. A palpable mass is present in the vast majority of patients. Pain and limited range of motion are each present in approximately 30% of patients.

Location. The vast majority of parosteal osteosarcomas involve the metaphyses of long bones. Most lesions are located at the posterior aspect of the distal femur. The next most frequent sites are the proximal tibia and proximal humerus.

Implications. Low-grade lesions tend to have a relatively good prognosis, but will recur if incompletely resected. For this reason, wide-margin excision has been advocated as the surgical treatment of choice. MR is the imaging modality of choice in detecting medullary involvement, which has important surgical implications. In these cases, wide excision is precluded and resection of the entire portion of the involved bone is necessary. Although medullary involvement does affect surgical management, there are conflicting reports as to whether invasion of the medullary cavity worsens the prognosis. There is a poor prognosis in lesions which undergo dedifferentiation, which has been reported in up to 16% of cases. In these cases, there is a coexisting high-grade spindle cell sarcoma. Dedifferentiation of the tumor markedly increases the risk of metastasis and accounts for the vast majority of deaths from parosteal osteosarcoma.

MRI Findings. The MR exam should not be interpreted without corresponding plain films, which are often diagnostic. On MRI, parosteal osteosarcomas appear as variably sized masses arising from the cortical surface of a long bone. The margin is typically lobulated, but may be smooth or irregular. As the mass grows, it tends to encircle the adjacent bone, remaining attached to the cortex by a small sessile base. A cleavage plane is often seen between the mass and the adjacent bone. The underlying cortex may be normal, thickened, or destroyed. In a recent review, parosteal osteosarcomas were associated with medullary involvement in 22% of cases, invasion of the adjacent soft tissue in 46% of cases, and invasion of the neurovascular bundle in 22% of cases. These lesions typically appear hypointense on T1-weighted sequences and heterogeneous on T2-weighted images with areas of low, intermediate, and high signal intensity.

Differential Diagnosis. Plain films are often characteristic for parosteal osteosarcoma, but the lesion may be confused for myositis ossificans or osteochondroma. On MRI, myositis ossificans typically remains separated from the underlying bone, which differentiates this entity from parosteal osteosarcoma. In the case of an osteochondroma, the spongiosa and cortex of the underlying bone are continuous with and extend into the lesion.

References

Okada K, Frassica F, Sim F, et al. Parosteal osteosarcoma: A clinicopathological study. *JBJS* 76A:366–378, 1994.

Hermann G, Abdelwahab I, Klein M, et al. Case report 711. *Skeletal Radiol* 21:69–71, 1992.

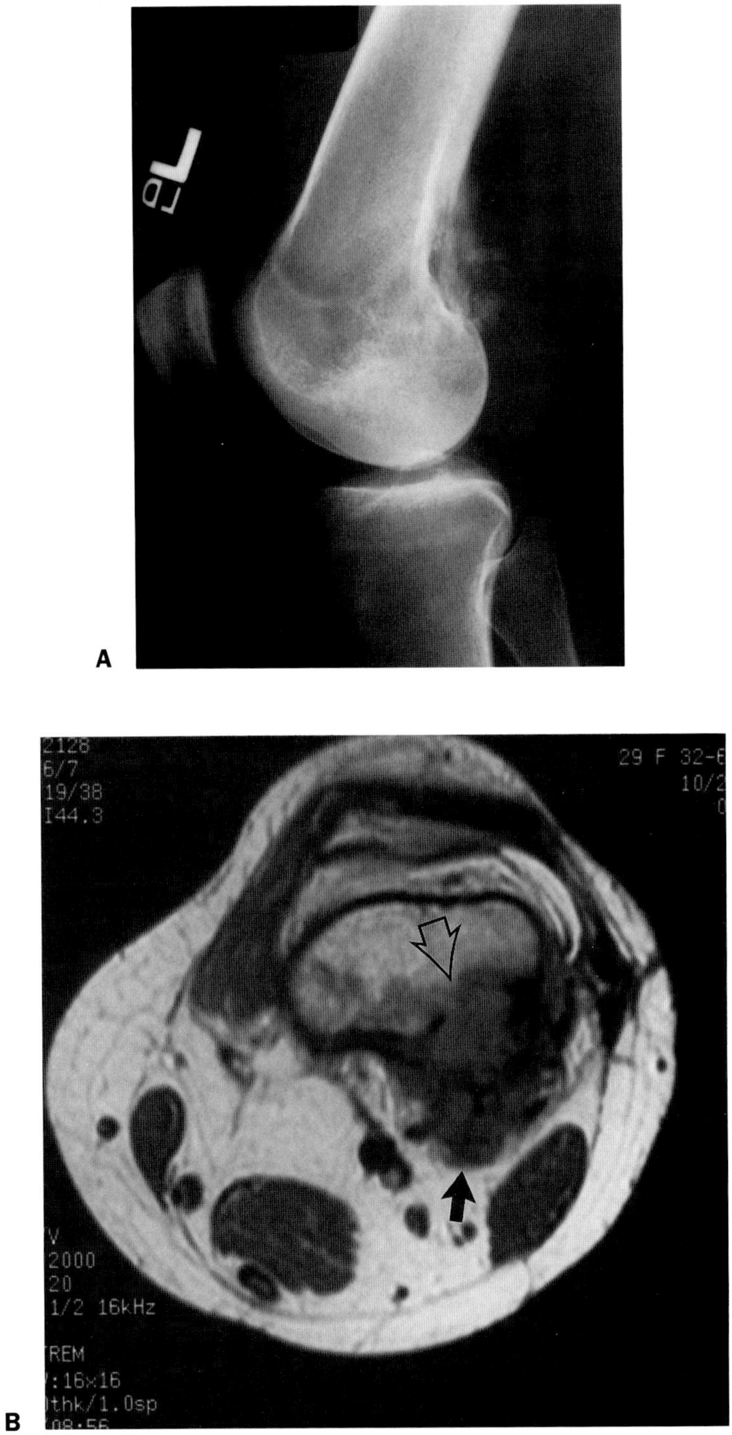

FIGURE 11.8 Parosteal osteosarcoma of the distal femur in a 29-year-old woman. (A) Lateral radiograph demonstrates an aggressive osteoid-producing mass arising from the posterior surface of the distal left femoral metaphysis. The location and appearance are classic for parosteal osteosarcoma. (B), (C) Axial proton density (2000/20) and T2-weighted (2000/80) images demonstrate a posterior soft tissue mass (arrows), cortical destruction, and extension into the medullary cavity (open arrows). Note the heterogeneous signal intensity with T2-weighting.

C

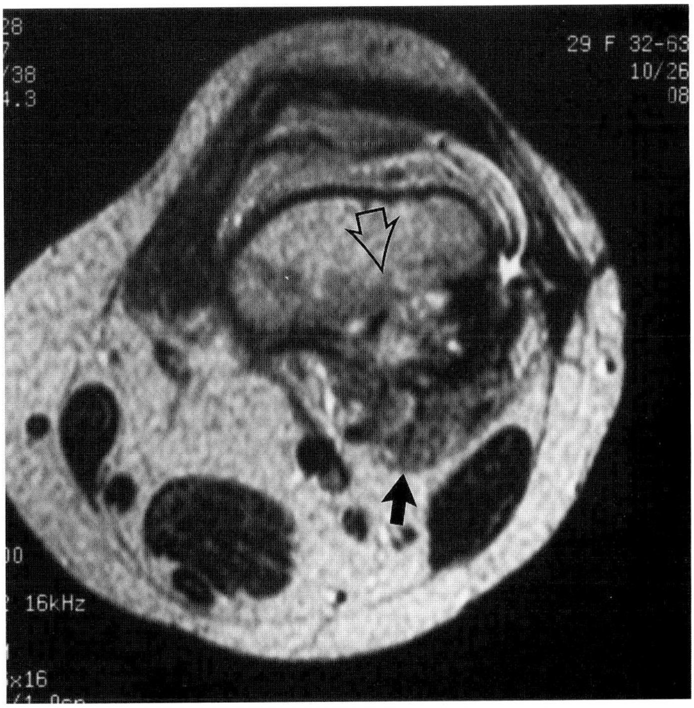

A

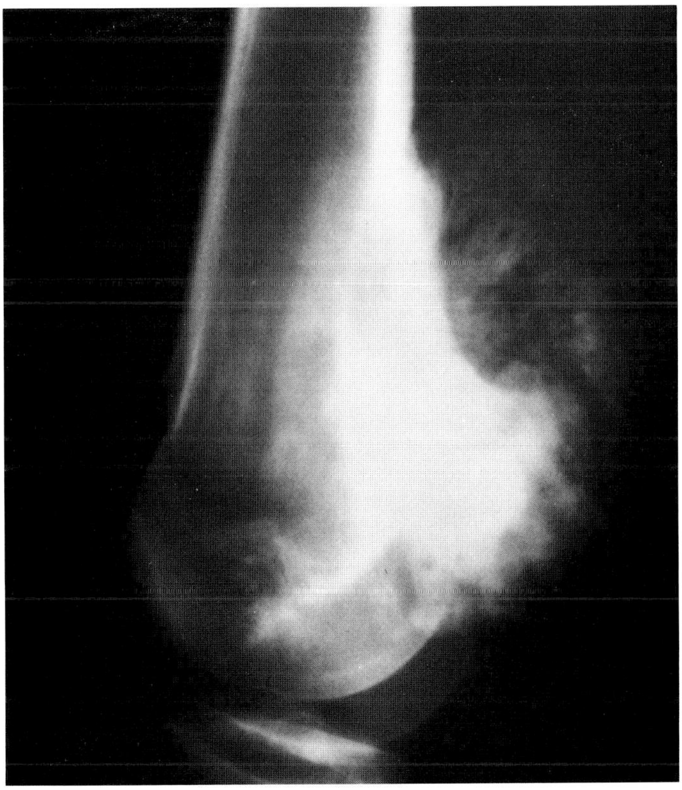

FIGURE 11.9 A 35-year-old male with a parosteal osteosarcoma of the distal femur. (A) Lateral radiograph reveals a large parosteal osteosarcoma arising from the posterior surface of the distal femoral metaphysis.

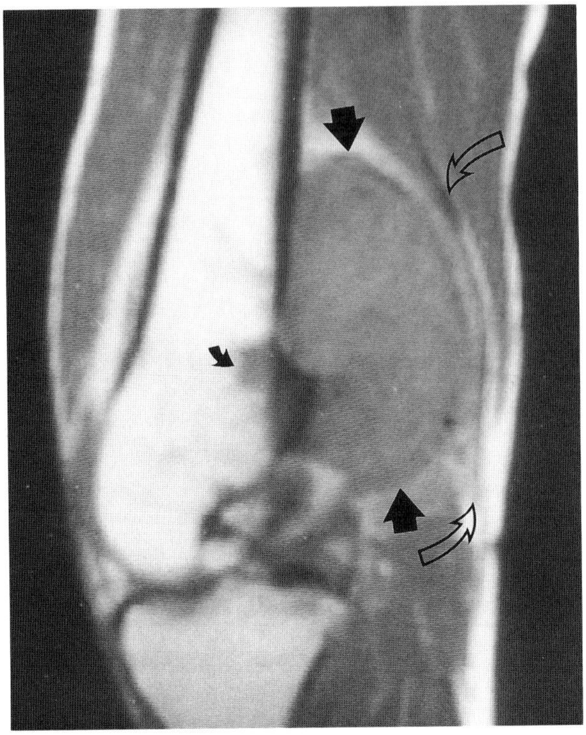

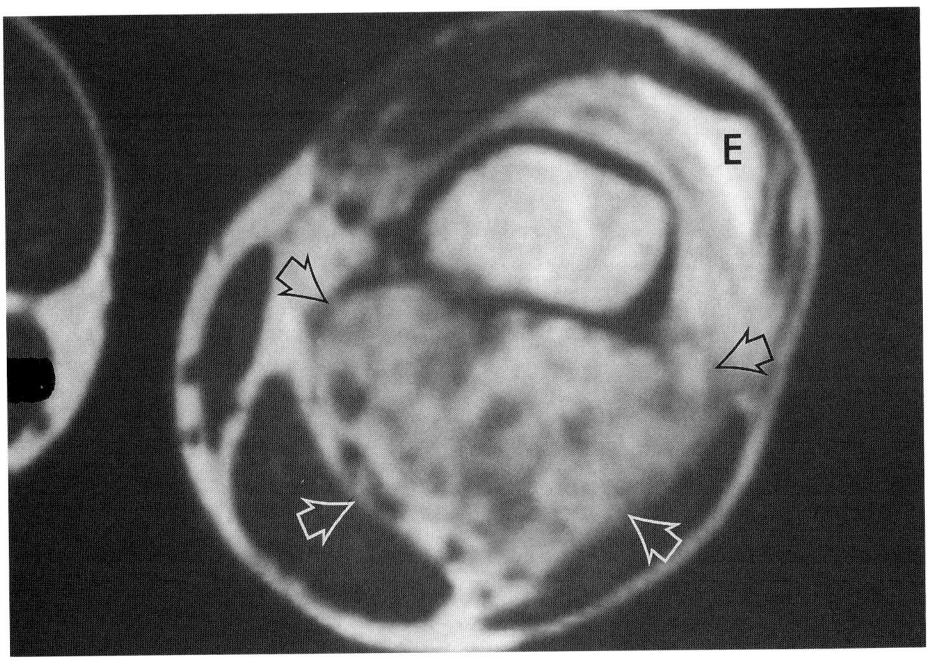

C

FIGURE 11.9 (continued) (B) Sagittal T1-weighted image (600/30) demonstrates a prominent soft tissue mass (arrows) which is of intermediate signal intensity. Note the extension into the medullary cavity (small curved arrow). There is significant posterior displacement of the popliteal artery (curved open arrows). (C) Axial T2-weighted image (2000/80) demonstrates heterogeneous signal intensity (open arrows). An associated joint effusion (E) is present.

12 Cartilaginous Tumors

Osteochondroma (Exostosis)

Definition. An osteochondroma (OC) is a benign osseous excrescence with a cartilaginous cap. The attachment to the underlying bone may be a narrow stalk (pedunculated) or broad-based (sessile). The precise etiology is unclear as to whether this lesion represents a true neoplasm or results from a developmental physeal defect. An OC may rarely arise in association with prior radiation therapy. The cortex and trabecular bone of an OC are in direct continuity with those of the underlying host bone. In the growing skeleton, there is a hyaline cartilage cap, which may gradually involute after skeletal maturation.

Clinical Features. OC is the most common benign bone tumor and is estimated to occur in 3% of individuals. Although these lesions may be found in individuals of all ages, about 75% of OCs are discovered in patients less than 20 years old. Most patients present with a palpable mass, with or without associated pain. There can be symptoms related to compression of neurovascular structures or adjacent bursal inflammation. OCs may continue to grow until the epiphyses are closed. Enlargement of a lesion after skeletal maturity is worrisome for the possibility of malignant transformation. Solitary OCs are much more common than multiple lesions (hereditary multiple exostoses). Hereditary multiple exostoses (osteochondromatosis) is an autosomal dominant and typically polyostotic condition in which symptoms develop during the first decade of life. Trevor's disease (dysplasia epiphysealis hemimelica) is a rare condition in which an osteochondroma arises from the epiphysis resulting in swelling, pain, deformity, and possibly secondary osteoarthritis.

Location. Although any bone may be affected, there is a predilection for the metaphysis of long bones. About half of all lesions occur in the bones about the knee and proximal humerus. About 10% of lesions involve the small bones of the hands or feet. The pelvis and scapula each account for about 5% of cases. Trevor's disease has a predilection for the talus, knee region, and distal tibia.

Implications. Numerous complications may occur in association with OCs including growth disturbance, skeletal deformity, limited range of motion, nerve compression, fracture of the bony stalk, vascular compression, pseudoaneurysm formation, bursitis, and spinal stenosis. The most serious complication associated with OCs is malignant transformation, typically in which a chondrosarcoma arises from the cartilage cap. The rate of malignant transformation in solitary OCs is about 1%, but may be as high as 10–30% in patients with hereditary multiple exostoses. The increased incidence of malignant transformation in these patients is thought to simply reflect the greater number of lesions (i.e., the more lesions, the greater the risk). Sessile OCs are much more likely to undergo malignant transformation than pedunculated lesions, presumably due to the increased surface area of the cartilaginous cap. In addition, lesions which are located centrally within the skeleton (pelvis, sternum, scapula, rib) are more prone to malignant transformation. The thickness of the cartilaginous cap has been used as a sign in predicting malignant transformation. As a general rule, although there are exceptions, benign osteochondromas typically have a cap thickness of less than 1 cm, whereas a thickness greater than 2 cm is concerning for the presence of secondary chondrosarcoma.

MRI Findings. An OC appears as an osseous protuberance in which the medullary and cortical bone components of the lesion are continuous with those of the adjacent host bone. The lesion is covered by a cartilage cap which is typically less than 1 cm in thickness in a benign OC. The cap may not be present in adult patients or may be difficult to identify if very thin (less than 2 mm). The cap typically appears approximately isointense to muscle on T1-weighted images and exhibits homogeneous high signal intensity on T2-weighted sequences, corresponding to lobules of hyaline cartilage found histologically. In tubular bones, OCs usually point away from the adjacent joint and are typically associated with widening of the underlying host bone (undertubulation). An adjacent fluid-filled bursa may be present, which would generally exhibit very high signal intensity on T2-weighted sequences, and may be difficult to delineate from the cartilage cap. In addition to clinical findings and cartilage cap thickness, other signs of malignant transformation include bone destruction and soft tissue invasion.

Differential Diagnosis. The diagnosis of OC is confirmed on MRI by demonstrating direct continuity of the host bone cortex and medullary space with the lesion. This may be important in the case of a sessile OC, in which the radiographic diagnosis may not be straightforward.

References

Giudici M, Moser R, Kransdorf M. Cartilaginous bone tumors. *Radiol Clin North Am* 31:237–259, 1993.

Griffiths H, Thompson R, Galloway H, et al. Bursitis in association with solitary osteochondromas presenting as mass lesions. *Skeletal Radiol* 20:513–516, 1991.

Cohen E, Kressel H, Frank T, et al. Hyaline cartilage-origin bone and soft-tissue neoplasms: MR appearance and histologic correlation. *Radiology* 167:477–481, 1988.

Recht M, Sachs P, LiPuma J, et al. Case report. Popliteal artery pseudoaneurysm in a patient with hereditary multiple exostoses: MRI and MRA diagnosis. *JCAT* 17:300–302, 1993.

A

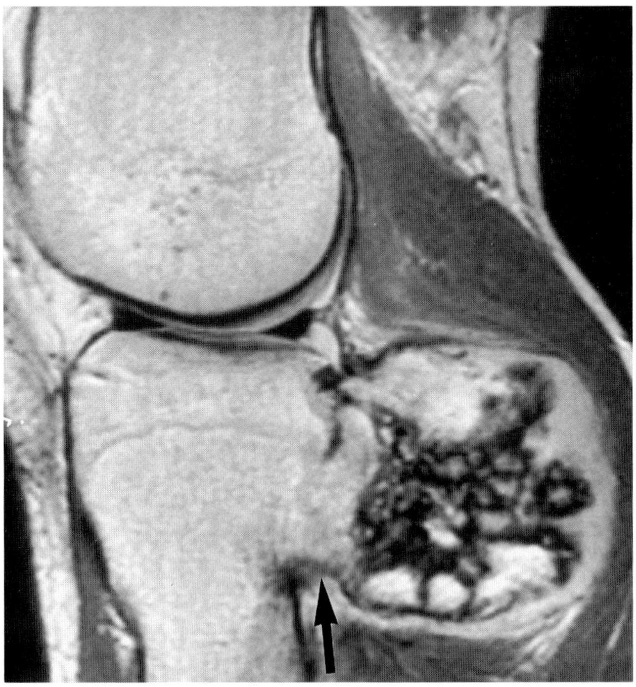

FIGURE 12.1 A 28-year-old male with hereditary multiple exostoses presented with knee pain and a palpable posterior mass. Sagittal (A) proton density (2700/25) and

(*continued*)

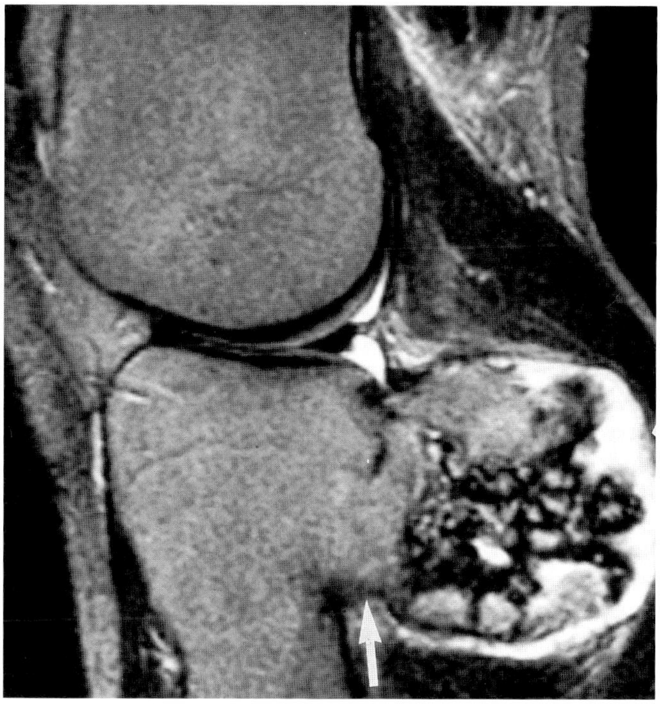

B

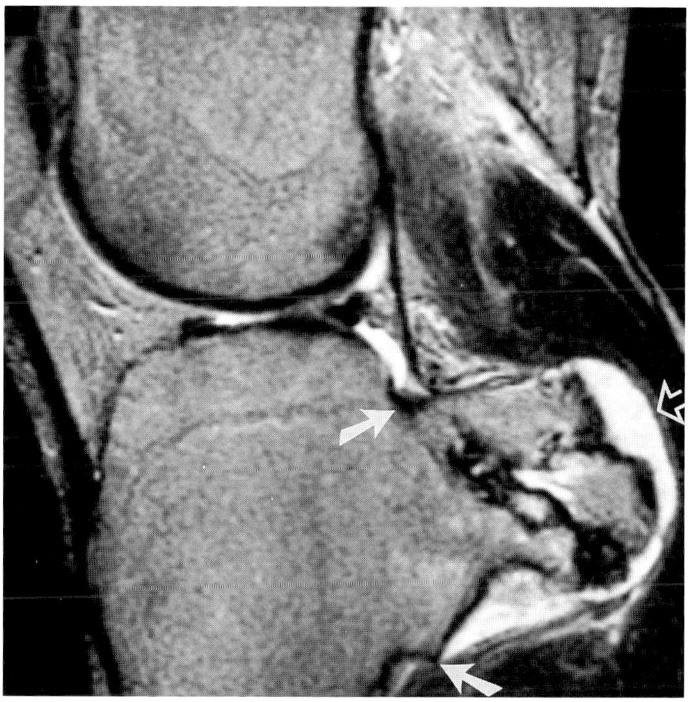

C

FIGURE 12.1 (continued) (B), (C) T2-weighted (2700/70) images reveal a large osteochondroma with heterogeneous signal intensity arising from the posterior metaepiphyseal region of the proximal tibia. Note that the cortex and medullary space of the lesion are in direct continuity with those of the host bone (arrows). With T2-weighting, the overlying cartilage cap exhibits very bright signal intensity (open arrows).

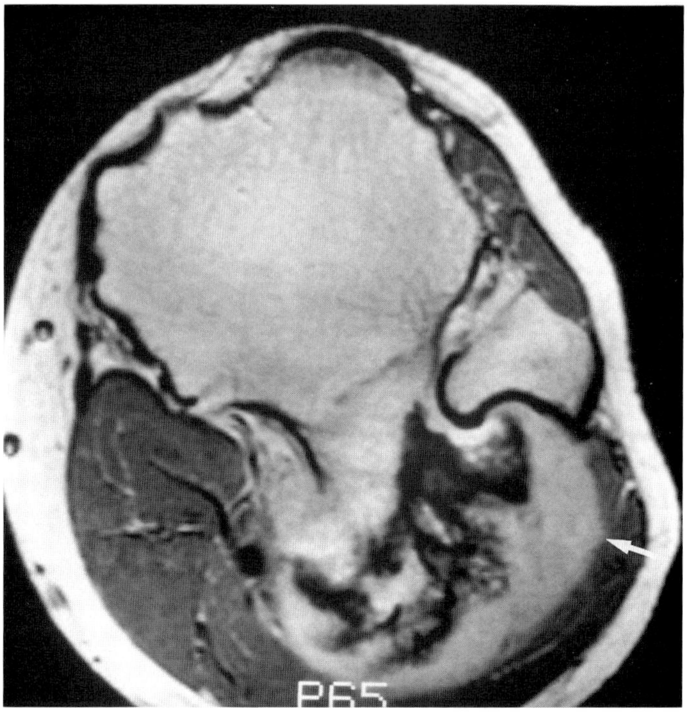

D

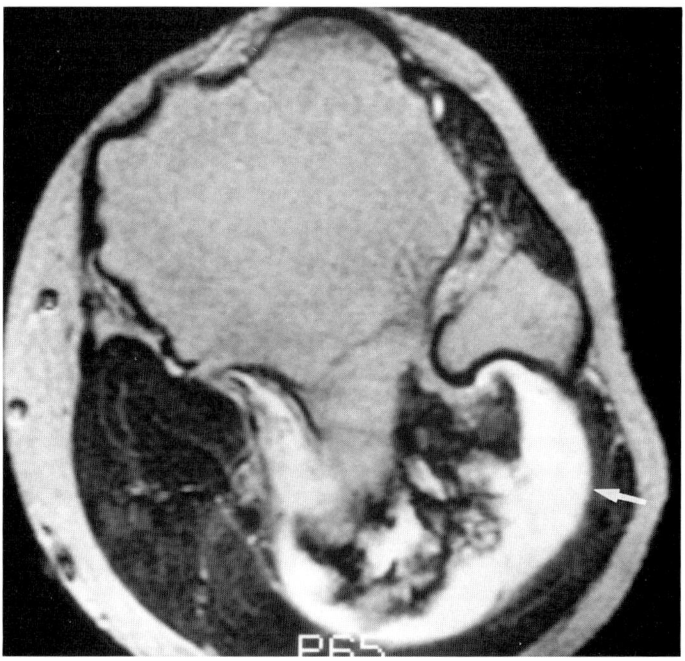

E

FIGURE 12.1 (continued) (D), (E) Axial dual-echo T2-weighted images (2500/20, 70) demonstrate increased thickness of the cartilaginous cap (thin arrows). This finding could indicate malignant transformation, although the history of pain in a skeletally mature patient is worrisome in and of itself. Note the presence of numerous smaller osteochondromas of the proximal tibia and fibula.

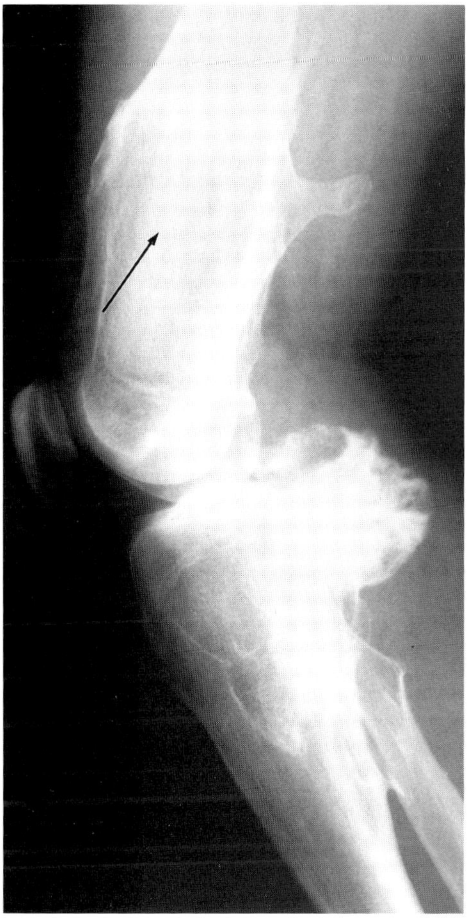

F

FIGURE 12.1 (continued) (F) Lateral radiograph demonstrates numerous sessile and pedunculated osteochondromas. There is pronounced undertubulation in the distal femur (long thin arrow). This is a classic appearance for hereditary multiple exostoses.

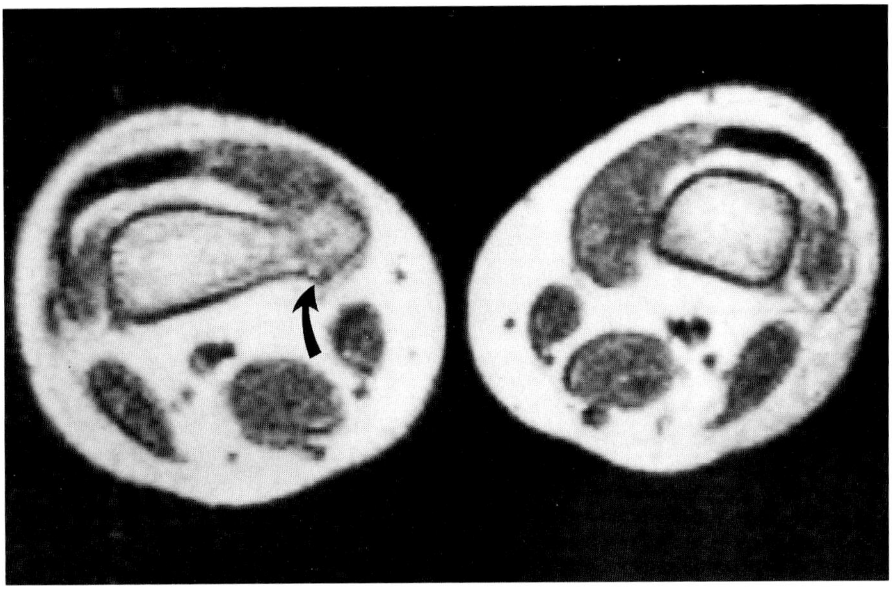

FIGURE 12.2 Benign osteochondroma of the distal femur in a 25-year-old woman. Axial proton density image demonstrates an osteochondroma arising from the medial aspect of the distal right femur (arrow). There is direct continuity of trabecular and cortical bone between the lesion and adjacent host bone.

Enchondroma

Definition. An enchondroma is a benign tumor of the medullary cavity which is composed of lobules of hyaline cartilage. Portions of the lesion may undergo necrosis, liquefaction, or cyst formation.

Clinical Features. Enchondromas occur most commonly between 10 and 40 years of age, although nearly all ages may be affected. These lesions are usually asymptomatic, but may be associated with swelling or pathologic fracture. The presence of pain, especially in an older patient, is concerning for the possibility of malignant transformation. Multiple enchondromas are present in Ollier's disease (enchondromatosis) and Maffucci's syndrome (enchondromatosis and soft tissue hemangiomas).

Location. About 50% of solitary enchondromas affect the hands, particularly the proximal phalanges. Approximately 25% of solitary enchondromas occur in the long tubular bones, with typical sites including the femur, tibia, and humerus. Enchondromas arise in the medullary space and are usually metaphyseal in the long tubular bones and diaphyseal in the short tubular bones of the hands and feet.

Implications. Enchondromas are not uncommonly detected as an incidental finding on knee and shoulder MR exams. The presence of growth after skeletal maturation or pain should heighten suspicion for malignant transformation, which is an infrequent complication, but more commonly noted about the shoulder or in the pelvis. This complication almost never occurs in the short tubular bones of the hands and feet. The risk of malignant transformation in Maffucci's syndrome is significantly higher than that of solitary enchondroma or Ollier's disease. It is important to note that it is frequently difficult to distinguish enchondroma from low-grade chondrosarcoma histologically.

MRI Findings. Typically, enchondromas appear as elongated or oval, multilobulated masses which demonstrate very bright signal intensity on T2-weighted sequences. These masses are of low signal intensity (approximately isointense to muscle) on T1-weighted sequences. Hypointense foci, representing calcification, may be present. Endosteal scalloping is common with larger lesions.

Differential Diagnosis. The identification of a multilobulated mass in the metaphysis of a long tubular bone with very bright signal intensity on T2-weighted sequences strongly suggests the diagnosis of enchondroma, especially if detected incidentally. The main differential diagnostic consideration for this lesion is low-grade chondrosarcoma, which is difficult to distinguish from an enchondroma radiographically and histologically. The most useful discriminator for suggesting low-grade chondrosarcoma is the presence of pain referrable to the mass. In addition, cortical destruction or soft tissue extension suggests the presence of chondrosarcoma (primary or secondary).

References

Giudici M, Moser R, Kransdorf M. Cartilaginous bone tumors. *Radiol Clin North Am* 31:237–259, 1993.

Cohen E, Kressel H, Frank T, et al. Hyaline cartilage-origin bone and soft-tissue neoplasms: MR appearance and histologic correlation. *Radiology* 167:477–481, 1988.

Aoki J, Sone S, Fujioka F, et al. MR of enchondroma and chondrosarcoma: Rings and arcs of Gd-DTPA enhancement. *JCAT* 15:1011–1016, 1991.

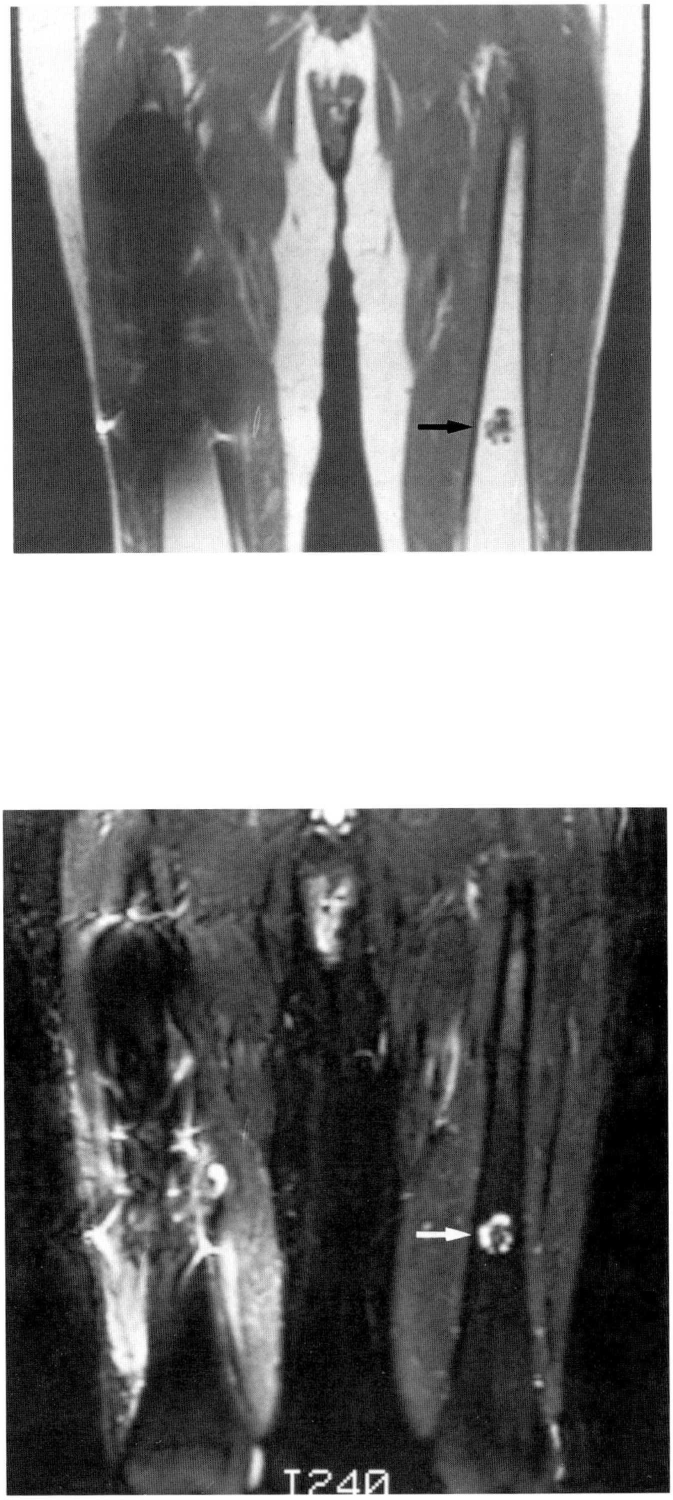

A

B

FIGURE 12.3 Incidentally detected left femur lesion in a 51-year-old male. The patient has had previous surgery for treatment of a malignant tumor of the right femur. Coronal (A) T1-weighted (600/10) and (B) FMPIR (4300/51, TI-150) images reveal an oval, lobulated medullary lesion in the left femoral diaphysis (arrows). There is prominent artifact related to right femoral hardware.

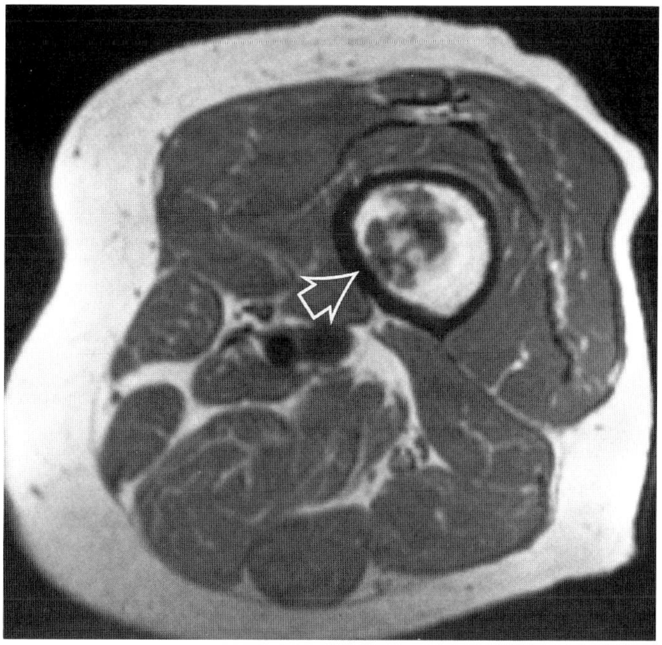

C

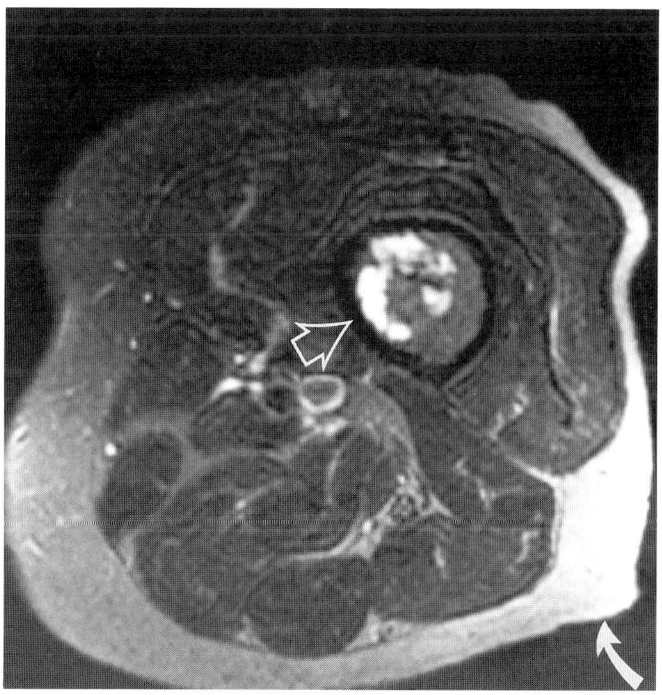

D

Figure 12.3 (continued) Axial (C) T1-weighted (500/12) and (D) FSE T2-weighted fat suppression (3000/102) images better depict the multilobulated lesion (open arrows). Note the bright signal intensity on the T2-weighted image. These findings are characteristic for an enchondroma, which was asymptomatic in this individual. Failure of fat suppression is present laterally (curved arrow).

Periosteal Chondroma (Juxtacortical Chondroma)

Definition. A periosteal (juxtacortical) chondroma is a slow growing benign cartilaginous tumor which arises beneath or within the periosteum. It is histologically identical to an enchondroma consisting of hyaline cartilage arranged in a lobular pattern. Hypercellularity and mild cellular atypia may be present.

Clinical Features. Periosteal chondroma is an uncommon tumor usually presenting with pain, swelling, and sometimes a palpable mass. Most lesions present before the age of 30 with a peak incidence in the second decade, although all ages may be affected. There is a slight male predominance.

Location. Most cases involve the metaphysis of tubular bones, particularly the proximal humerus, femur, and phalanges of the hand. The lesion can occasionally extend into the medullary cavity.

Implications. The treatment of choice is marginal or intralesional excision, which should be curative. Similar to an enchondroma, this lesion may be difficult to distinguish histologically from a low-grade chondrosarcoma due to hypercellularity.

MRI Findings. This lesion appears as a periosteal mass with hypointense signal (approximately isointense to muscle) on T1-weighted images and hyperintense signal on T2-weighted sequences. The mass may be lobulated. Foci of hypointense signal, representing calcification, may be seen. Scalloping of the adjacent cortex is typically present and the lesion occasionally extends into the medullary space.

Differential Diagnosis. A periosteal chondroma must be differentiated from a periosteal chondrosarcoma, which is usually larger and occurs in an older age group than periosteal chondroma. A heterogeneous mass or large soft tissue component should raise the possibility of a periosteal chondrosarcoma. Plain radiographs should also be examined for signs of an aggressive lesion.

References

Varma D, Kumar R, Carrasco C, et al. MR imaging of periosteal chondroma. *JCAT* 15:1008–1010, 1991.

Lewis M, Kenan S, Yabut S, et al. Periosteal chondroma. A report of ten cases and review of the literature. *Clin Orthop* 256:185–192, 1990.

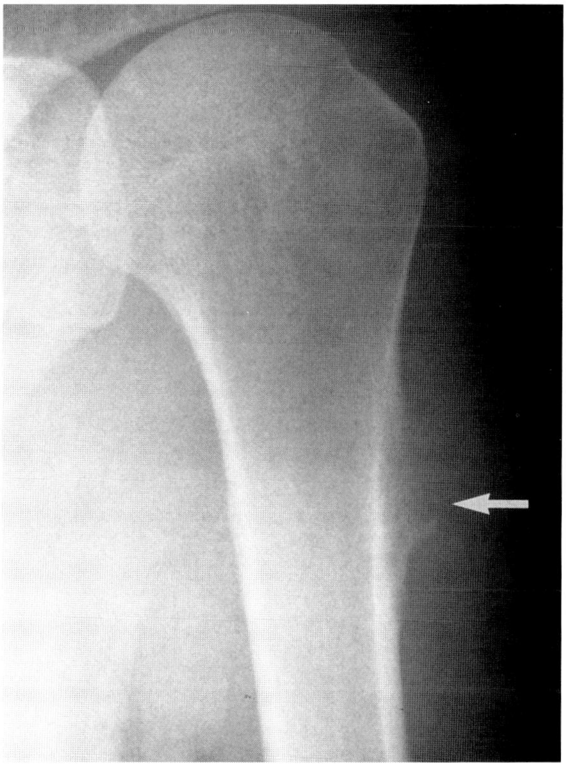

A

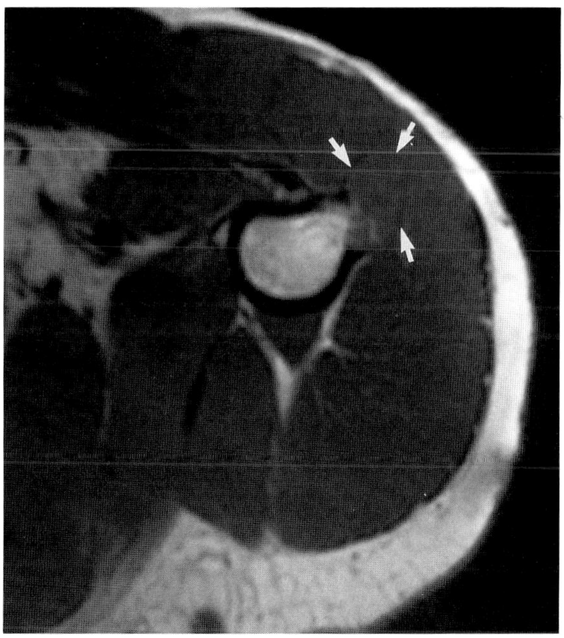

B

FIGURE 12.4 A 26-year-old woman with left shoulder pain. (A) AP radiograph demonstrates a periosteal lesion arising from the lateral aspect of the proximal diaphysis of the left humerus (arrow). (B) Axial T1-weighted image (700/16) shows that the periosteal lesion (short arrows) is isointense to muscle.

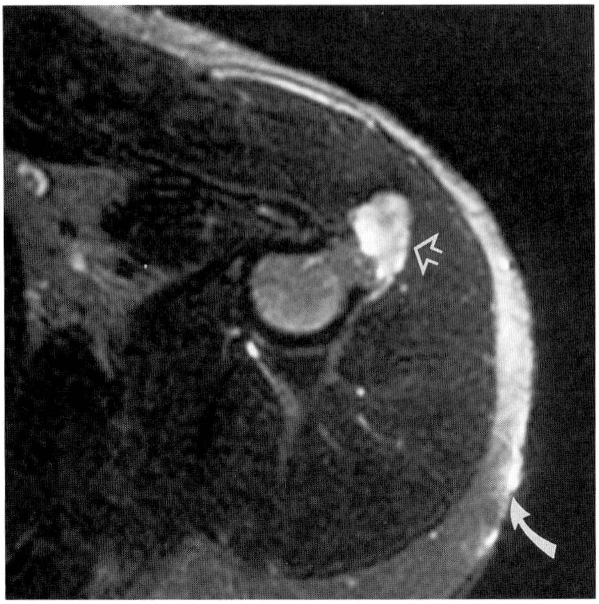

C

FIGURE 12.4 (continued) (C) Axial FSE T2-weighted fat suppression image (3850/102) reveals some small lobulations as well as predominantly bright signal intensity (open arrow). Radiographic and MRI findings are characteristic of a periosteal chondroma. Note the failure of fat suppression laterally (curved arrow).

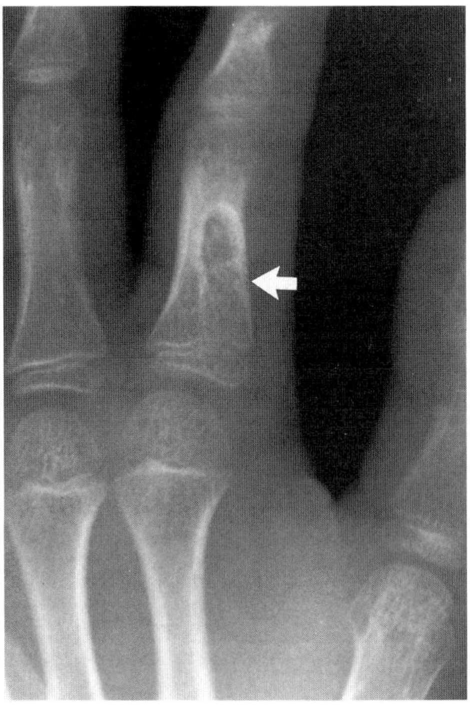

A

FIGURE 12.5 Periosteal chondroma of the finger in a 7-year-old male. (A) Oblique radiograph demonstrates a periosteal lesion (arrow) with a thin rim of reactive sclerosis arising from the metadiaphyseal region of the left second proximal phalanx.

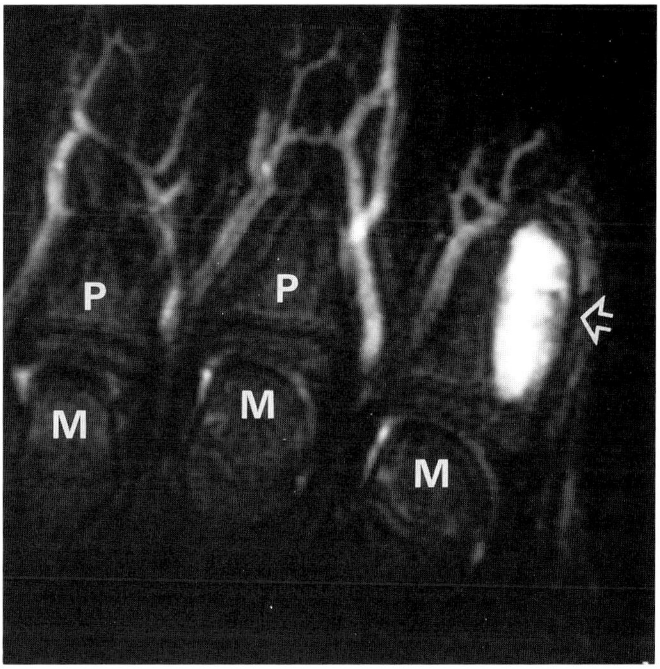

B

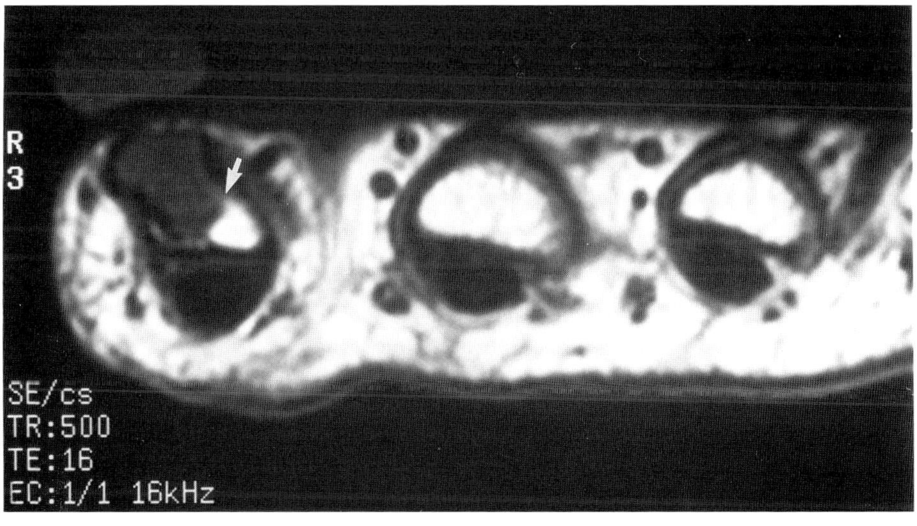

C

FIGURE 12.5 (continued) (B) Coronal FSE T2-weighted fat suppression image (3000/110) demonstrates hyperintense signal within the lesion (open arrow). Metacarpal heads (M), proximal phalanges (P). (C) Axial T1-weighted (500/16) and

(*continued*)

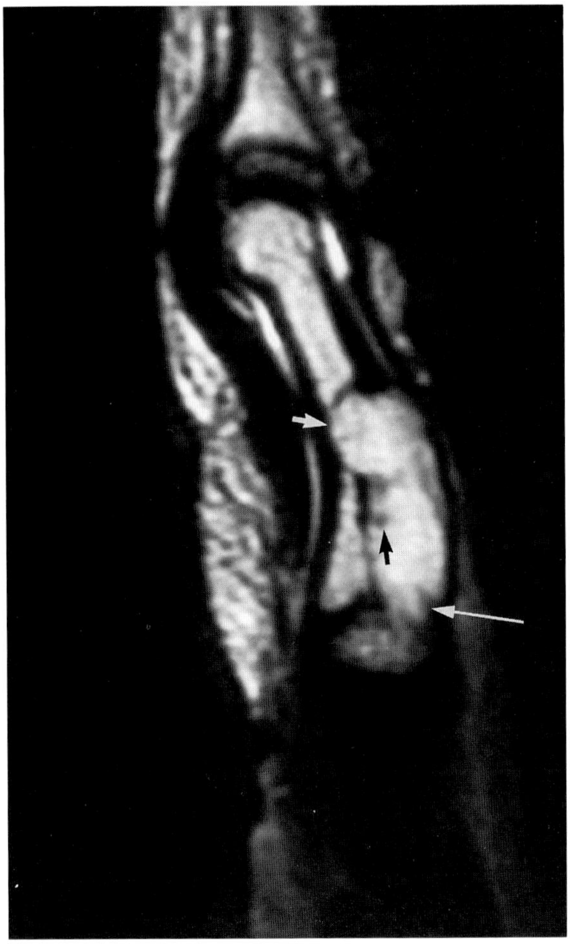

D

FIGURE 12.5 (continued) (D) sagittal FSE T2-weighted (3000/110) images reveal extension of the mildly lobulated lesion into the medullary cavity (short arrows). A focus of hypointense signal is present which may represent calcification (short black arrow). Note extension to the physis (long thin arrow).

Chondroblastoma

Definition. Chondroblastoma is a benign cartilaginous tumor which has also been referred to as Codman's tumor. It is characterized histologically by the presence of chondroblasts surrounded by variable amounts of chondroid matrix and scattered multinucleated giant cells.

Clinical Features. Chondroblastomas are uncommon, representing only about 1% of all bone tumors. The vast majority of lesions occur between 5 and 25 years of age and present with pain, tenderness, and swelling. There is a 2–3:1 male predominance.

Location. Most chondroblastomas occur in the epiphyses of long bones, especially around the knee (distal femur and proximal tibia, 50%) and proximal humerus (20%). The lesion may arise in an apophysis, which is an epiphysis-equivalent, such as the greater trochanter. About 10% of cases involve the small bones of the hands and feet, particularly the talus and calcaneus.

Implications. Surgical treatment is usually limited to curettage, which is most often curative. However, recurrence following surgery is not uncommon. Some authors advocate conservative therapy, citing evidence that chondroblastomas heal spontaneously. The fact that nearly all chondroblastomas are seen in young individuals does suggest that undetected lesions undergo spontaneous involution.

MRI Findings. These lesions typically appear as oval or round lobulated masses which are hypointense (isointense to muscle) on T1-weighted images and are of mixed signal intensity on T2-weighted sequences. Alternating foci of low, intermediate, and high signal intensity seen on T2-weighted sequences correspond to areas of calcification, chondroid matrix (hyaline cartilage), and fluid and/or hemorrhage. This heterogeneous appearance has been described as a "cobblestone" pattern. The MR appearance depends on the percentage of calcification, cartilage, and hemorrhage/fluid within a particular lesion. Calcifications, which appear hypointense (signal void) on all pulse sequences, are seen in approximately half of all lesions (range: 25–60%). Fluid-fluid levels may be present. Associated periosteal reaction is commonly present (about half of cases) and is typically located in the diametaphyseal region, away from the lesion. Periostitis appears as cortical thickening and/or bright signal on T2-weighted sequences. Prominent adjacent marrow and soft tissue edema are commonly present. These areas exhibit low signal on T1-weighted images and high signal on T2-weighted sequences, and also enhance following gadolinium administration. Endosteal erosion may be seen as well as penetration through the cortex.

Differential Diagnosis. The differential diagnosis of a solitary epiphyseal lesion in a young patient consists primarily of chondroblastoma, infection, and less commonly, eosinophilic granuloma and aneurysmal bone cyst. The MR images should be correlated with plain radiographs. The diagnosis of chondroblastoma can often be made based upon the plain films if calcified chondroid matrix is visualized. If calcification is not seen on plain film, MRI suggests the diagnosis if a mass with small lobulations (2–5 mm) is seen with a heterogeneous "cobblestone" appearance on T2-weighted sequences. The presence of adjacent marrow and soft tissue edema is characteristic of chondroblastoma, but not specific for this entity and may be seen with numerous other lesions including infection, eosinophilic granuloma, osteoid osteoma, osteoblastoma, and various malignant lesions. In a skeletally mature individual, an additional diagnostic consideration is giant cell tumor, which does not typically show small lobulations on MRI. A chondroblastoma can also be distinguished from a giant cell tumor on plain radiographs by the identification of a sclerotic border or calcifications. On MRI, it may be difficult to distinguish chondroblastoma from clear cell chondrosarcoma, but the latter typically occurs in an older age group (3rd–5th decades).

References

Weatherall P, Maale G, Mendelsohn D, et al. Chondroblastoma: Classic and confusing appearance at MR imaging. *Radiology* 190:467–474, 1994.

Brower A, Moser R, Kransdorf M. The frequency and diagnostic significance of periostitis in chondroblastoma. *AJR* 154:309–314, 1990.

Giudici M, Moser R, Kransdorf M. Cartilaginous bone tumors. *Radiol Clin North Am* 31:237–259, 1993.

Fobben E, Dalinka M, Schiebler M, et al. The magnetic resonance imaging appearance at 1.5 Tesla of cartilaginous tumors involving the epiphysis. *Skeletal Radiol* 16:647–651, 1987.

Cohen E, Kressel H, Frank T, et al. Hyaline cartilage-origin bone and soft-tissue neoplasms: MR appearance and histologic correlation. *Radiology* 167:477–481, 1988.

A

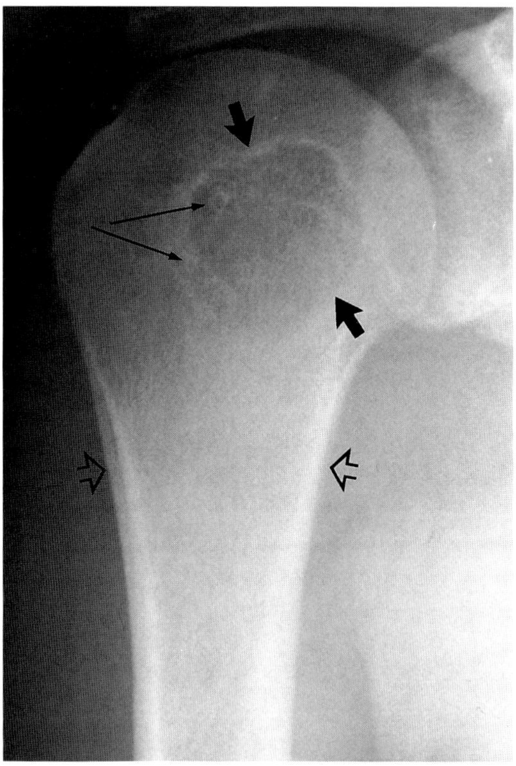

Figure 12.6 An 18-year-old male baseball player with shoulder pain. (A) AP radiograph demonstrates a well-marginated lytic lesion in the proximal humeral epiphysis surrounded by a thin sclerotic border (arrows). Two small ring-like calcifications are present (thin arrows). There is associated periosteal reaction in the metadiaphyseal region (open arrows). These findings are characteristic for chondroblastoma.

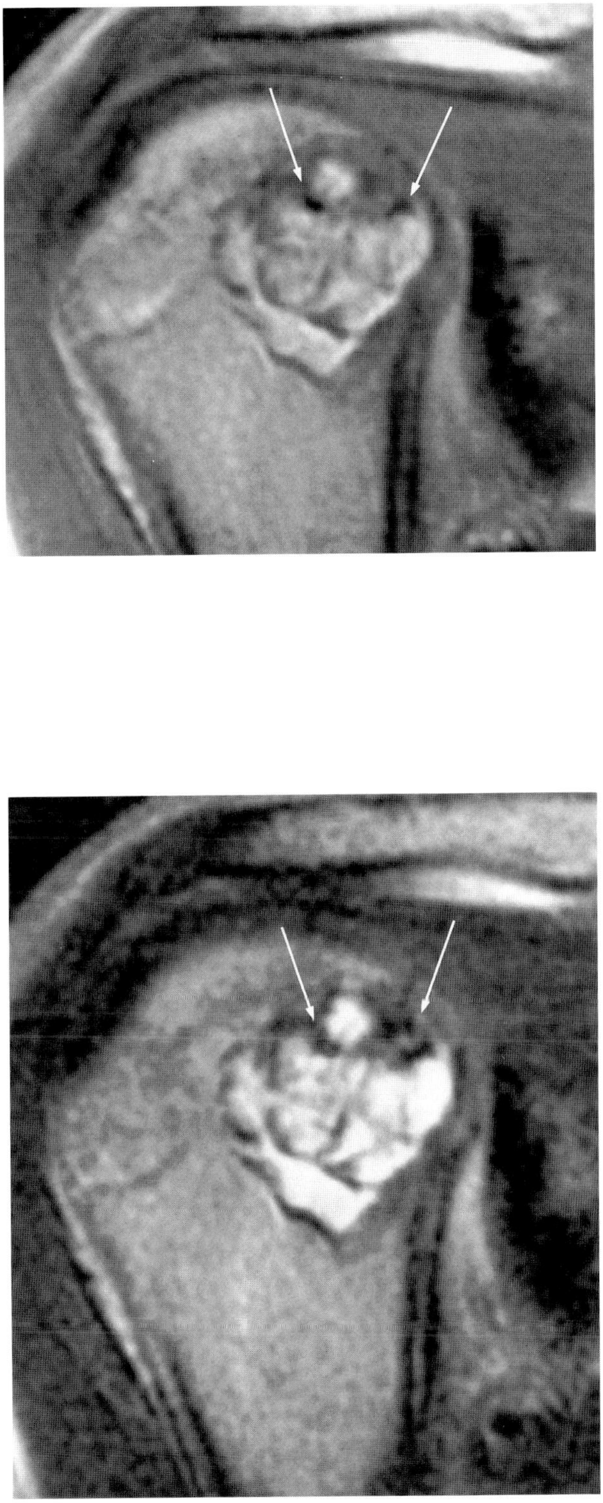

B

C

FIGURE 12.6 (continued) (B), (C) Coronal dual-echo T2-weighted images (2000/30, 70) reveal a multilobulated epiphyseal lesion, which has heterogeneous, predominantly high signal intensity with T2-weighting. The lesion extends into the metaphysis. The hypointense foci (thin white arrows) likely represent calcification.

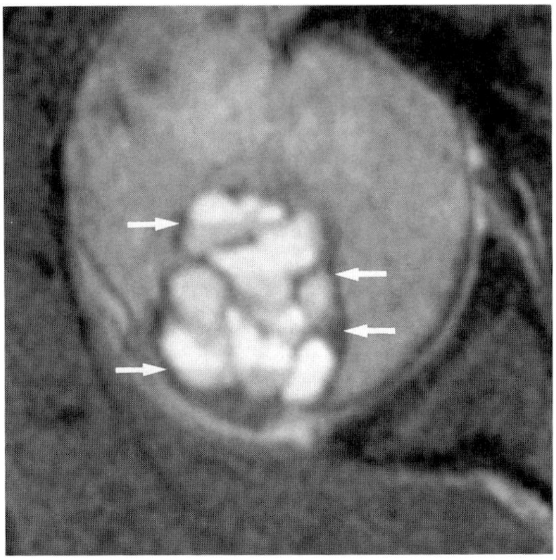

D

FIGURE 12.6 (continued) (D) Axial FMPIR image (3700/28, TI-150) reveals numerous fluid-fluid levels (short arrows) consistent with hemorrhage.

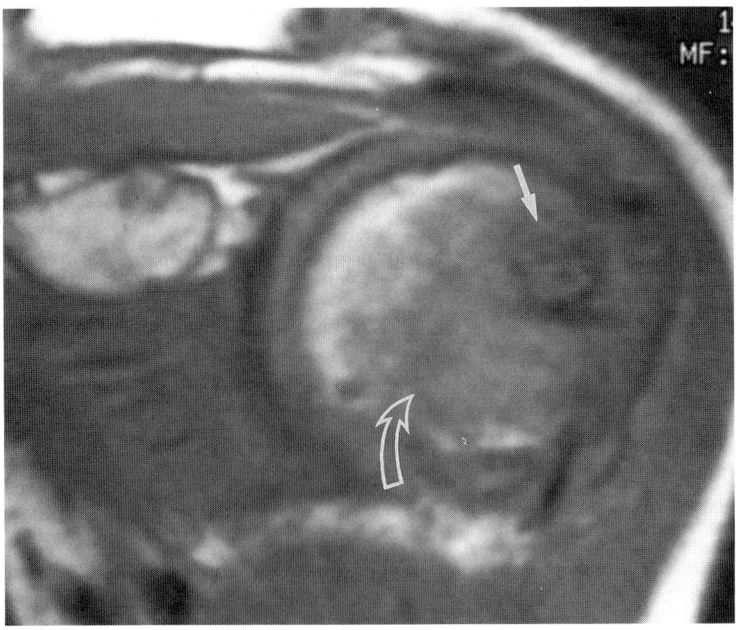

A

FIGURE 12.7 Chondroblastoma of the proximal left humerus in a 14-year-old male. Coronal (A) T1-weighted (600/18) and

(*continued*)

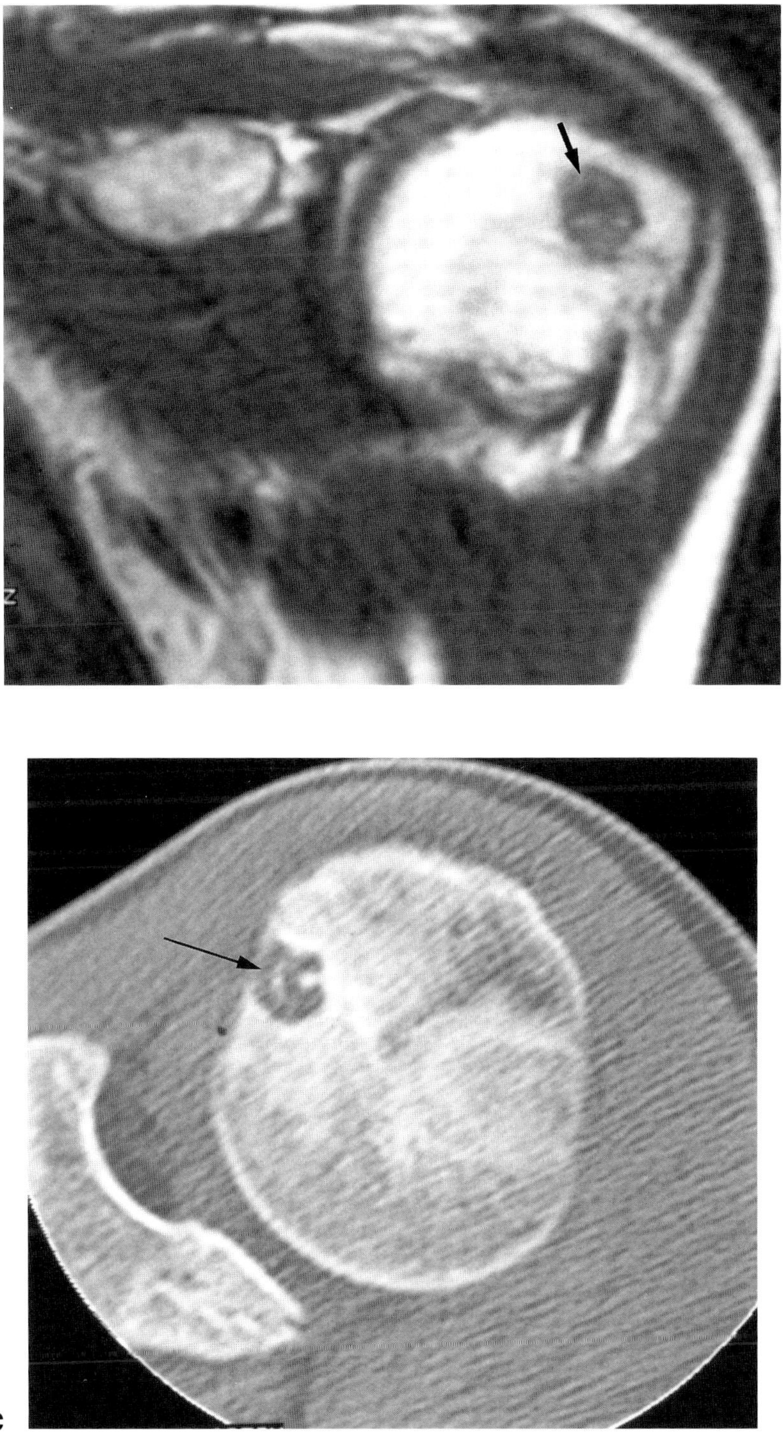

B

C

FIGURE 12.7 (continued) (B) FSE T2-weighted (2500/80) images reveal a small epiphyseal lesion in the proximal humerus. There is heterogeneous, predominantly low signal intensity on the T2-weighted image. Internal foci of hypointense signal are consistent with calcification (arrows). There is a peripheral rim of low signal intensity corresponding to a thin sclerotic border. Note the prominent surrounding bone marrow edema, which is better delineated on the T1-weighted image (open arrow). (C) Axial CT image confirms the presence of internal foci of calcification (long arrow).

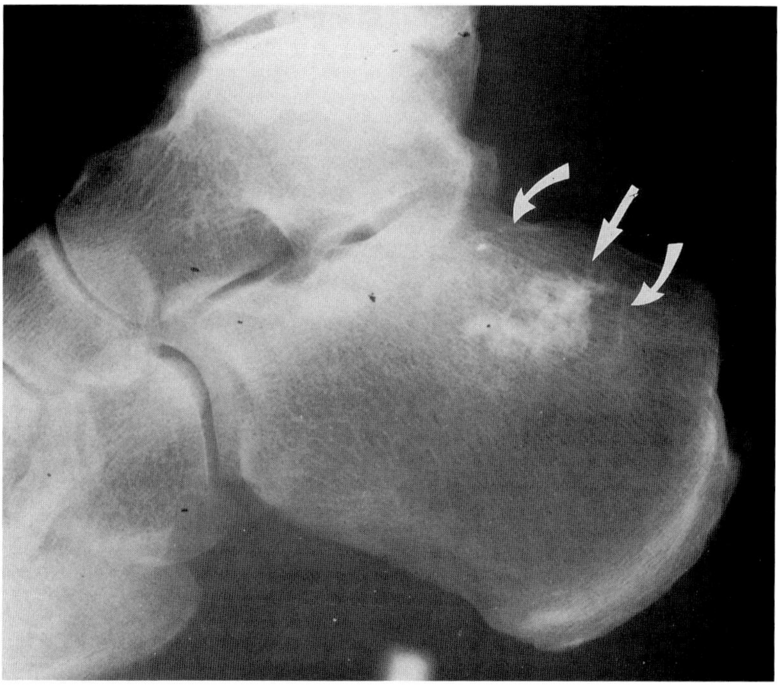

A

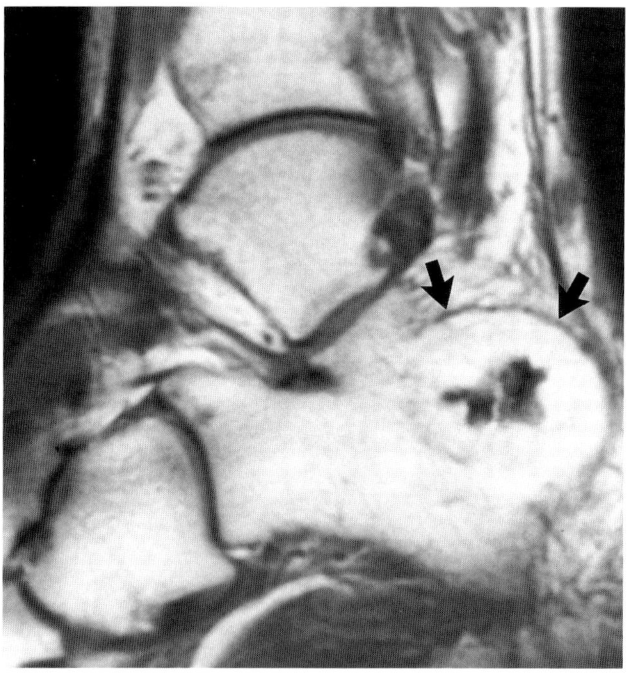

B

FIGURE 12.8 A 54-year-old male with an old "burned-out" chondroblastoma of the calcaneus resulting in a palpable mass. The lesion was resected due to its mass effect on the peroneal tendons. (A) Lateral radiograph demonstrates coarse calcification in the superior calcaneus (arrow). There are remnants of a thin sclerotic border (curved arrows). (B) Sagittal T1-weighted image (600/13) demonstrates prominent hypointense signal centrally due to calcification. Note a remnant of the thin sclerotic border appearing as a rim of low signal intensity (black arrows).

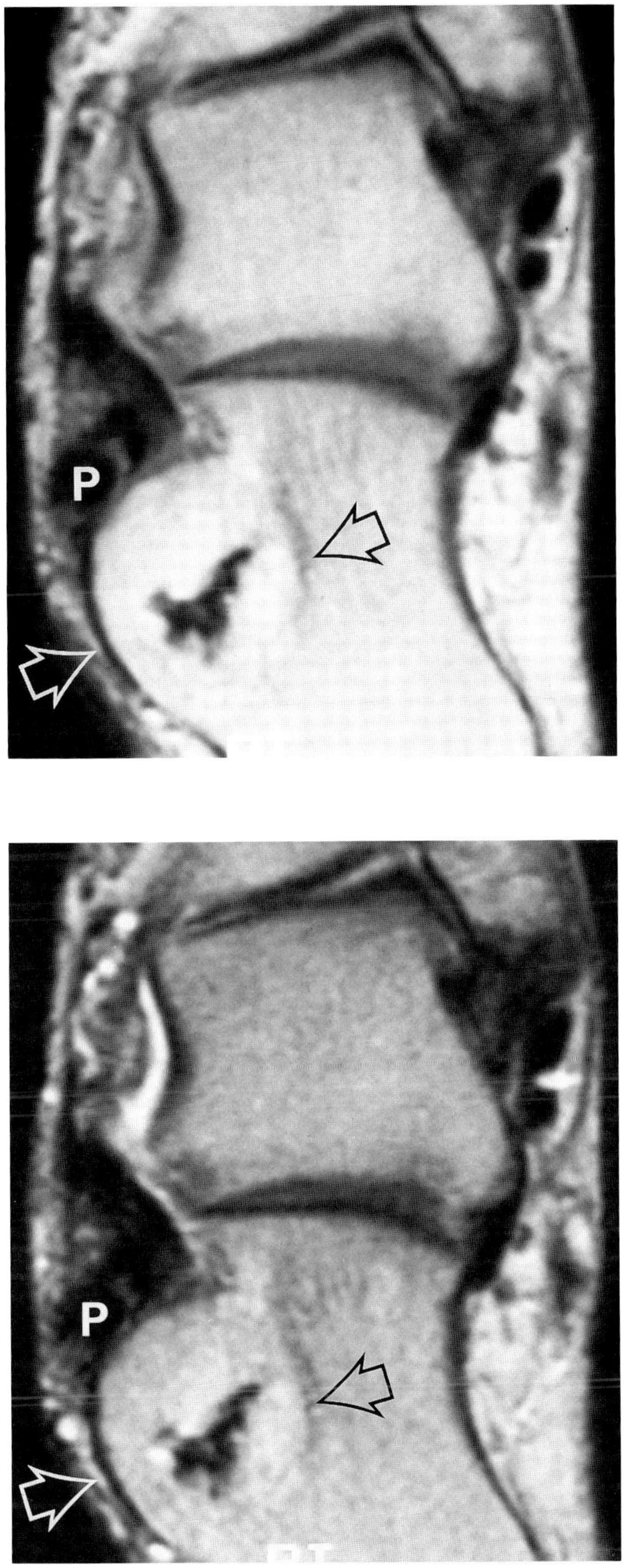

C

D

FIGURE 12.8 (continued) (C), (D) Coronal dual-echo T2-weighted images (2000/30, 80) reveal the eccentric, expansile nature of the mass (open arrows). The signal intensity is isointense with the adjacent marrow consistent with fatty replacement of this old, healed lesion. There is mass effect on the peroneal tendons (P).

Chondrosarcoma

Definition. Chondrosarcoma (CS) is a malignant cartilaginous tumor which can be primary or secondary in nature. Primary lesions arise de novo, whereas secondary lesions arise from a pre-existing benign tumor such as enchondroma or osteochondroma. CS may also be categorized according to whether it arises from the medullary cavity (central, intramedullary) or from the bone surface (juxtacortical, peripheral). The vast majority of lesions are central. Most juxtacortical lesions arise from preexisting osteochondromas. Histologically, CS is composed of lobules of hyaline cartilage surrounded by fibrovascular bundles. Calcification, myxoid change, and necrosis may be present. Clear cell CS is an interesting histologic variant which is discussed separately (*see* Index for listing).

Clinical Features. CS is the third most common primary malignant bone neoplasm with only multiple myeloma and osteosarcoma occurring more frequently. Most patients present in adulthood with an average age of about 45 years old. The most common presenting symptoms (frequently of 1–2 years duration) are pain, swelling, tenderness, and a palpable mass.

Location. Although nearly any bone may be affected, the most frequently involved sites are the pelvis, femur, humerus, rib, and tibia. The vast majority of CSs are intramedullary (central) in position.

Implications. The most effective treatment of CS consists of radical excision or en bloc resection. The prognosis of CS is inversely proportional to histologic grade. Most central CSs are low-grade with a ten-year survival rate of about 85%. More than half of high-grade lesions are associated with metastasis. Dedifferentiated CS, in which there is a highly aggressive sarcomatous component coexistent with a lower-grade CS component, occurs in about 10% of cases and is associated with a poor prognosis. Compared with extremity lesions, CS involving the axial skeleton is associated with a poorer prognosis, presumably because these lesions tend to be larger than appendicular lesions at the time of presentation. It is important to note that it may be difficult to histologically distinguish low-grade CS from an active enchondroma or osteochondroma. Clinical and radiographic correlation are critical in these patients.

MRI Findings. On MRI, CS typically appears as a lobulated mass exhibiting isointense or slightly hyperintense signal in relation to muscle on T1-weighted images and high signal on T2-weighted sequences. However, the MR appearance is variable depending on the histologic composition. Low-grade lesions typically exhibit lobules of homogeneous signal intensity separated by thin curvilinear fibrous septa of low signal intensity on all pulse sequences. High-grade CSs tend to appear more heterogeneous, possibly secondary to myxoid change or necrosis. Areas of calcified matrix will appear as foci of signal void on all pulse sequences. Endosteal scalloping is typically present. Often, the adjacent cortex is thinned and there may be cortical disruption with soft tissue extension.

Differential Diagnosis. The MRI findings of CS are variable and must be correlated with radiographs. On plain films, low-grade CSs can be confused with bone infarcts. MRI should enable this distinction since bone infarcts typically possess a serpiginous peripheral rim of low signal intensity on all pulse sequences. It may not be possible to differentiate low-grade CS from enchondroma on radiographs or MRI. In fact, this distinction may be difficult histologically. Clinical history is also important in making this distinction since uncomplicated enchondromas are typically not painful. Both of these lesions typically appear as homogeneous lobulated masses of high signal intensity on T2-weighted sequences with thin curvilinear septa of low signal intensity. Features suggesting malignancy include cortical thinning and especially cortical disruption with soft tissue extension. High-grade lesions have a more varied appearance which may resemble numerous other aggressive bone lesions.

References

Varma D, Ayala A, Carrasco C, et al. Chondrosarcoma: MR imaging with pathologic correlation. *RadioGraphics* 12:687–704, 1992.

Giudici M, Moser R, Kransdorf M. Cartilaginous bone tumors. *Radiol Clin North Amer* 31:237–259, 1993.

Cohen E, Kressel H, Frank T, et al. Hyaline cartilage-origin bone and soft-tissue neoplasms: MR appearance and histologic correlation. *Radiology* 167:477–481, 1988.

Aoki J, Sone S, Fujioka F, et al. MR of enchondroma and chondrosarcoma: Rings and arcs of Gd-DTPA enhancement. *JCAT* 15:1011–1016, 1991.

Geirnaerdt M, Bloem J, Eulderink F, et al. Cartilaginous tumors: Correlation of gadolinium-enhanced MR imaging and histopathologic findings. *Radiology* 186:813–817, 1993.

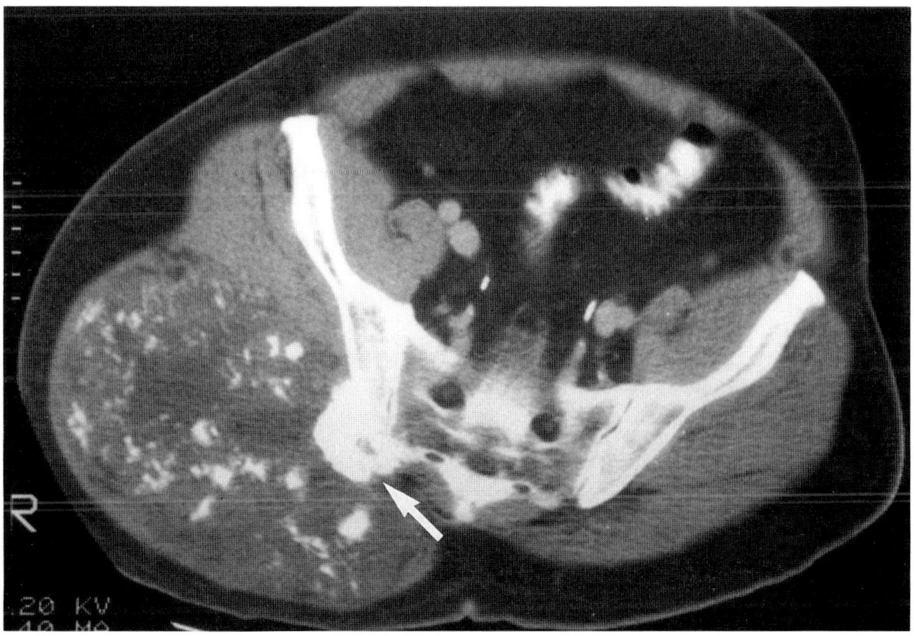

A

FIGURE 12.9 A 55-year-old male with a juxtacortical chondrosarcoma arising from an osteochondroma of the right ilium. (A) Axial CT image demonstrates a very large calcified mass in the right gluteal region arising from an osteochondroma (arrow) at the posteromedial aspect of the right ilium.

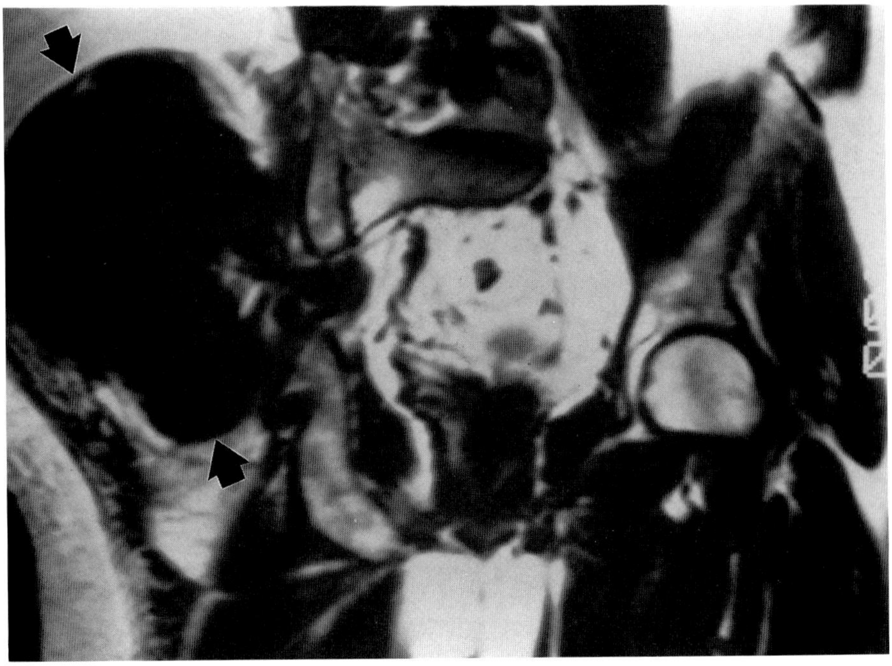

B

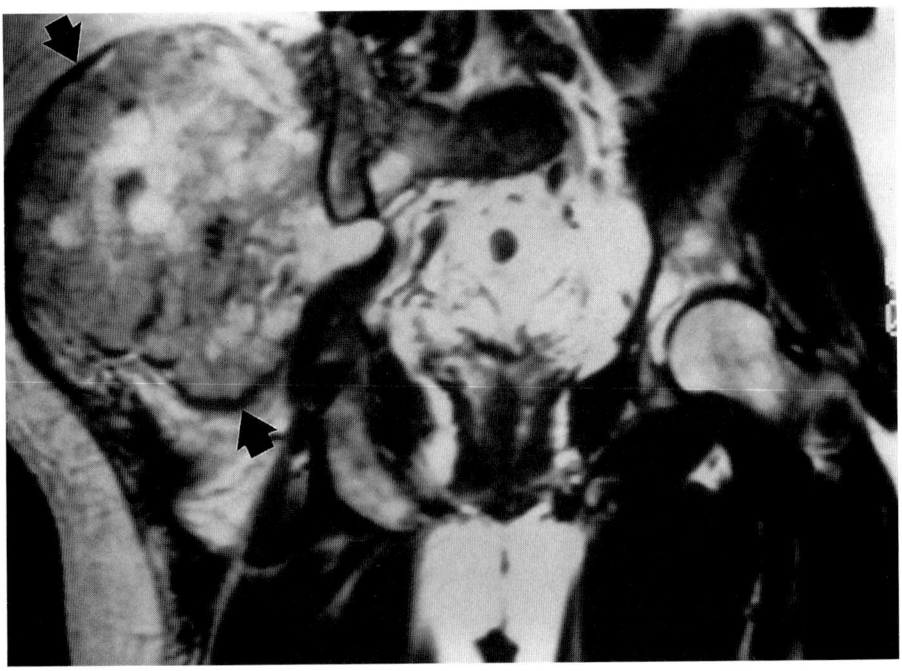

C

FIGURE 12.9 (continued) (B) Coronal T1-weighted image (650/20) shows that the large mass (black arrows) is approximately isointense to muscle. (C) Coronal FSE T2-weighted image (3000/68) reveals heterogeneous signal intensity including numerous foci of very low signal representing calcification. In addition, there are numerous internal septations of low signal intensity.

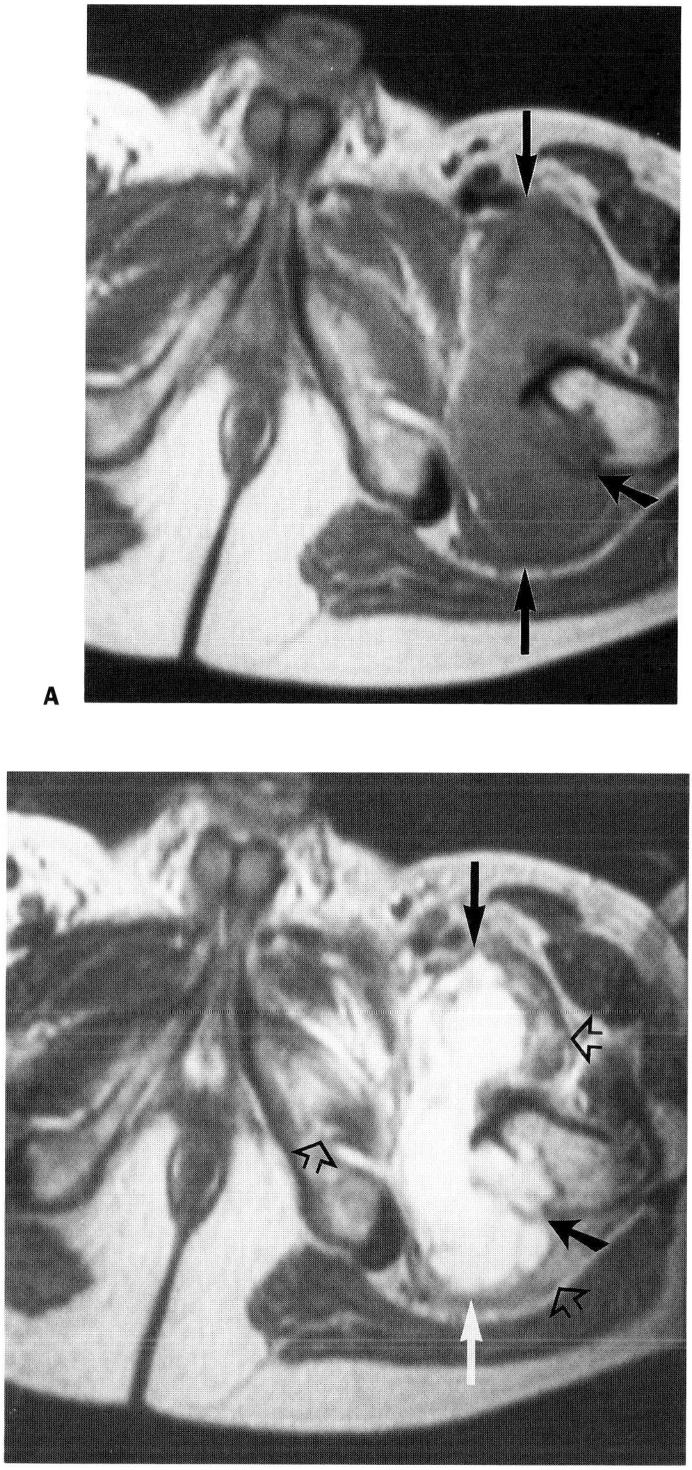

Figure 12.10 Chondrosarcoma of the proximal left femur in a 69-year-old male. (A), (B) Axial dual-echo T2-weighted images (2000/20, 80) reveal a mass arising from the lesser trochanter with cortical disruption (arrows) and a large soft tissue mass (long arrows). Note the very bright signal intensity with T2-weighting as well as internal septations of low signal. There is edema involving the surrounding muscles (open arrows).

Clear Cell Chondrosarcoma

Definition. Clear cell chondrosarcoma is a slow-growing, low-grade malignant chondroid neoplasm. It accounts for approximately 2% of all chondrosarcomas. Histologically, clear cells are always identified and are the hallmark of the tumor. These cells are arranged in a microlobular pattern and separated by a fibrovascular stroma. Focal areas of necrosis are common and calcification may be present. In most cases, areas of coexisting conventional chondrosarcoma are also identified.

Clinical Features. Clear cell chondrosarcoma is a rare tumor which occurs most commonly in the 3rd–5th decades of life. There is a male predominance. Patients typically present with localized pain of long duration. Pathologic fracture may be present.

Location. These lesions occur in the epiphysis, with a predilection for the upper end of long bones, especially the proximal femur (approximately two-thirds of all cases) and also the proximal humerus and proximal tibia. Large lesions may extend into the metaphysis.

Implications. The treatment of choice is en bloc resection, which is usually curative. Incomplete resection frequently results in recurrence and metastasis. Overall, the mortality rate is about 15%.

MRI Findings. On MRI, these lesions typically appear as mildly expansile epiphyseal masses measuring less than 5 cm. There may be small lobulations or endosteal scalloping. The cortex is usually intact, but is frequently thinned. Less commonly, soft tissue extension is seen. Amorphous calcification, which appears as hypointense signal on all pulse sequences, is present in approximately 30% of cases. These lesions are generally hypointense or isointense to muscle on T1-weighted images. The T2-weighted signal characteristics are variable, depending on the percentage of clear cells, calcified matrix, necrosis, and coexisting conventional chondrosarcoma. Therefore, these masses may appear predominantly hypointense, isointense, hyperintense, or heterogeneous on T2-weighted sequences.

Differential Diagnosis. The differential diagnosis consists mainly of the other more commonly occurring epiphyseal lesions. Chondroblastoma can have a similar appearance, although it usually occurs in a younger age group than clear cell chondrosarcoma. In addition, clear cell chondrosarcoma is more frequently associated with extension into the metaphysis. A giant cell tumor can be excluded by the identification of calcified matrix or a sclerotic border on plain films. Geodes typically appear as homogeneous lesions with very bright signal on T2-weighted sequences (similar to that of joint fluid) and in association with intra-articular abnormalities. If the lesion is large and unusually aggressive, it may resemble various other malignant lesions. The MR images must be interpreted in the presence of corresponding radiographs.

References

Present D, Bacchini P, Pignatti G, et al. Clear cell chondrosarcoma of bone. A report of 8 cases. *Skeletal Radiol* 20:187–191, 1991.

Leggon R, Unni K, Beabout J, et al. Mayo Clinic tumor rounds. Clear cell Chondrosarcoma. *Orthopedics* 13:593–596, 1990.

Bagley L, Kneeland J, Dalinka M, et al. Unusual behavior of clear cell chondrosarcoma. *Skeletal Radiol* 22:279–282, 1993.

Fobben E, Dalinka M, Schiebler M, et al. The magnetic resonance imaging appearance at 1.5 Tesla of cartilaginous tumors involving the epiphysis. *Skeletal Radiol* 16:647–651, 1987.

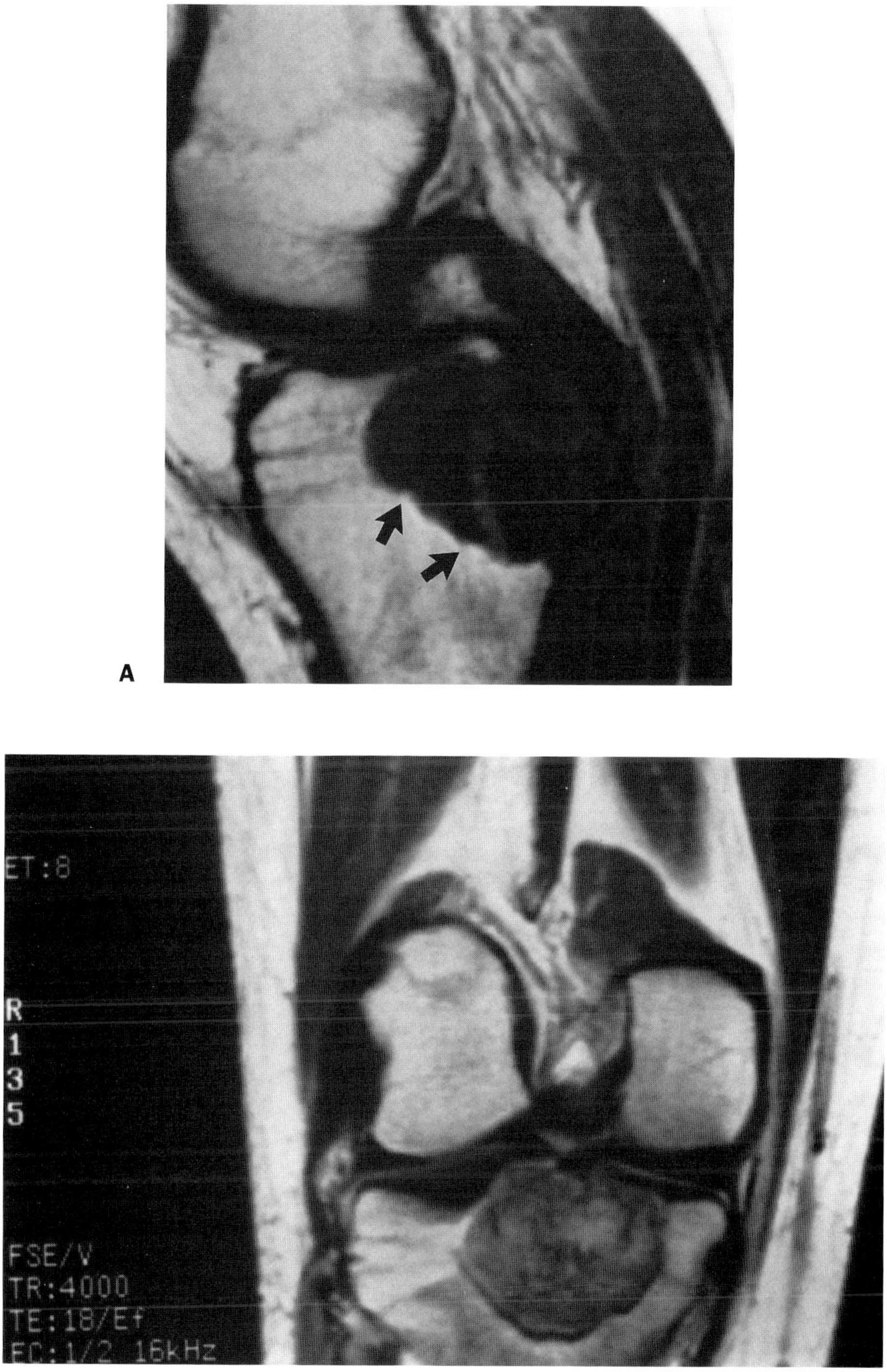

FIGURE 12.11 A 20-year-old woman with a clear cell chondrosarcoma of the proximal tibia. (A) Sagittal T1-weighted image reveals a well-marginated mass within the epiphysis and metaphysis of the proximal tibia. The signal intensity is approximately isointense to muscle. There is a slightly lobulated border (arrows). (B) Coronal FSE proton density image reveals heterogeneous signal intensity within the lesion.

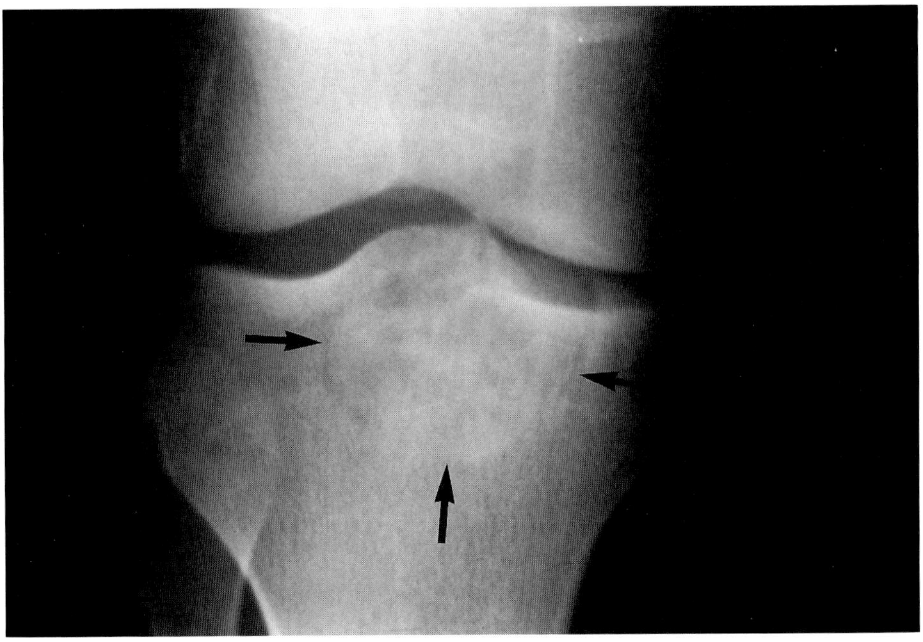

C

Figure 12.11 (continued) (C) AP radiograph demonstrates a predominantly sclerotic appearance of the lesion (long arrows) related to calcified chondroid matrix. (Courtesy of James O. Johnston, MD).

13 Fibrous Lesions

Fibrous Cortical Defect/Nonossifying Fibroma

Definition. Fibrous cortical defect (FCD) and nonossifying fibroma (NOF) are histopathologically identical tumors consisting of spindle-shaped fibroblasts arranged in whorls and bundles. Small amounts of hemorrhage and hemosiderin are present in many of these lesions. The term FCD is generally reserved for smaller masses and the term NOF is used when they enlarge and grow into the medullary cavity.

Clinical Features. FCDs are very common and have been reported to occur in approximately 1/3 of patients in the first and second decades of life. FCD and NOF are generally not seen after the age of 30. FCDs are asymptomatic lesions. NOFs should also be pain-free unless there is associated pathologic fracture (complete fracture or stress fracture).

Location. The vast majority of these lesions occur in the long tubular bones, especially the tibia and femur. They arise in the metaphysis and may move towards the diaphysis with skeletal growth. FCDs are not uncommonly multiple. Multiple NOFs are much less common.

Implications. FCD and NOF are benign and involute spontaneously. They are nearly always detected as incidental findings on imaging studies. Intense uptake may be present on scintigraphy. Multiple NOFs can be seen with neurofibromatosis. FCDs require no treatment. Large NOFs may be treated with curettage and bone grafting to prevent pathologic fracture.

MRI Findings. These lesions exhibit variable signal characteristics on MRI. The signal intensity may be homogeneous or heterogeneous. On all pulse sequences, the lesions are typically surrounded by a low signal intensity rim, corresponding to the sclerotic border on radiographs. They may demonstrate predominantly marked hypointense signal in relation to muscle on both T1- and T2-weighted sequences due to the presence of large amounts of collagen and/or hemosiderin. Those lesions containing abundant cellular material may exhibit hypointense signal on T1-weighted sequences and hyperintense signal with T2-weighting.

Differential Diagnosis. The MRI findings of FCD and NOF are variable and nonspecific. Corresponding plain radiographs should be obtained and are nearly always diagnostic.

Reference

Kransdorf M, Utz J, Gilkey F. MR appearance of fibroxanthoma. *JCAT* 12:612–15, 1988.

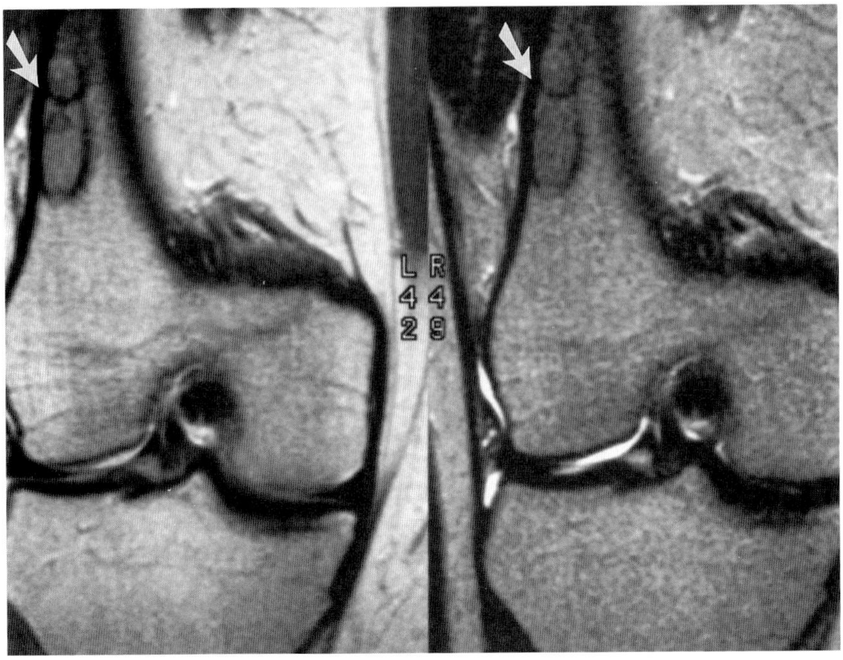

A

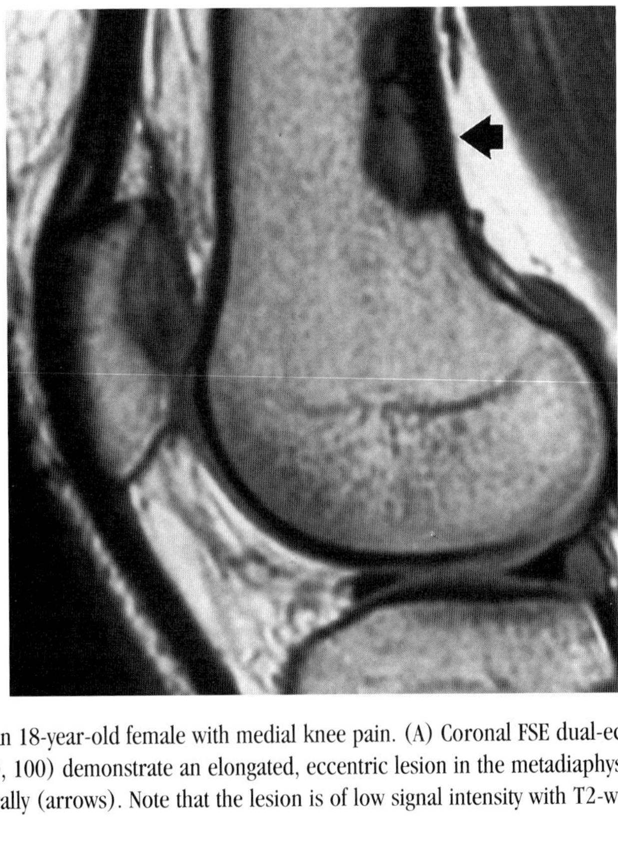

B

Figure 13.1 An 18-year-old female with medial knee pain. (A) Coronal FSE dual-echo T2-weighted images (4000/20, 100) demonstrate an elongated, eccentric lesion in the metadiaphyseal region of the distal femur laterally (arrows). Note that the lesion is of low signal intensity with T2-weighting.

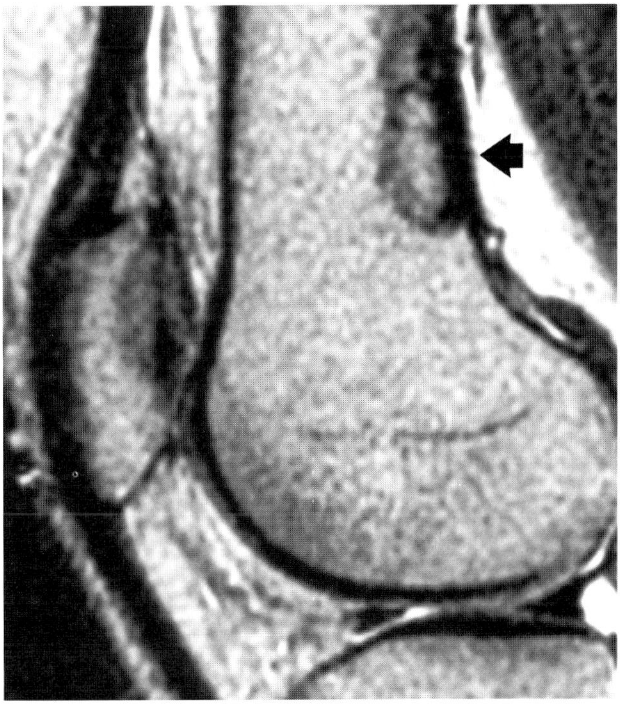

C

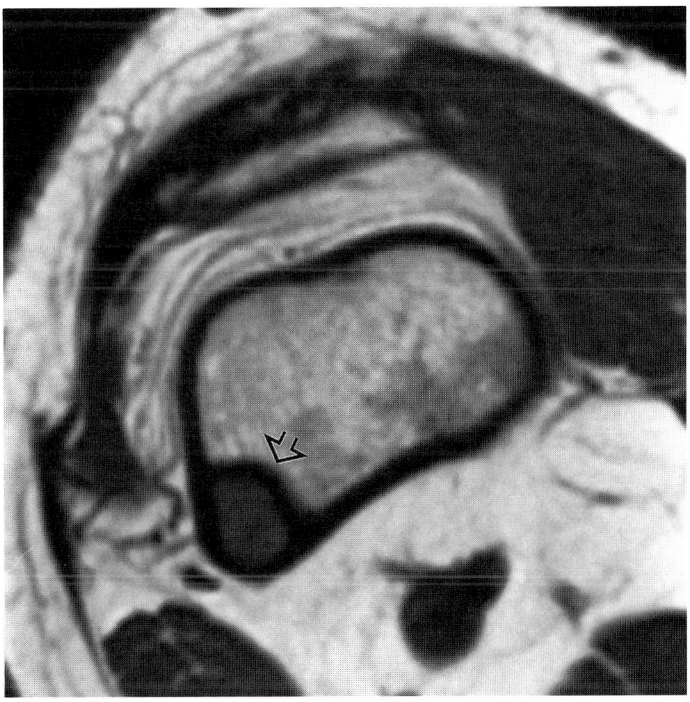

D

FIGURE 13.1 (continued) (B), (C) Sagittal proton density (2400/16) and T2-weighted (2400/70) images reveal that the lesion involves the posterior medullary space and cortex (black arrows). There are internal septations of low signal intensity. On both of these images, the predominant signal intensity is between that of muscle and fat. Axial (D) T1-weighted (800/16) and

(continued)

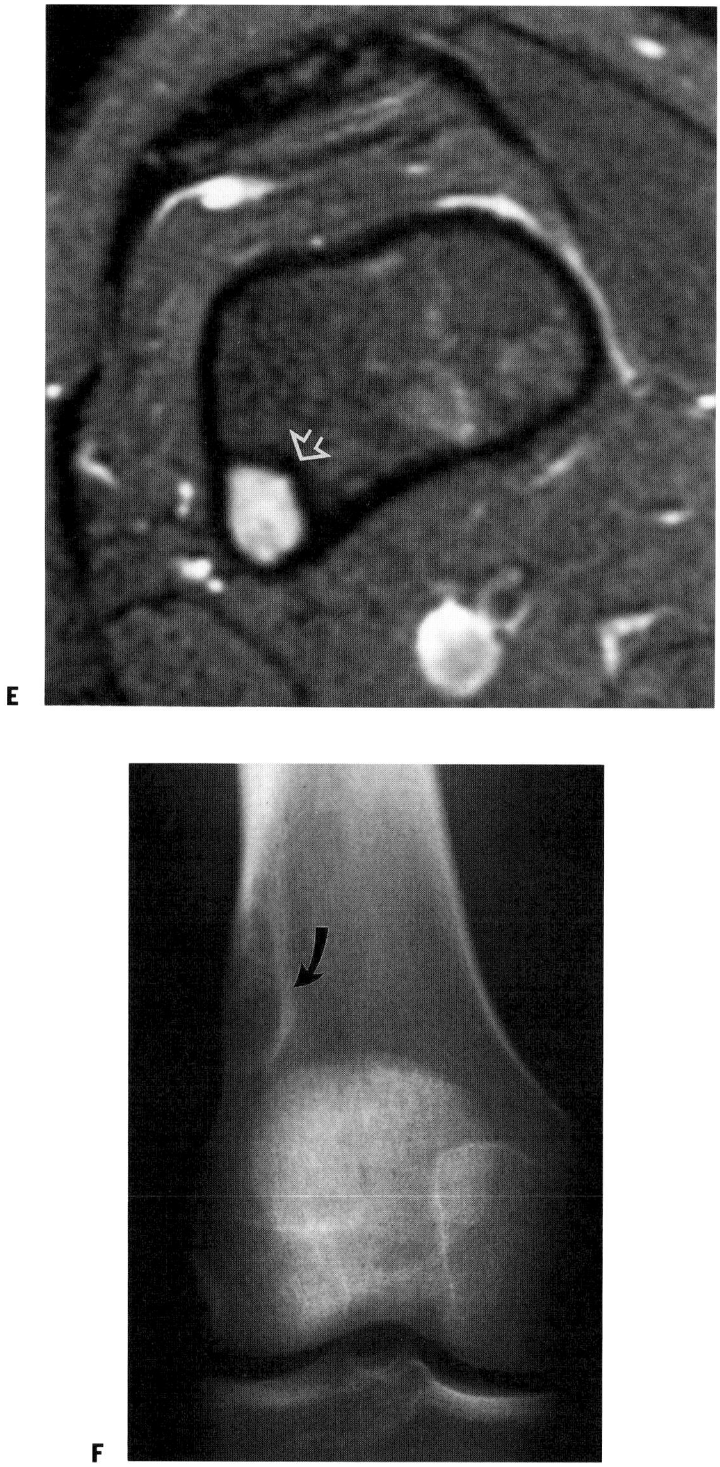

Figure 13.1 (continued) (E) FSE T2-weighted fat suppression (4500/54) images demonstrate a peripheral rim of low signal intensity (open arrows). Interestingly, the lesion becomes bright when fat suppression technique is used. (F) AP radiograph shows a characteristic appearance of a small nonossifying fibroma, which was detected incidentally in this patient. The lesion is slightly expansile and contains a sclerotic border (curved arrow).

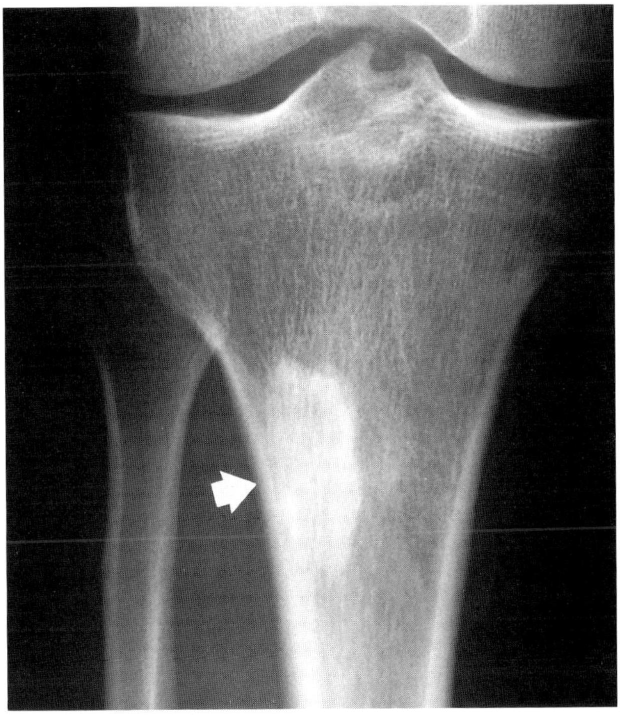

A

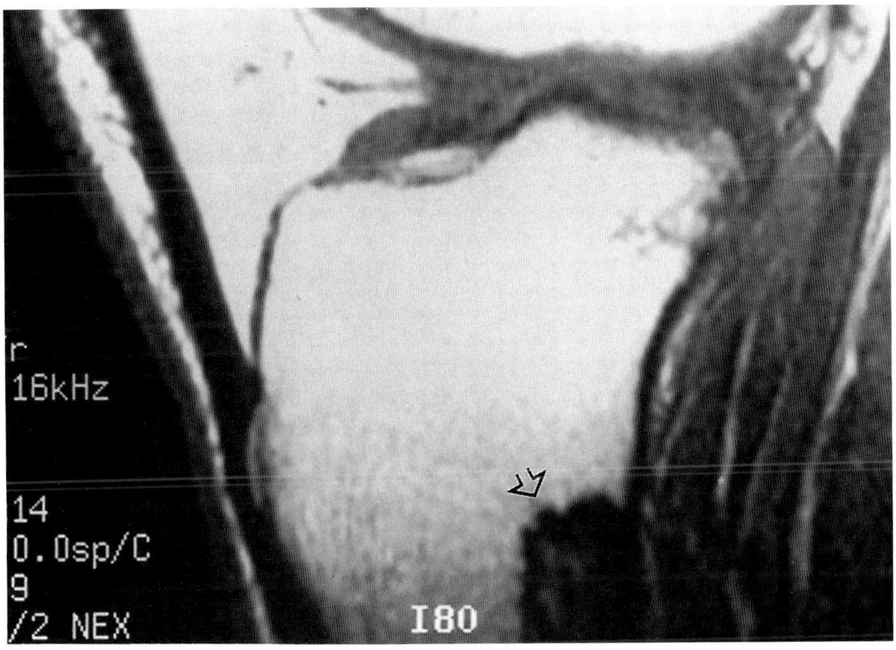

B

FIGURE 13.2 A 29-year-old male with an incidentally detected sclerotic right tibial lesion. (A) AP radiograph shows the typical appearance of a sclerotic (healing) nonossifying fibroma in the lateral metadiaphyseal region of the proximal tibia (arrow). (B) Sagittal T1-weighted (650/12) and

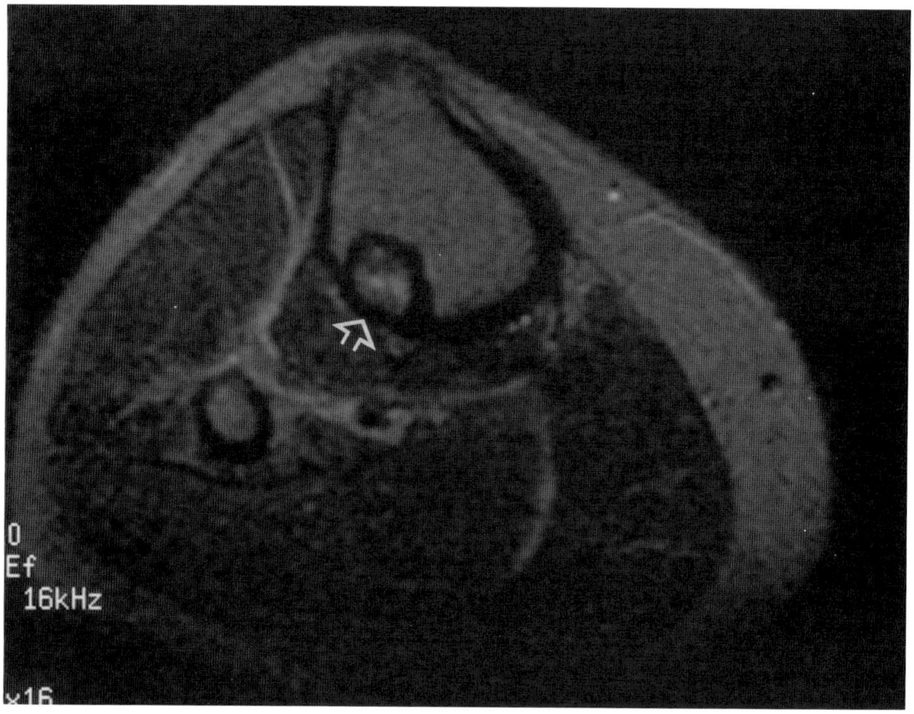

C

FIGURE 13.2 (continued) (C) axial FSE T2-weighted fat suppression (3500/68) images reveal that there is heterogeneous, but predominantly very low signal intensity within the lesion (open arrows) due to sclerosis. Note the peripheral rim of signal void corresponding to the sclerotic border.

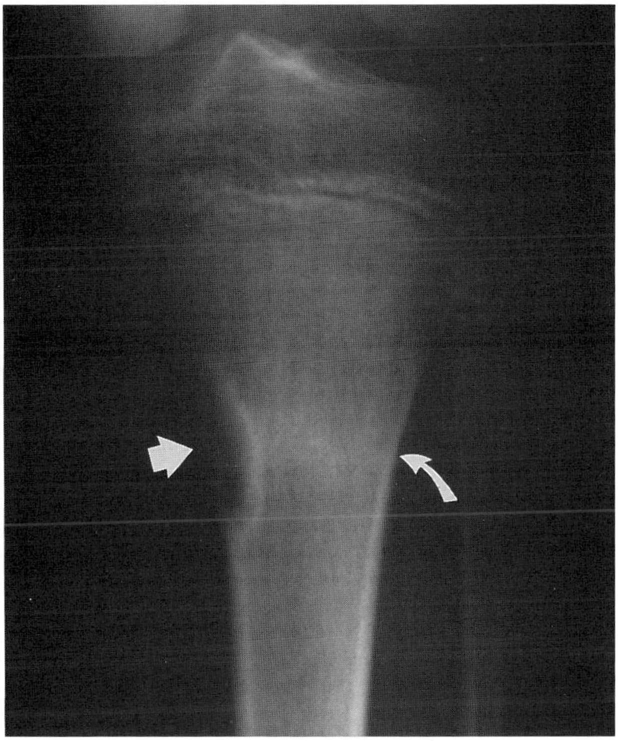

A

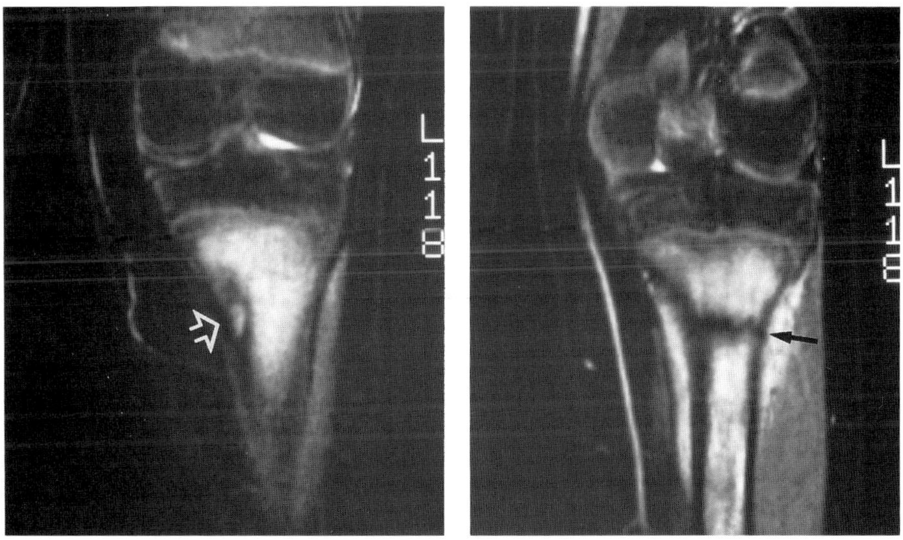

B

FIGURE 13.3 A 9-year-old girl with pain in the proximal tibial region. (A) AP radiograph demonstrates an elongated well-marginated lytic lesion with a thin sclerotic border in the medial metadiaphyseal region of the proximal tibia (arrow). This appearance is characteristic for a nonossifying fibroma. Note the adjacent transverse area of faint, ill-defined sclerosis (curved arrow). (B) Coronal FMPIR images (3000/13, TI-150) clearly depict a transverse fracture line (thin arrow) adjacent to the lesion (open arrow). There is surrounding bone marrow and soft tissue edema. This case nicely depicts a nonossifying fibroma associated with a stress fracture. It is important to note that these lesions should be asymptomatic in the absence of an associated fracture.

Fibrous Dysplasia

Definition. Fibrous dysplasia (FD) is a benign developmental disorder in which normal bone marrow is replaced by proliferating fibro-osseous tissue with variable amounts of stroma and bone. Trabeculae composed of immature woven bone are present within a fibrous tissue stroma. Hemorrhage and cystic change are occasionally present. Secondary aneurysmal bone cyst formation may occur. In addition, small foci of cartilage, which can calcify, are occasionally identified within the lesion (fibrocartilaginous dysplasia). FD may affect one (monostotic) or multiple (polyostotic) bones.

Clinical Features. FD is a relatively common disorder, typically encountered in adolescents and young adults. About 75% of patients are less than 30 years of age at the time of diagnosis, although all ages may be affected. Monostotic FD is usually asymptomatic and detected incidentally on radiographs. If present, symptoms include pain, swelling, tenderness, and pathologic fracture (stress or complete). Polyostotic FD is six times less common than the monostotic form and has a more aggressive clinical course. Patients with polyostotic FD typically present early, with two-thirds of patients becoming symptomatic by 10 years of age. About 75% of patients with polyostotic FD are symptomatic. Numerous endocrine abnormalities have been reported in association with FD, most notably McCune-Albright syndrome, which consists of the classic triad of polyostotic FD (usually unilateral), cutaneous cafe-au-lait spots (typically ipsilateral to the FD with irregular "coast of Maine" borders), and endocrine dysfunction (particularly precocious puberty in girls). Extensive osseous involvement may be associated with marked deformity such as leg length discrepancy, "shepherd's crook" deformity of the proximal femur, tibial bowing, and craniofacial asymmetry.

Location. FD may occur throughout the skeletal system. The most common sites of monostotic FD are the ribs, proximal femur, craniofacial bones, and tibia, respectively. Polyostotic FD most commonly affects the femur, tibia, pelvis, and foot. A pelvic lesion is almost invariably accompanied by a lesion in the ipsilateral proximal femur. In long bones, FD has a predilection for the diaphysis and may be central or eccentric in position. The lesion may extend into the epiphysis, but isolated epiphyseal involvement is rare.

Implications. Often times, a presumptive diagnosis of FD can be made on radiographs and biopsy is not required. The most common complication related to FD is pathologic fracture and large lesions may be treated prophylactically with curettage and bone grafting. Pathologic fractures have been reported to occur in as many as 85% of patients with polyostotic FD. Pregnancy or estrogen therapy may increase the size and exacerbate symptoms of pre-existing FD. FD may rarely undergo secondary aneurysmal bone cyst formation or even malignant transformation (most commonly to osteosarcoma followed by fibrosarcoma and chondrosarcoma). The incidence of malignant conversion has been reported to be 0.5%, however, the spontaneous rate may be considerably lower since many of the reported patients received prior radiation therapy. In addition, the cartilaginous foci which are sometimes present within FD can be mistaken pathologically for low-grade chondrosarcoma, which may account for some other reported cases. Malignant transformation typically manifests with increasing pain and/or a soft tissue mass. There is a rare association between FD (especially polyostotic) and intramuscular myxomas (typically multiple) known as Mazabraud's syndrome.

MRI Findings. FD can vary in size from a small focal abnormality to a lesion extending from one end of a bone to the other. In general, polyostotic FD lesions tend to be more extensive. On T1-weighted images, FD tends to exhibit homogeneous low signal (hypointense or isointense to muscle), unless complicated by pathologic fracture. The signal intensity on T2-weighted sequences tends to be heterogeneous and is highly variable depending on the fibro-osseous content and cellularity as well as the presence of cystic change, hemorrhage, and cartilaginous tissue. Therefore, areas ranging from very low signal to very bright signal intensity may be identified. The margins of the lesions tend to be sharply demarcated. There may be a well-defined peripheral rim of low signal (on all pulse sequences) corresponding to a sclerotic margin. Endosteal scalloping, cortical thinning, and bony expansion may be present. FD may even demonstrate focal or multifocal areas of full-thickness cortical bone destruction. In cases requiring surgical intervention, MR is the imaging modality of choice for characterizing the internal structure and delineating the extent of the lesion(s).

Differential Diagnosis. The MRI findings of FD are nonspecific and highly variable depending on the histologic content of the specific lesion. The radiographic appearances of FD are also numerous, with a spectrum ranging from lytic to sclerotic. Nevertheless, the plain film findings frequently permit a presumptive diagnosis of FD to be made. However, there are many instances in which the radiographic differential diagnosis of FD includes numerous additional benign lesions.

References

Kransdorf M, Moser R, Gilkey F. Fibrous dysplasia. *RadioGraphics* 10:519–537, 1990.

Utz J, Kransdorf M, Jelinek J, et al. MR appearance of fibrous dysplasia. *JCAT* 13:845–851, 1989.

Fisher A, Totty W, Kyriakos M. Case report. MR appearance of cystic fibrous dysplasia. *JCAT* 18:315–318, 1994.

Yao L, Eckardt J, Seeger L. Fibrous dysplasia associated with cortical bony destruction: CT and MR findings. *JCAT* 18:91–94, 1994.

Gober G, Nicholas R. Case report 800. *Skeletal Radiol* 22:452–455, 1993.

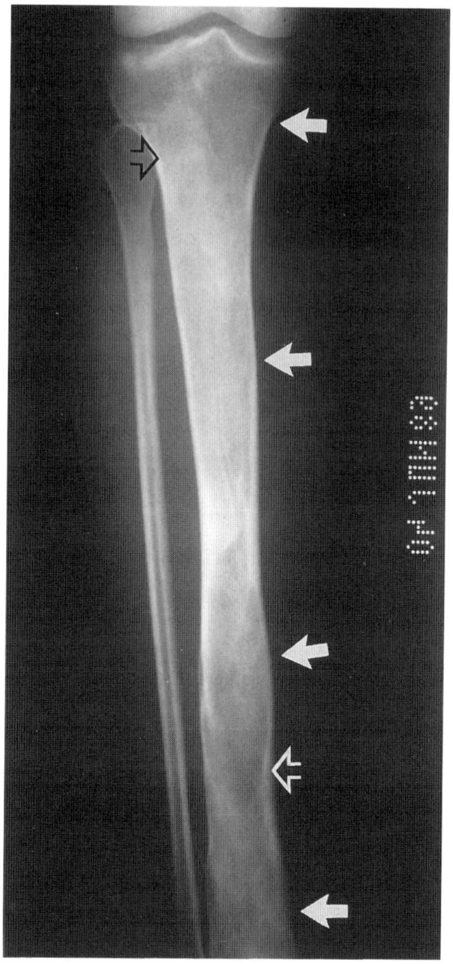

A

FIGURE 13.4 Fibrous dysplasia of the tibia in a 29-year-old woman. (A) AP radiograph demonstrates extensive fibrous dysplasia involving nearly the entire length of the tibia (arrows). There is a mixed lytic (open white arrow) and sclerotic (open black arrow) appearance representing both fibrous and osseous components. Note the presence of endosteal scalloping, cortical thinning, and osseous expansion, which is most prominent distally. This appearance is characteristic of fibrous dysplasia.

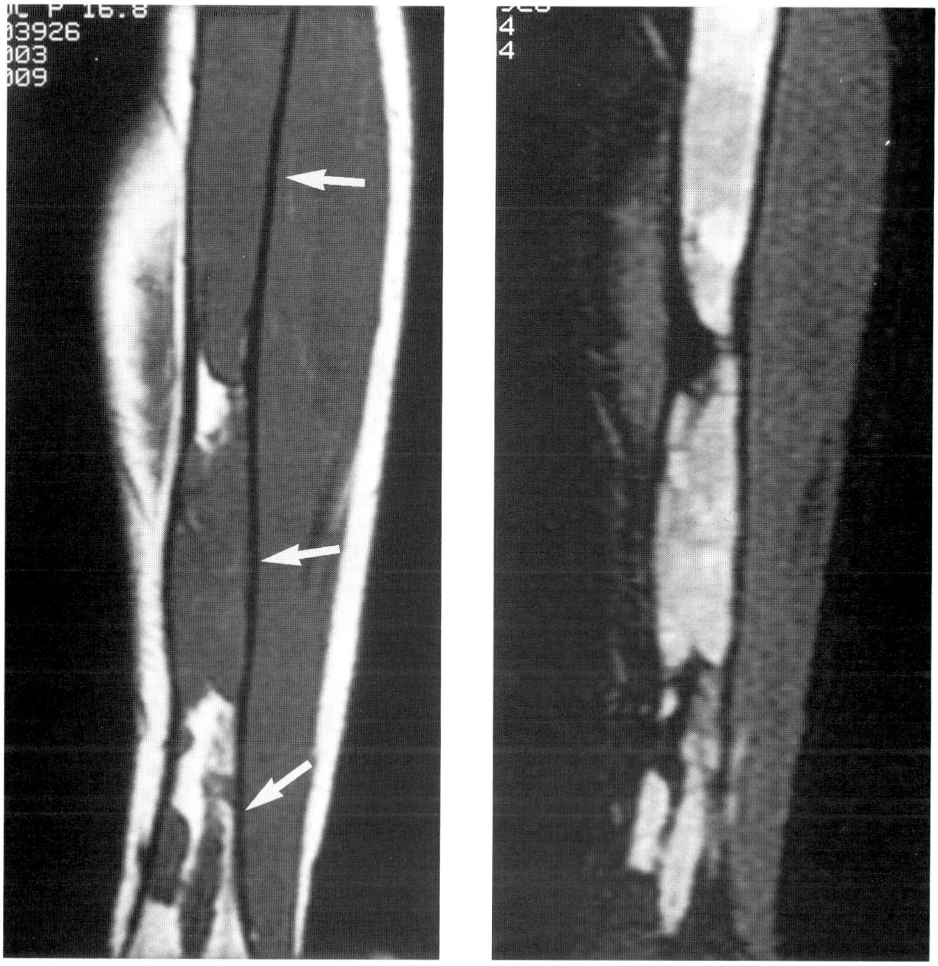

B C

FIGURE 13.4 (continued) (B) Coronal T1-weighted (500/13) image shows that the lesion (long arrows) is predominantly isointense to muscle. (C) Coronal inversion recovery image (2000/30, TI-160) reveals heterogeneous, predominantly high signal intensity throughout the lesion.

Desmoplastic Fibroma (Desmoid Tumor) of Bone

Definition. Desmoplastic fibroma (DF) of bone is a locally aggressive tumor which is histologically identical to a soft tissue desmoid tumor, consisting of fibroblasts within a nonmineralized, collagen matrix. There may be areas of cystic necrosis. Gross pathologic examination reveals a firm, rubbery tumor which varies from white to tan in color. It is also referred to as intraosseous desmoid tumor or desmoid tumor of bone.

Clinical Features. DF of bone is a rare tumor (less common than its soft tissue counterpart) with a peak incidence in the second and third decades of life, although it may occur at any age. Common clinical manifestations include pain (present in 65–90%), swelling, and a palpable mass. Pathologic fracture is present in about 10% of cases. It may also be detected as an incidental finding on imaging studies.

Location. DF has been reported in nearly all bones, but is most common in the mandible, femur, pelvis, tibia, humerus, and radius. In long bones, it is usually metaphyseal in location but may extend into the epiphysis and can be central or eccentric in position. DF may rarely arise from the periosteum.

Implications. DF does not metastasize, but is locally aggressive and has a high recurrence rate following curettage. The treatment of choice is en bloc resection (if possible) or wide surgical excision. Careful long-term follow-up is necessary since local recurrence has been described up to 15 years following presentation. It is important to note that DF may be difficult to distinguish from low-grade fibrosarcoma histologically. It may also resemble nonossifying fibroma on pathologic examination.

MRI Findings. In long bones, DF typically appears as an oval or elongated lesion with its long axis aligned longitudinally with the host bone. There is usually fusiform expansion of the bone. The signal intensity of the mass may be low to intermediate on T1-weighted images. The T2-weighted appearance is variable, ranging from low to high signal intensity. The mass appears heterogeneous containing radiating folds of very low signal intensity on all pulse sequences, corresponding to residual ridges of bone known as pseudotrabeculae. These trabeculations can be thin or coarse. Typically, there is a thin low signal intensity rim surrounding the lesion representing a fibrous pseudocapsule. This peripheral rim remains of low signal intensity on all pulse sequences. Endosteal scalloping is frequent. Cortical destruction is present in about 30% of cases and there may be a soft tissue mass present.

Differential Diagnosis. Although the signal characteristics of DF are nonspecific, there are some fairly unique MR characteristics which when used in conjunction with the radiographic findings, may enable the correct diagnosis to be made. Internal radiating folds of very low signal on all pulse sequences is a fairly distinctive feature and is the plain film correlate of a lace-like or reticular pattern of pseudotrabeculae. A similar appearance can be seen with hemangioma of bone. In addition, some DFs are predominantly low in signal intensity on T2-weighted sequences, which is atypical for the vast majority of osseous lesions, but can be seen with other fibrous masses. Nevertheless, the presence of these features in a metaphyseal lesion with fusiform bone expansion is suggestive of the diagnosis. If the pseudotrabeculae are thick and coarsened, the appearance may resemble Paget's disease.

References

Crim J, Gold R, Mirra J, et al. Desmoplastic fibroma of bone: radiographic analysis. *Radiology* 172:827–832, 1989.

Haney J, Olson P, Griffiths H. The clinical and radiologic features of desmoplastic fibroma of bone. *Orthopedics* 17:77–88, 1994.

Savy J, Laredo J, Prier A, et al. Case report 723. *Skeletal Radiol* 21:388–391, 1992.

Dong P, Seeger L, Eckardt J, et al. Case report 847. *Skeletal Radiol* 23:560–563, 1994.

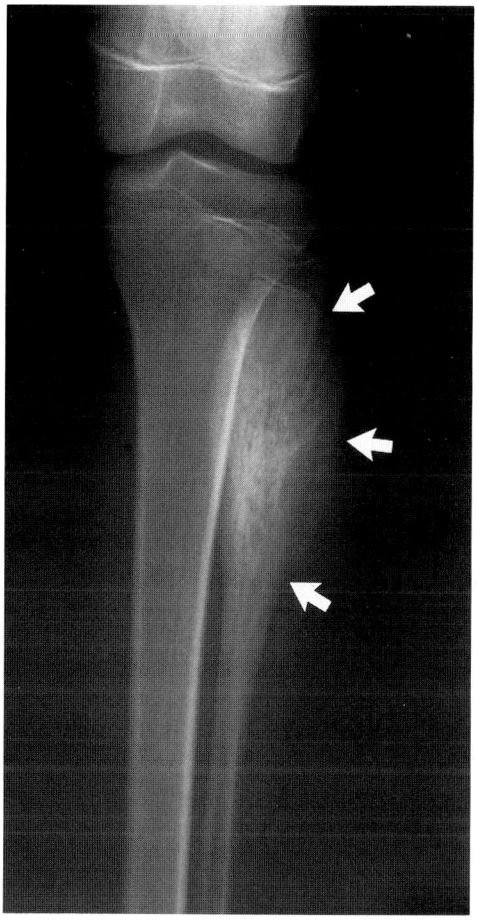

A

Figure 13.5 Desmoid tumor of the proximal fibula in a 13-year-old girl who presented with pain and swelling below the knee laterally. (A) AP radiograph shows a fusiform expansile lesion involving the metadiaphyseal region of the proximal left fibula (arrows). Note the radiating sclerotic appearance of the pseudotrabeculae. (B) Axial T1-weighted image (550/10) reveals signal which is isointense to muscle as well as foci of low signal within the mass (open arrows).

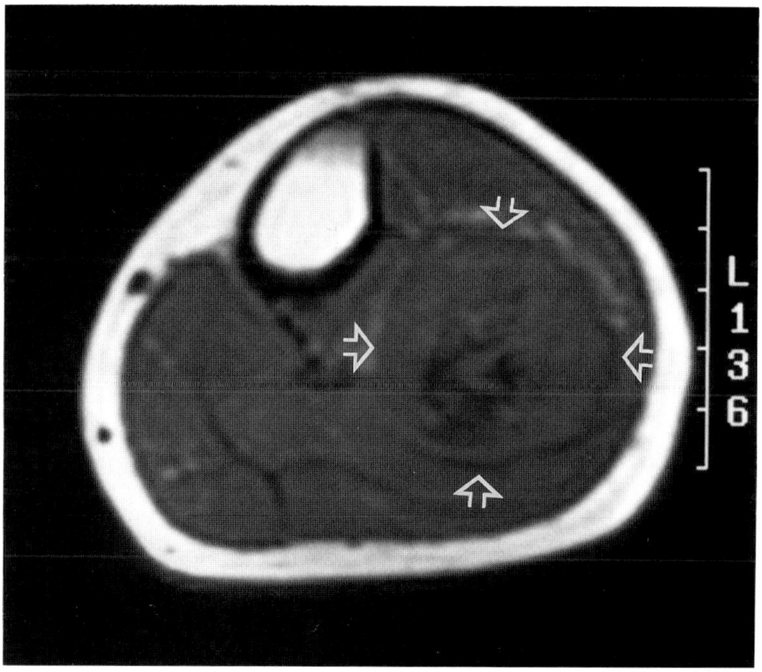

B

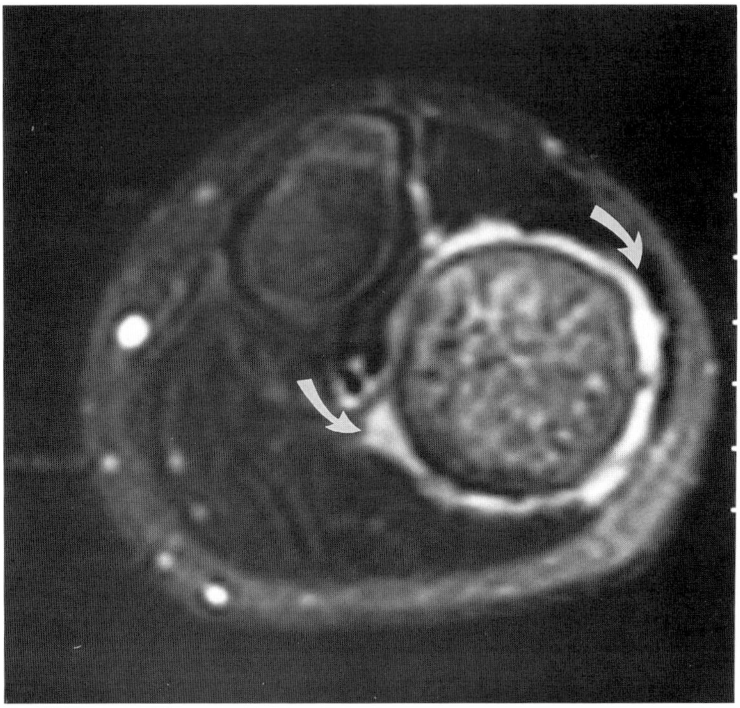

C

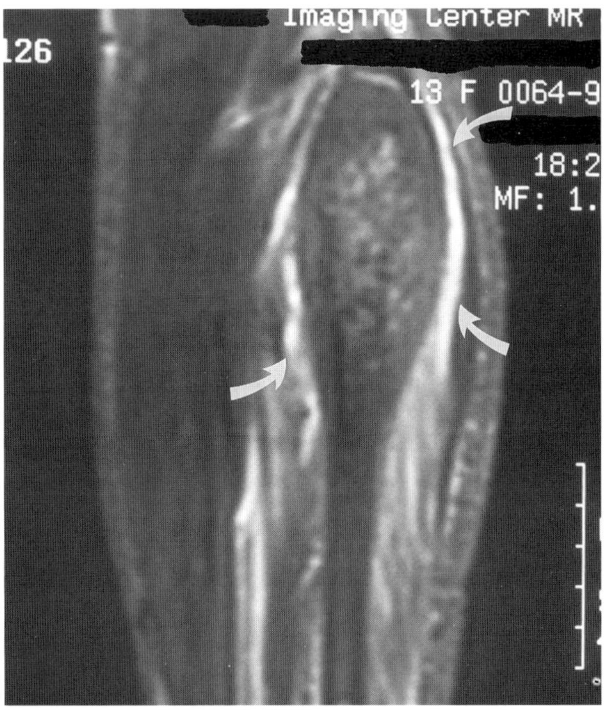

D

FIGURE 13.5 (continued) (C) Axial FSE T2-weighted fat suppression (3450/102) and (D) coronal FMPIR (4216/48, TI-120) images demonstrate heterogeneous signal intensity within the lesion. The predominantly low and intermediate signal intensity is atypical for the vast majority of bone lesions. There are internal foci of very low signal corresponding to pseudotrabeculae. Note the surrounding soft tissue edema (curved arrows).

Malignant Fibrous Histiocytoma of Bone

Definition. Malignant fibrous histiocytoma (MFH) of bone may be primary (arising de novo) or secondary (20%), occurring in association with entities such as bone infarction, Paget's disease, radiation therapy, and fibrous dysplasia. Histologically, the majority of lesions consist of disorganized deposits of dense fibrous tissue in a "storiform" or "cartwheel" pattern. Areas of hemorrhage and necrosis are commonly present.

Clinical Features. MFH of bone accounts for about 5% of primary malignant bone neoplasms and usually occurs in the 4th–7th decades of life, although all ages may be affected. It is typically associated with pain, tenderness, and an enlarging mass. Pathologic fracture has been reported in 20–50% of cases.

Location. The majority of lesions occur in the metaphyses of long bones, especially the femur, proximal tibia, and proximal humerus. There is frequent extension into the epiphysis or diaphysis. The pelvis is the next most frequent location. Any bone may be affected.

Implications. MFH of bone is an aggressive lesion frequently associated with recurrence and metastasis. Treatment typically consists of chemotherapy and surgical resection, sometimes with radiation therapy as well.

MRI Findings. On MRI, MFH of bone typically appears as an infiltrative mass with ill-defined margins, extensive medullary involvement, cortical destruction, and soft tissue extension. A "storiform-wormy" pattern consisting of numerous thick, curved stripes and septa has been described on T1- and T2-weighted sequences, corresponding to the disorganized dense fibrous deposits seen histologically. Other lesions will show nonspecific signal characteristics (hypointense with T1-weighting, hyperintense with T2-weighting) and variable heterogeneity depending on the amount of hemorrhage and necrosis present. These lesions could also appear predominantly hypointense on T2-weighted sequences if a large amount of dense fibrous tissue is present.

Differential Diagnosis. MR images should be interpreted in the presence of corresponding plain films, since radiography remains the modality of choice for bone tumor diagnosis. One may be able to suggest the diagnosis of MFH if a "storiform wormy" MR pattern is seen and the plain films are compatible with the diagnosis. In addition, the presence of predominantly hypointense signal on T2-weighted images suggests a fibrous lesion, although there are exceptions. In many cases, the MR signal characteristics will be nonspecific and the differential diagnosis will depend primarily on the plain film findings.

References

Murphey M, Gross T, Rosenthal H. Musculoskeletal malignant fibrous histiocytoma: Radiologic-pathologic correlation. *RadioGraphics* 14:807–826, 1994.

Golfieri R, Baddeley H, Pringle J, et al. Primary bone tumors: MR morphologic appearance correlated with pathologic examinations. *Acta Radiologica* 32:290–298, 1991.

Resnick D. *Bone and Joint Imaging*. Philadelphia, PA, W.B. Saunders Company; 1989: pp 1153–1154.

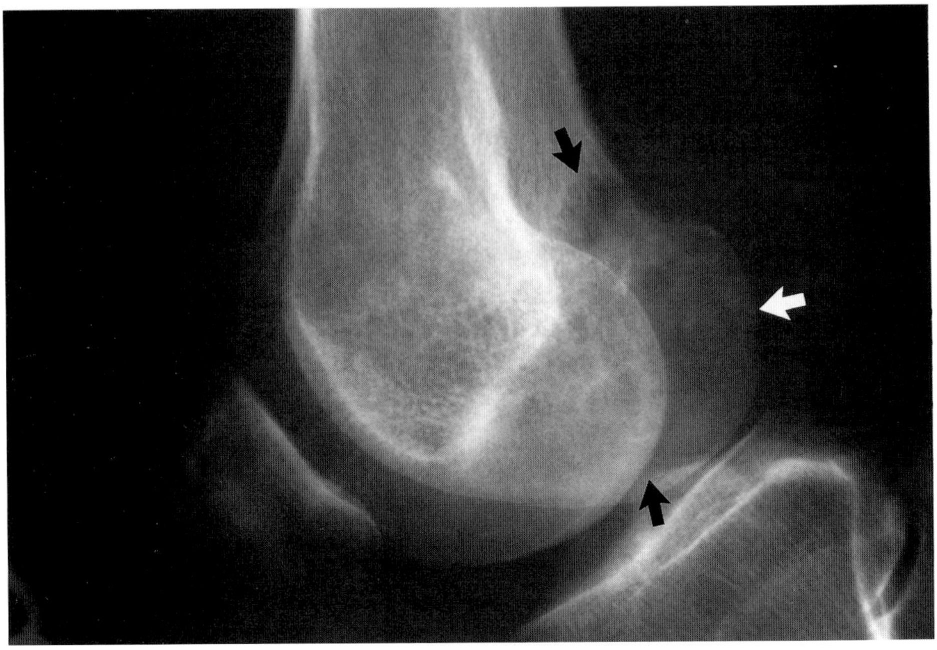

A

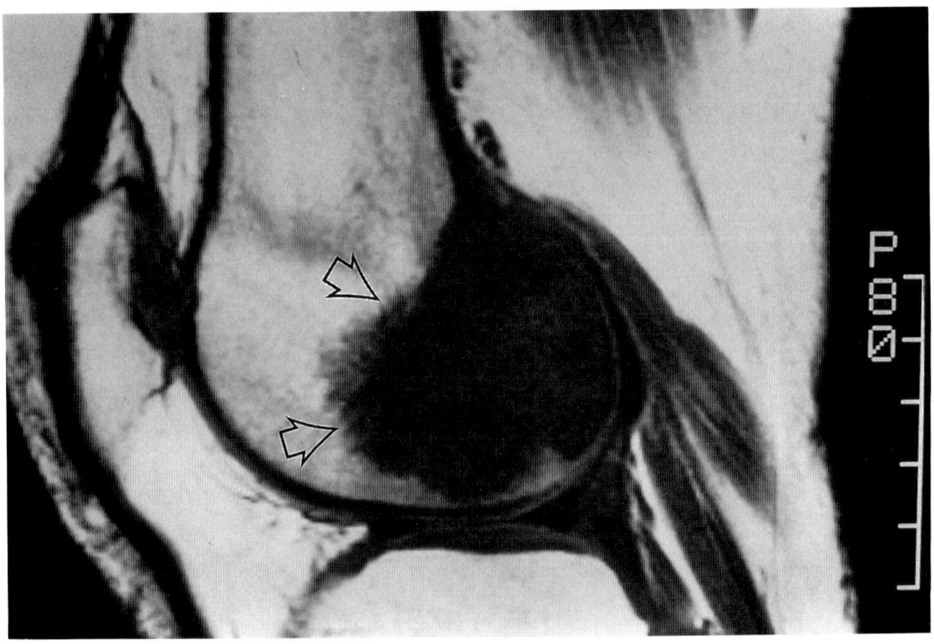

B

FIGURE 13.6 A 36-year-old male with a malignant fibrous histiocytoma of the distal femur. (A) Lateral radiograph demonstrates an ill-defined lytic lesion within the posterior aspect of the distal femur (arrows). Sagittal (B) T1-weighted and

(*continued*)

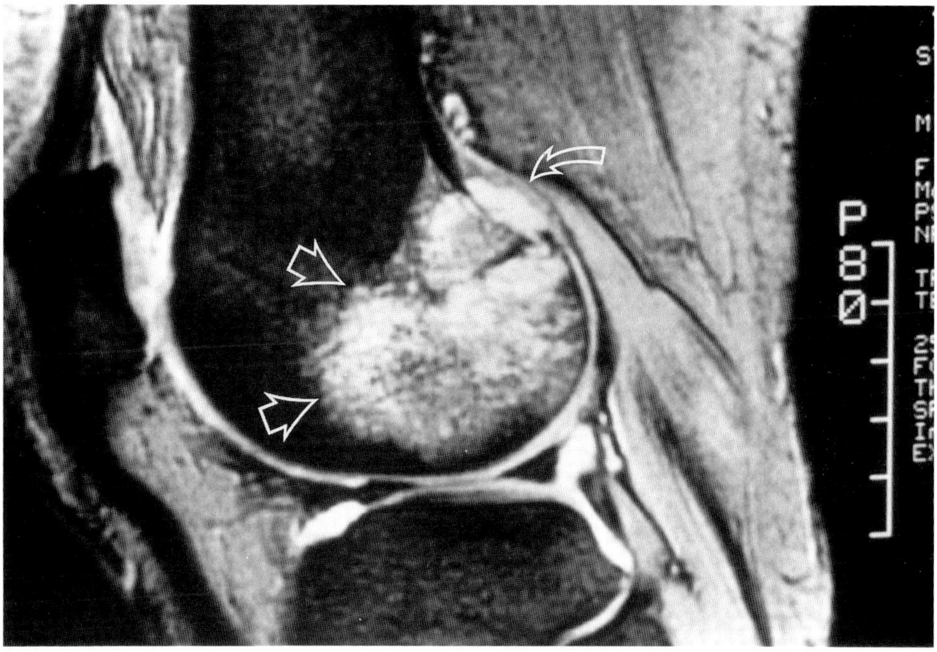

C

FIGURE 13.6 (continued) (C) gradient-recalled echo images delineate the extent of the lesion (open arrows) within the metaphysis and epiphysis. The signal characteristics are nonspecific. Note that a portion of the lesion extends through the cortex (curved open arrow). (Courtesy of James O. Johnston, MD).

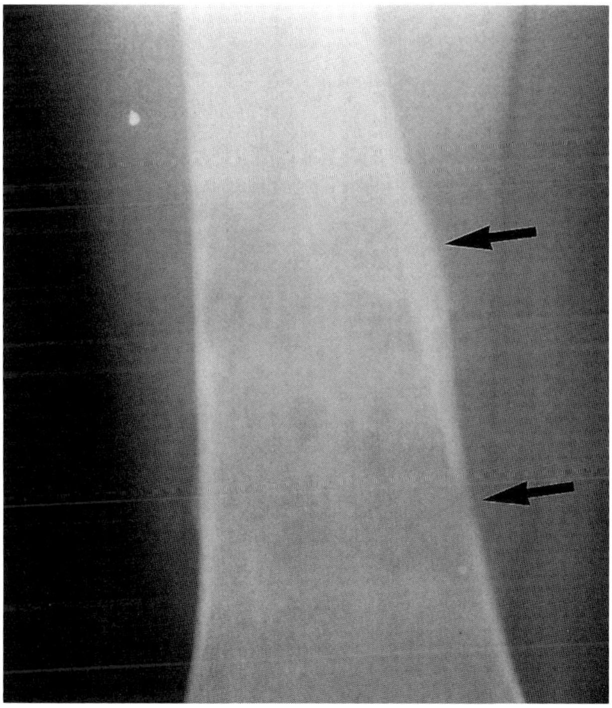

A

FIGURE 13.7 Malignant fibrous histiocytoma of the distal femur in a 31-year-old woman. (A) AP radiograph shows a poorly-defined aggressive lytic lesion within the distal femoral diaphysis (arrows).

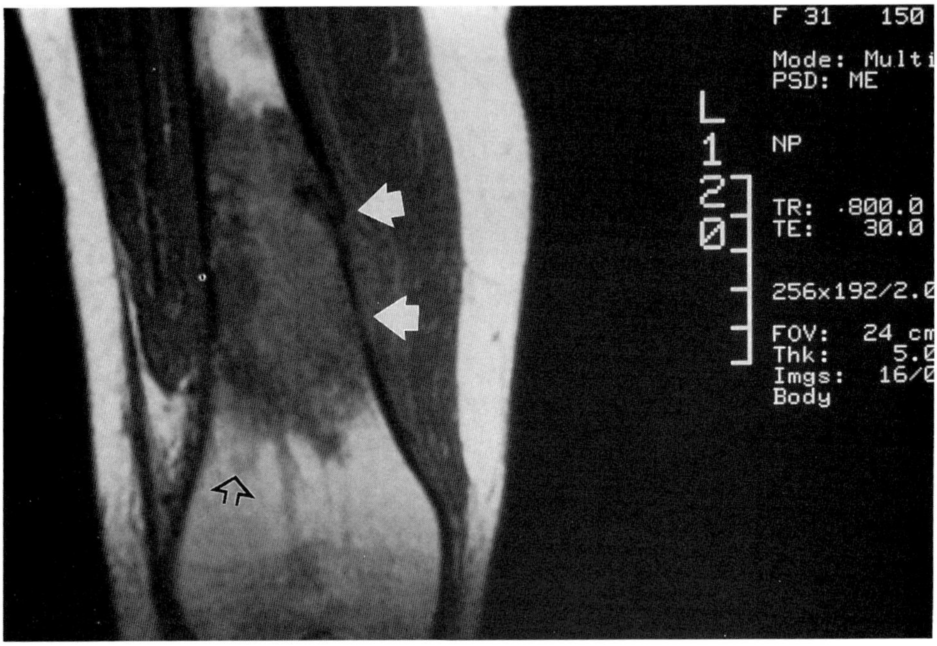

B

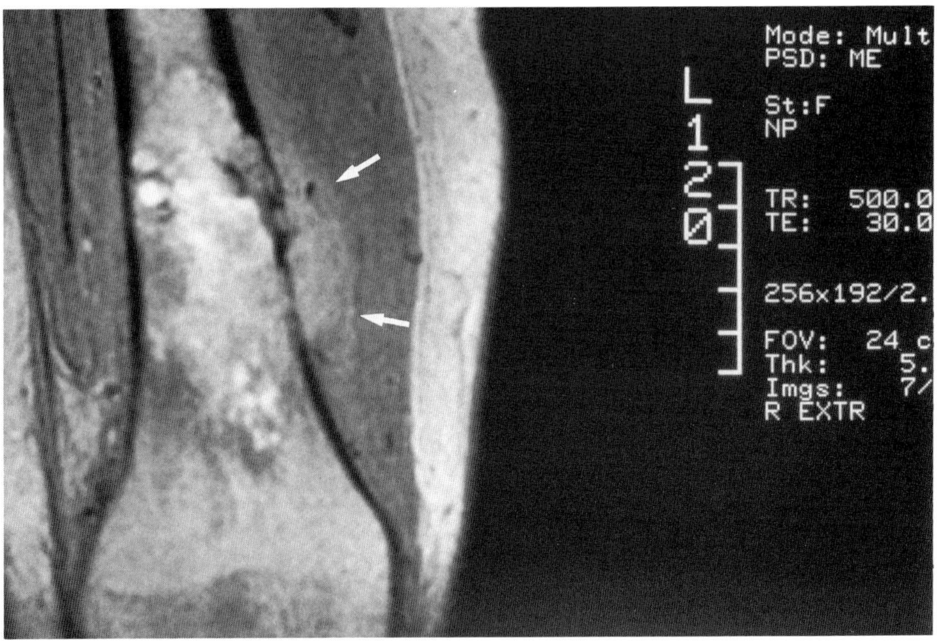

C

Figure 13.7 (continued) (B) Coronal T1-weighted image (800/30) reveals extension of the lesion through the cortex medially (white arrows). Note the ill-defined inferior margin (open arrow). There is heterogeneous signal intensity including scattered hyperintense areas likely representing hemorrhage. (C), (D) Gadolinium-enhanced coronal T1-weighted fat suppression images (500/30) demonstrate heterogeneous enhancement and delineate the medial soft tissue mass (thin white arrows). Incomplete fat suppression is present. (Courtesy of James O. Johnston, MD).

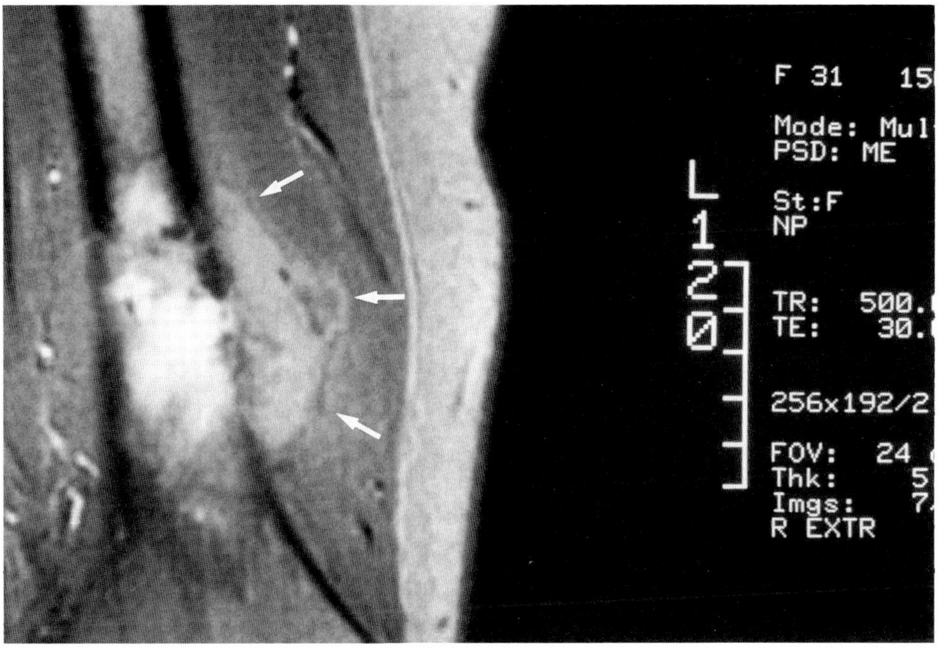
F 31 15
Mode: Mul
PSD: ME
L120
St:F
NP
TR: 500.
TE: 30.
256x192/2
FOV: 24
Thk: 5
Imgs: 7
R EXTR

D

Fibrosarcoma of Bone

Definition. Fibrosarcoma of bone is a malignant neoplasm which may be primary (arising de novo) or secondary, occurring in association with bone infarction, radiation therapy, Paget's disease, or chronic osteomyelitis. Histologically, the lesion is characterized by collagen-producing spindle cells.

Clinical Features. Fibrosarcoma of bone is a rare tumor occurring most frequently in the 3rd–6th decades of life, although all ages may be affected. It typically presents with pain and swelling. Pathologic fracture occurs in approximately one-third of cases.

Location. Most lesions occur in the long bones, especially around the knee. In the long bones, the lesion typically involves the metaphysis and may extend into the diaphysis or epiphysis.

Implications. The histologic grade ranges from well-differentiated to poorly-differentiated and the prognosis varies accordingly. However, most lesions are aggressive with a tendency for recurrence and/or metastasis.

MRI Findings. Fibrosarcoma of bone frequently appears as an infiltrative mass with ill-defined margins, extensive medullary involvement, cortical destruction, and soft tissue extension. These lesions could appear predominantly hypointense on T2-weighted sequences if a large amount of fibrous tissue is present. Other lesions will exhibit nonspecific signal characteristics (hypointense with T1-weighting, hyperintense with T2-weighting) and variable heterogeneity depending on the histologic grade and the amount of hemorrhage and necrosis present.

Differential Diagnosis. MR images should be interpreted in the presence of corresponding plain films, since radiography remains the modality of choice for bone tumor diagnosis. The presence of predominantly hypointense signal on T2-weighted sequences suggests a fibrous lesion, although there are exceptions. In many cases, the MR signal characteristics are nonspecific and the differential diagnosis depends primarily on the plain film findings.

References

Resnick D. *Bone and Joint Imaging.* Philadelphia, PA, W.B. Saunders Company; 1989; pp 1146–1147.

Golfieri R, Baddeley H, Pringle J, et al. Primary bone tumors: MR morphologic appearance correlated with pathologic examination. *Acta Radiologica* 32:290–298, 1991.

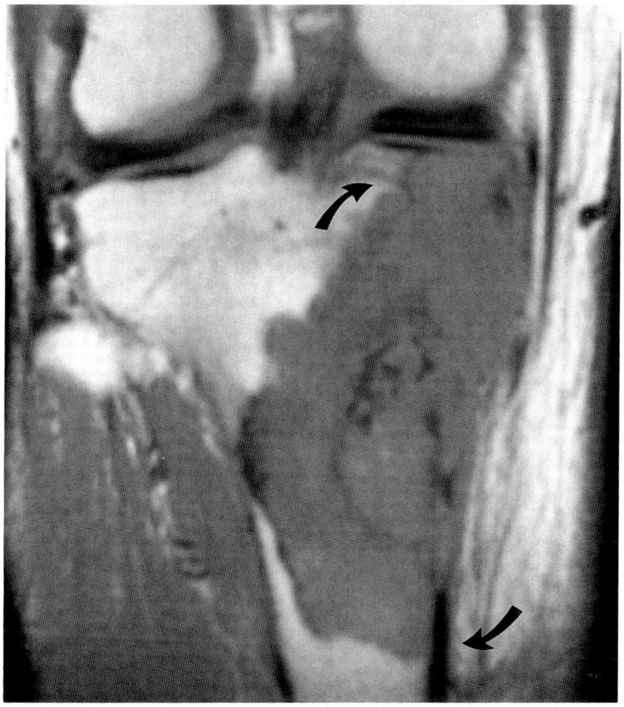

A

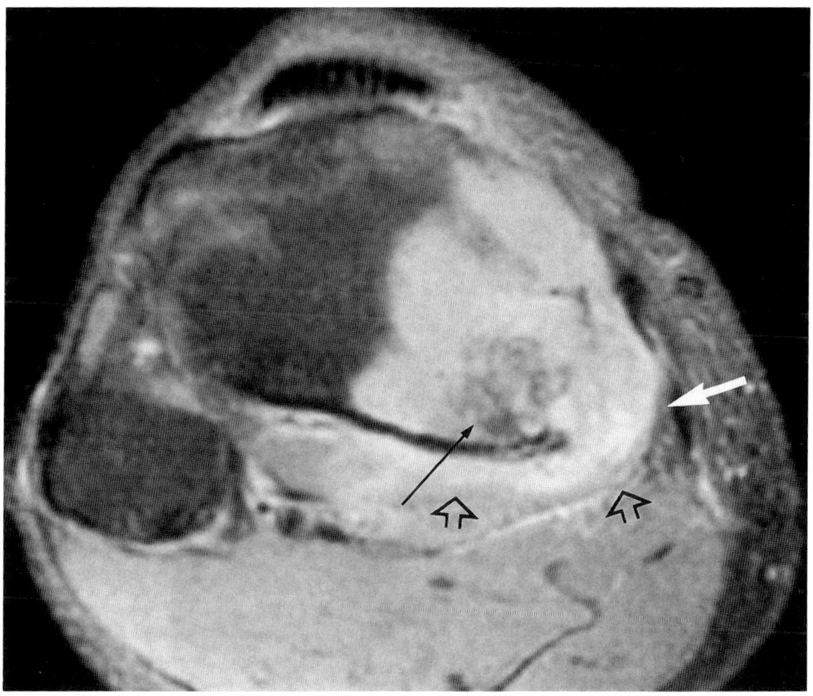

B

FIGURE 13.8 A 34-year-old male with knee pain. (A) Coronal T1-weighted image (850/16) demonstrates a mass arising from the medial metaphyseal region of the proximal tibia with extension into the epiphysis and proximal diaphysis (curved arrows). The predominant signal intensity is approximately isointense to muscle, but there are multiple areas of very hypointense signal within the lesion.

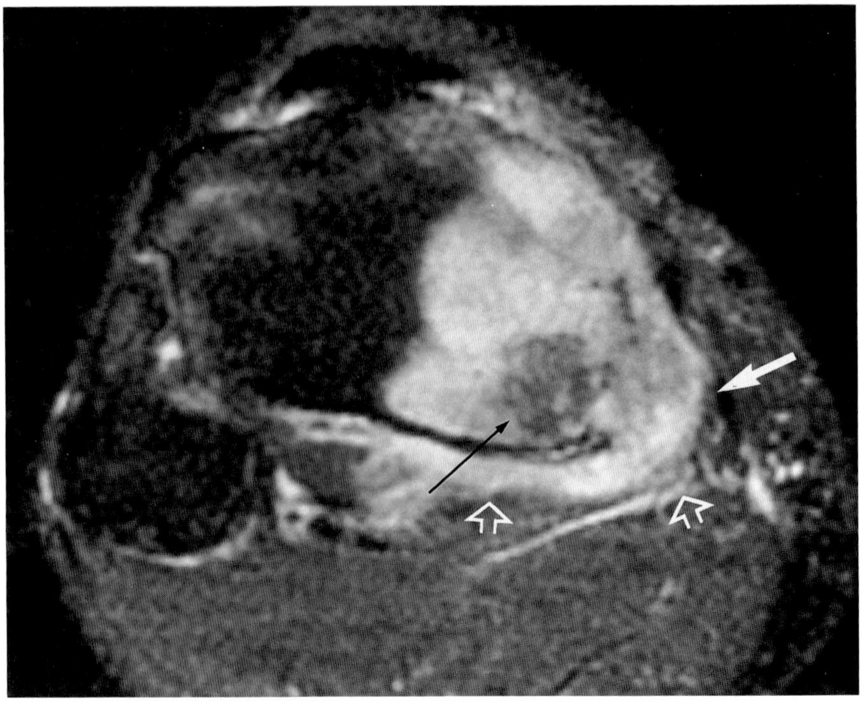

C

FIGURE 13.8 (continued) (B), (C) Axial dual-echo T2-weighted fat suppression images (2800/19, 70) reveal associated cortical destruction (arrows) and soft tissue extension (open arrows). Note the areas of low signal intensity (thin arrows), which likely correspond to deposits of dense fibrous tissue. Pleomorphic fibrosarcoma was diagnosed pathologically.

14 Cystic/Fluid-Filled Masses

Geode (Subchondral Cyst)

Definition. Geodes are juxta-articular cystic lesions which have also been termed subchondral cysts and subarticular pseudocysts. Geodes occur in association with osteoarthritis, calcium pyrophosphate dihydrate deposition disease (CPPD), rheumatoid arthritis, and osteonecrosis. Geodes typically contain myxoid material and fibrous tissue. Those associated with rheumatoid arthritis are typically filled with granulomatous inflammatory tissue. There may or may not be an identifiable communication with the joint space. Cysts associated with osteoarthritis and CPPD are thought to arise from either synovial fluid intrusion or bone contusion. The cysts of rheumatoid arthritis occur as a result of erosion by inflammatory synovial tissue or pannus. In osteonecrosis, cysts occur as a result of osteoclastic resorption of necrotic trabeculae with fibrous replacement of bone.

Clinical Features. The clinical presentation is variable, depending on the underlying disease process. Geodes associated with osteoarthritis are commonly asymptomatic and detected incidentally on radiographic examination.

Location. These lesions occur in the juxta-articular subchondral bone. In rheumatoid arthritis, geodes initially occur at the chondro-osseous junctions.

Implications. The geodes themselves do not require treatment. Therapy and prognosis depend on the underlying disease process. It is important to recognize geodes and not confuse them with true neoplasms. These lesions should not be biopsied. They may enlarge over time.

MRI Findings. In general, geodes appear as round or oval well-marginated masses which demonstrate homogeneous, low to intermediate signal intensity on T1-weighted images and uniform bright signal intensity on T2-weighted sequences. Lesions related to rheumatoid arthritis may be of more intermediate signal intensity due to pannus. Geodes may contain internal debris. Cysts related to osteoarthritis are commonly multiple and typically range from 2 mm to 2 cm in diameter. Associated findings of osteoarthritis should be seen including articular cartilage loss and osteophytosis. Eburnation may also be seen which appears as marked hypointense signal on all pulse sequences. The cysts of rheumatoid arthritis are often multiple, occur initially at the chondro-osseous junctions, and are associated with early cartilage loss. In CPPD, the cysts are typically larger and more numerous than those with osteoarthritis. Adjacent evidence of osteonecrosis should be seen with a geode caused by this process.

Differential Diagnosis. The differential diagnosis of a geode includes other epiphyseal lesions such as infection (Brodie's abscess), giant cell tumor, chondroblastoma, and intraosseous ganglion. An active Brodie's abscess should be distinguishable based upon clinical grounds. Also, a Brodie's abscess would be suggested by the identification of a serpiginous tract extending from the lesion. It may also contain internal debris. A giant cell tumor would not typically have signal as bright as joint fluid on T2-weighted images, as would be expected with a geode. Additionally, plain radiographs would be helpful in this distinction because a giant cell tumor possesses a nonsclerotic border whereas a geode has a sclerotic margin. Chondroblastoma typically occurs in a younger age group (less than 20) than geodes. In addition, approximately half of chondroblastomas will demonstrate calcification, which appears as hypointense foci on all pulse sequences. Geodes should be seen in the presence of additional findings associated with the underlying disease process (i.e., osteoarthritis, CPPD, rheumatoid arthritis, osteonecrosis). If a subchondral cystic lesion is seen without other abnormalities, an intraosseous ganglion should be suggested. Intraosseous ganglia are usually solitary and are most common in the hip, medial malleolus, proximal tibia, and carpus.

References

Dahlin D, Unni K. *Bone Tumors*. 4th ed. Springfield, Ill, Charles C. Thomas Publishing; 1986, pp 446–448.

Resnick D. *Bone and Joint Imaging*. Philadelphia, PA, W.B. Saunders Company; 1989, pp 383–384.

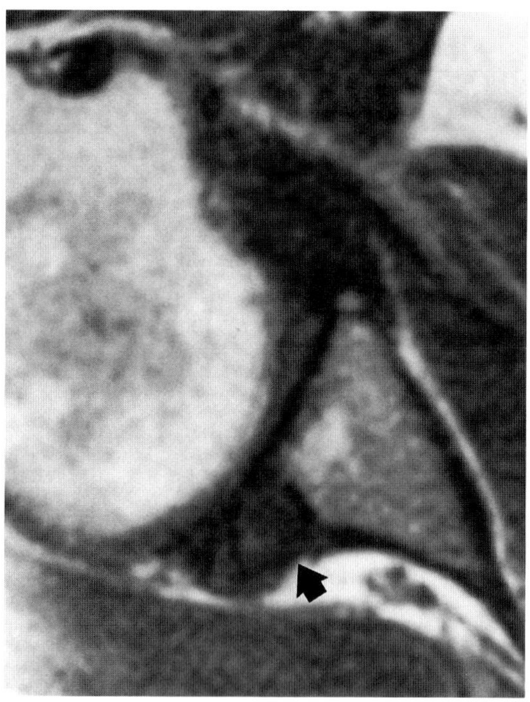

A

FIGURE 14.1 A 49-year-old male who sustained a shoulder injury one year prior presented with worsening pain. Radiographs revealed glenohumeral degenerative joint disease. Axial (A) T1-weighted (400/20) and (B) MPGR (400/20, 25 degrees) images reveal a well-marginated round lesion within the posterior glenoid (arrows). There is uniformly bright signal intensity within the lesion on the gradient-echo image. These findings are consistent with a geode associated with osteoarthritis.

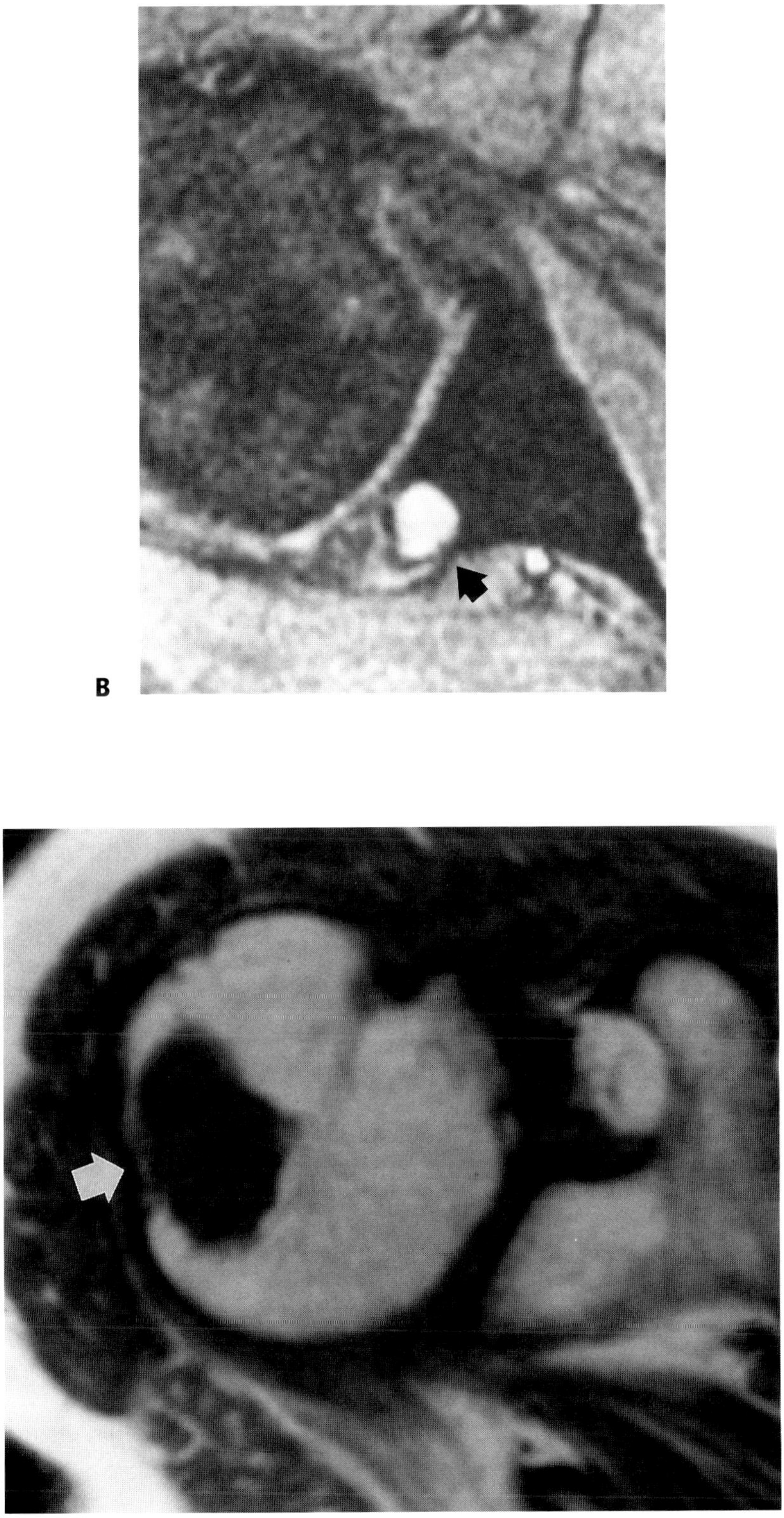

B

A

FIGURE 14.2 A 50-year-old woman with rheumatoid arthritis presented with shoulder pain. (A) Axial T1-weighted image (400/20) demonstrates an oval-shaped lesion within the lateral aspect of the right humeral head (arrow). The signal is isointense to muscle.

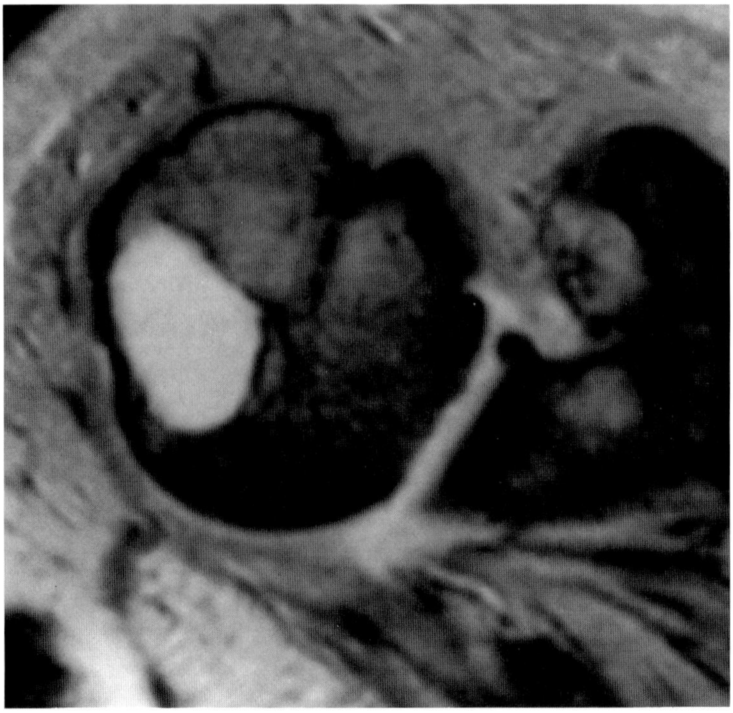

B

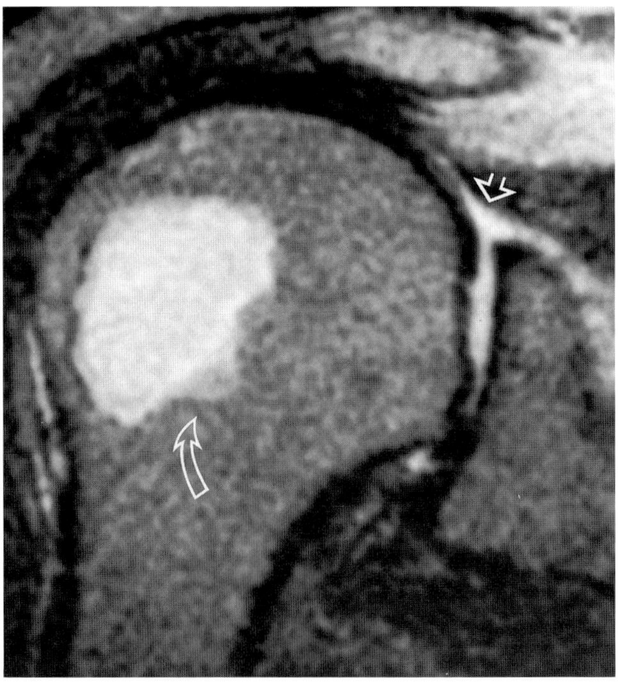

C

FIGURE 14.2 (continued) (B) Axial MPGR image (400/20, 25 degrees) shows that the lesion exhibits uniform hyperintense signal similar to the adjacent joint fluid. (C) Coronal T2-weighted image (2000/70) demonstrates a partially irregular border (curved open arrow) of the lesion. With this sequence, the signal of the lesion is slightly less intense than that of the adjacent joint fluid (open arrow). This lesion represents a geode associated with rheumatoid arthritis. Additional images revealed an extensive rotator cuff tear.

Intraosseous Ganglion

Definition. An intraosseous ganglion is a benign subchondral cystic lesion which is histologically identical to a soft tissue ganglion. This cystic lesion is surrounded by a fibrous membrane and filled with a viscous, mucoid jelly-like material. It lacks a synovial lining and generally has no identifiable communication with the articular surface or joint space. It may be uniloculated or multiloculated. In general, there is no significant degenerative change in the adjacent joint which distinguishes this lesion from a subchondral cyst of osteoarthritis. There are two types of intraosseous ganglia: one originates from the penetration of an extraosseous ganglion into the underlying bone; the other is idiopathic. Proposed theories for the idiopathic variety include herniation of capsular and ligamentous structures into bone, and repetitive minor trauma resulting in a focal area of avascular necrosis which undergoes cystic degeneration.

Clinical Features. Intraosseous ganglia are rare lesions usually occurring between the ages of 20 and 60 years, but nearly all ages may be affected. There is a slight male predominance. Many lesions are asymptomatic and discovered incidentally during radiographic examination, although approximately 60% of patients present with pain, which may increase with exercise. The duration of the pain ranges from months to years.

Location. These juxta-articular, subchondral lesions occur more commonly in long tubular bones. The most common sites of involvement are the hip, ankle (medial malleolus), knee (proximal tibia), and carpus. The lesions are usually solitary, but multiple lesions (often bilateral and symmetrical) have been reported.

Implications. Incidental lesions need not have therapy. The most definitive treatment is curettage, and excision with bone grafting may be performed if the lesion is large. Segmental resection may be used for large lesions in a nonweight-bearing bone. The recurrence rate following any treatment is very low. These lesions may grow, which should not raise concern for a more aggressive process. Pathologic fracture has not been reported. Large lesions may induce secondary osteoarthritis.

MRI Findings. On MRI, an intraosseous ganglion appears as a well-defined oval or round subchondral lesion. The adjacent cortex may be thinned or even expanded. The lesion may be unilocular or multilocular and the size is typically 1–5 cm. It demonstrates homogeneous low to intermediate signal intensity on T1-weighted images and uniform high signal intensity with T2-weighting. The lesion may be septated. Typically, there are no associated joint changes.

Differential Diagnosis. The differential diagnosis includes other epiphyseal lesions such as subchondral cyst secondary to osteoarthritis, geode associated with rheumatoid arthritis or osteonecrosis, infection (Brodie's abscess), giant cell tumor, and chondroblastoma. If there are no associated degenerative changes in the adjacent joint, a subchondral cyst related to osteoarthritis can be excluded. The presence of osteoarthritis does not completely exclude an intraosseous ganglion, because this lesion may occasionally result in secondary osteoarthritis. If a large subchondral cystic lesion is seen in the presence of degenerative joint disease in a younger patient (less than 30), the possibility of an intraosseous ganglion with secondary osteoarthritis should be considered. An intraosseous ganglion may be distinguished from a geode related to rheumatoid arthritis or osteonecrosis by the presence or absence of associated findings of these processes. An active Brodie's abscess should be able to be differentiated based upon clinical grounds. A Brodie's abscess would be suggested by the identification of a serpiginous tract extending from the lesion; it may also contain internal debris. A giant cell tumor would not typically have signal as bright as joint fluid on T2-weighted images, as would be expected with an intraosseous ganglion. Also, plain radiographs would be helpful in this distinction because a giant cell tumor would have a nonsclerotic border, whereas an intraosseous ganglion usually has a thin sclerotic border. Chondroblastoma typically occurs in a younger age group (less than 20) than intraosseous ganglion. In addition, approximately half of chondroblastomas demonstrate calcification, which appears as hypointense foci on all pulse sequences.

References

Schagowicz F, Sainz M, Slullitel J. Juxta-articular bone cysts (intra-osseous ganglia). *JBJS* 61(B):107–116, 1979.

Pope T, Fechner R, Keats T. Intra-osseous ganglion. *Skeletal Radiol* 18:185–187, 1989.

Tanaka H, Araki Y, Yamamoto H, et al. Intraosseous ganglion. *Skeletal Radiol* 24:155–157, 1995.

Magee T, Rowedder A, Degnan G. Intraosseous ganglia of the wrist. *Radiology* 195:517–520, 1995.

A

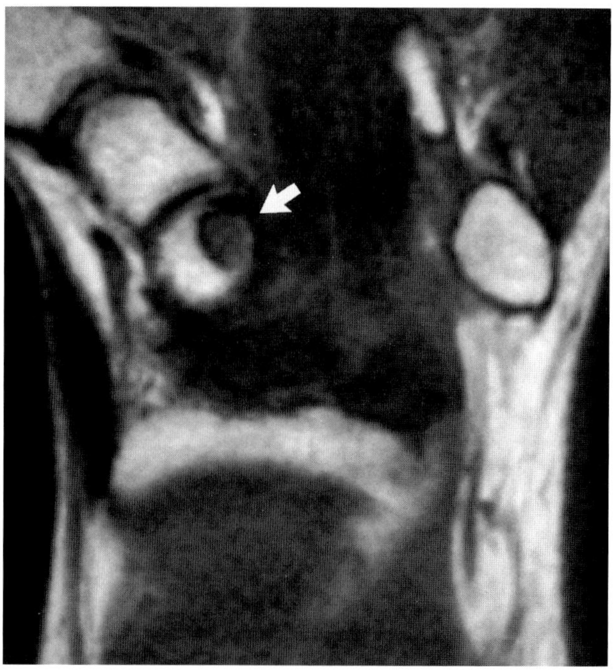

FIGURE 14.3 Intraosseous ganglion of the carpus in a 33-year-old woman. (A) Coronal T1-weighted image (550/25) demonstrates a small, round, well-marginated lesion within the distal pole of the scaphoid (arrow). The signal of the lesion is isointense to muscle.

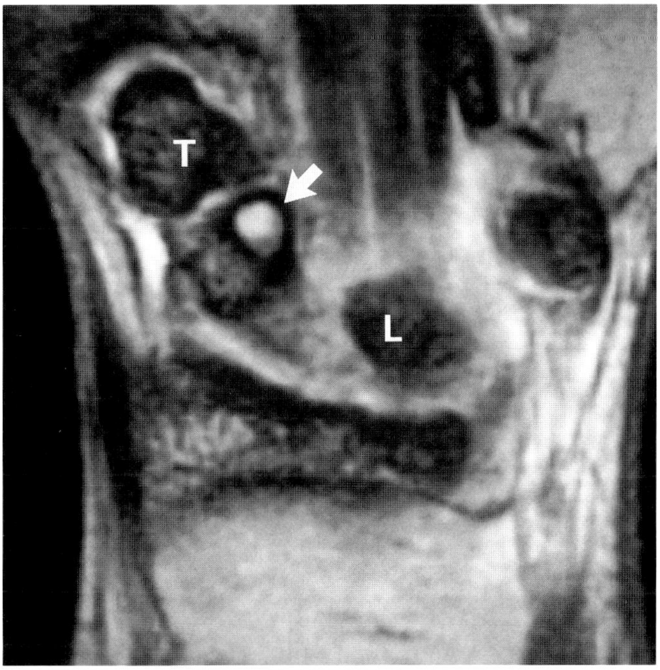

B

FIGURE 14.3 (continued) (B) Coronal MPGR image (400/20, 25 degrees) reveals bright signal intensity within the lesion (arrow). Note the absence of degenerative changes in the adjacent joint. Trapezium (T), lunate (L).

Synovial Herniation Pit

Definition. This lesion is also known as "Pitt's pit" and refers to a subcortical pit or cavity formed by the herniation of soft tissue (synovium or adjacent retinacula) through defects in the anterolateral cortex of the femoral neck. It is postulated that with excessive hyperextension of the hip, single or multiple defects/perforations develop within the anterior femoral neck cortex due to abrasive action from the overlying hip capsule. Herniation of soft tissue through these defects into the medullary cavity may then occur.

Clinical Features. Herniation pits are benign and incidental with an estimated incidence of approximately 5% in normal adults.

Location. These lesions are characteristically located in the anterior subcortical region of the proximal superior quadrant of the femoral neck, projecting 5–15 mm below the superior femoral neck margin. They may be present bilaterally but are not symmetric.

Implications. A synovial herniation pit is nearly always an incidental finding. The lesion may increase in size and possibly even grow rapidly. Although not proven, it is postulated that a herniation pit could be symptomatic in some individuals. It is also postulated that a herniation pit may weaken the cortex of the femoral neck, predisposing to hip fracture in the elderly. In general, the main importance of diagnosing this entity is not mistaking it for a more worrisome process.

MRI Findings. A synovial herniation pit appears as a well-marginated round or oval lesion in the proximal superior quadrant of the femoral neck anteriorly. It typically exhibits hypointense signal on T1-weighted images and hyperintense signal on T2-weighted sequences consistent with the presence of fluid. Occasionally, the signal intensity is low with T2-weighting corresponding to fibroconnective tissue. There is generally a thin peripheral rim of signal void on all pulse sequences representing a sclerotic border. The connection between the cavity and the cortex is best identified on axial images. These lesions are usually less than one cm in size. Uncommonly, a lobulated appearance may be seen.

Differential Diagnosis. The typical location of this lesion should suggest the diagnosis. However, the MR signal characteristics are nonspecific. Therefore, if such a lesion is identified within a symptomatic hip, plain films should be obtained and should allow differentiation from other entities which may appear similar on MRI such as stress fracture, Brodie's abscess, or osteoid osteoma. In addition, identification of an anterior connection with the cortex may help in distinguishing a herniation pit from these processes.

References

Pitt M, Graham A, Shipman J, et al. Herniation pit of the femoral neck. *AJR* 138:1115–1121, 1982.

Nokes S, Vogler J, Spritzer C, et al. Herniation pits of the femoral neck: Appearance at MR imaging. *Radiology* 172:231–234, 1989.

Crabbe J, Martel W, Matthews L. Case report. Rapid growth of femoral herniation pit. *AJR* 159:1038–1040, 1992.

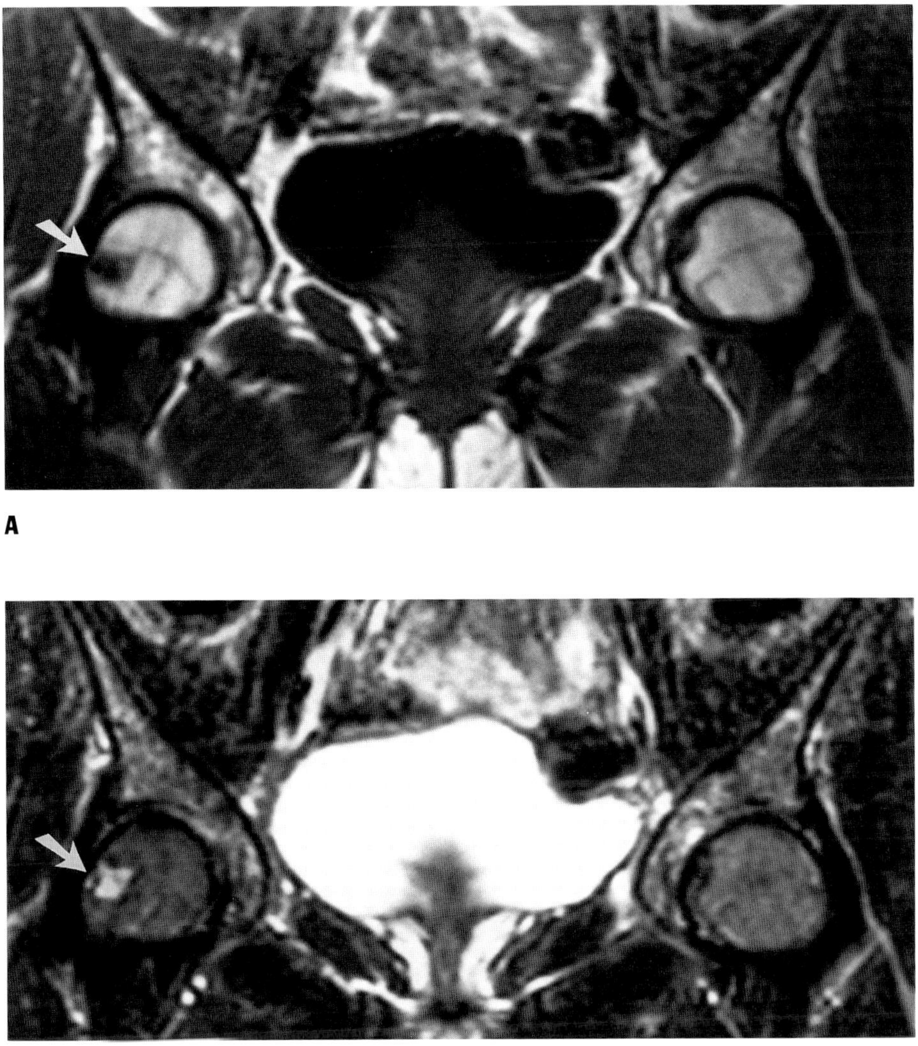

A

B

FIGURE 14.4 A 35-year-old woman with an incidental synovial herniation pit of the right hip. Coronal (A) T1-weighted (700/11) and (B) FSE T2-weighted fat suppression (3500/100) images reveal a small well-marginated lesion (arrows) in the superolateral aspect of the right femoral neck with fluid-like signal characteristics. The location and appearance are characteristic of a synovial herniation pit.

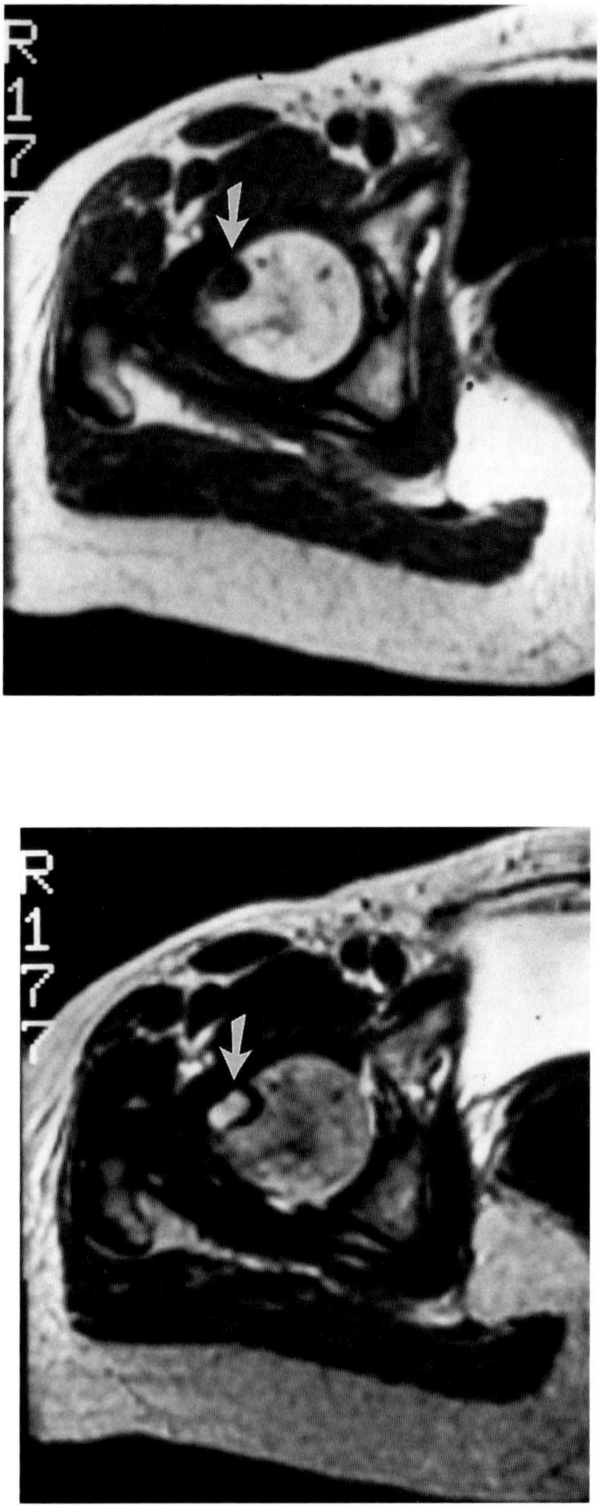

A

B

FIGURE 14.5 Synovial herniation pit in a 60-year-old woman. Axial (A) T1-weighted (600/10) and (B) FSE T2-weighted (2800/102) images reveal a small, oval, subcortical lesion in the anterolateral aspect of the proximal right femoral neck (arrows). Note the fluid-like signal characteristics and the peripheral rim of signal void.

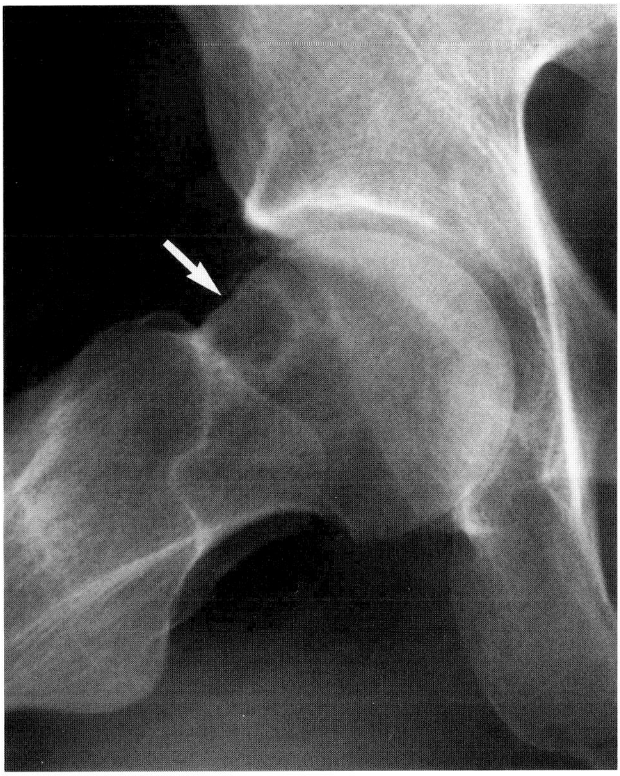

FIGURE 14.6 Classic radiographic appearance of a synovial herniation pit. Plain film of the right hip reveals a small, round, well-marginated lytic lesion with a thin sclerotic border in the anterolateral subcortical region of the proximal femoral neck (arrow).

Solitary Bone Cyst (Simple or Unicameral Bone Cyst)

Definition. Solitary bone cyst (SBC) is a fluid-filled lesion of unknown etiology. The cystic cavity is lined by a thin rim of fibrous connective tissue, rather than a true endothelial lining. The cyst is usually unilocular, but internal septations may be present. The cystic fluid is usually straw-colored, but may be bloody in the setting of prior trauma or pathologic fracture. Within the lesion, there may be a fibrin coagulum, which can undergo ossification.

Clinical Features. SBCs are relatively common lesions and the vast majority are detected in patients less than 20 years of age. These lesions are usually asymptomatic unless there is associated pathologic fracture. About half of patients present with pathologic fracture.

Location. The vast majority of lesions occur centrally within long bones, with a predilection for the metaphysis and proximal diaphysis. The most common sites are the proximal humerus, proximal femur, and proximal tibia, in order of decreasing frequency. Most of the lesions detected after the age of 20 occur in the calcaneus and ilium. In the calcaneus, these lesions invariably occur in the antero-middle region, centered below the anterior aspect of the posterior subtalar facet.

Implications. SBCs are benign lesions, but they may recur following surgery. They may be treated with curettage and bone grafting or by intralesional steroid injection. Although pathologic fracture is common with long bone lesions, this complication is very rare for SBCs of the calcaneus.

MRI Findings. A SBC would generally appear as a well-marginated oval long bone lesion in association with cortical thinning and mild bony expansion. Internal septations may be present. Typically, there would be a thin peripheral rim of very low signal intensity on all pulse sequences, corresponding to a sclerotic margin. Uncomplicated lesions would be expected to have fluid-like signal characteristics (i.e., low signal with T1-weighting and very bright signal with T2-weighting). However, this may be altered by the presence of hemorrhage related to previous trauma or pathologic fracture. Fluid-fluid levels have been reported.

Differential Diagnosis. Plain films continue to be the imaging standard for establishing the diagnosis of SBC. The "fallen fragment" sign within a pathologically-fractured lesion is virtually pathognomonic. The MRI findings of SBC are nonspecific and should be correlated with radiographs.

References

Burr B, Resnick D, Syklawer R, et al. Case report. Fluid-fluid levels in a unicameral bone cyst: CT and MR findings. *JCAT* 17:134–136, 1993.

Sanerkin N. Old fibrin coagula and their ossification in simple bone cysts. *JBJS* 61(B):194–199, 1979.

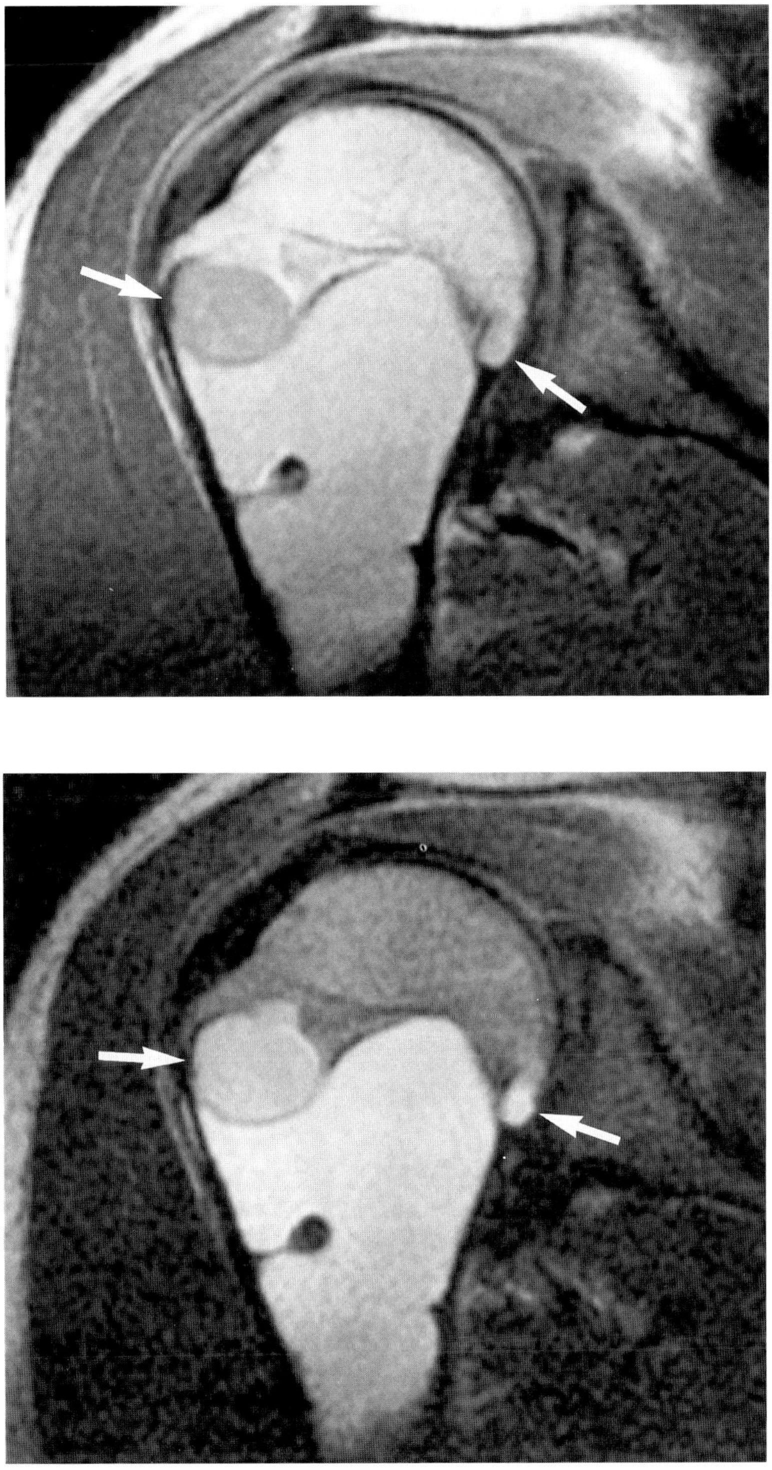

A

B

FIGURE 14.7 A 34-year-old male presented with impingement syndrome. (A), (B) Coronal dual-echo T2-weighted images (2000/30, 70) reveal a well-marginated mass involving the metaphysis and proximal diaphysis of the right humerus. Note the presence of smaller loculations (arrows) and internal septations. The main portion of the lesion exhibits homogeneously bright signal with T2-weighting.

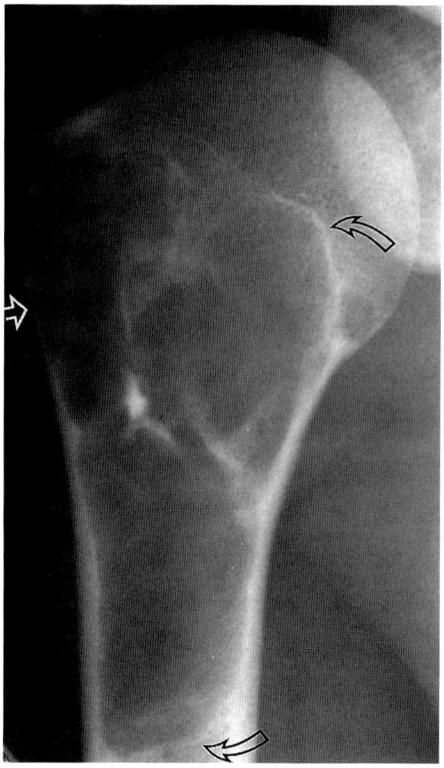

C

FIGURE 14.7 (continued) (C) AP radiograph reveals a well-marginated lytic lesion with a thin sclerotic border (curved open arrows) with some associated cortical thinning (open arrow). The appearance is characteristic of a solitary bone cyst.

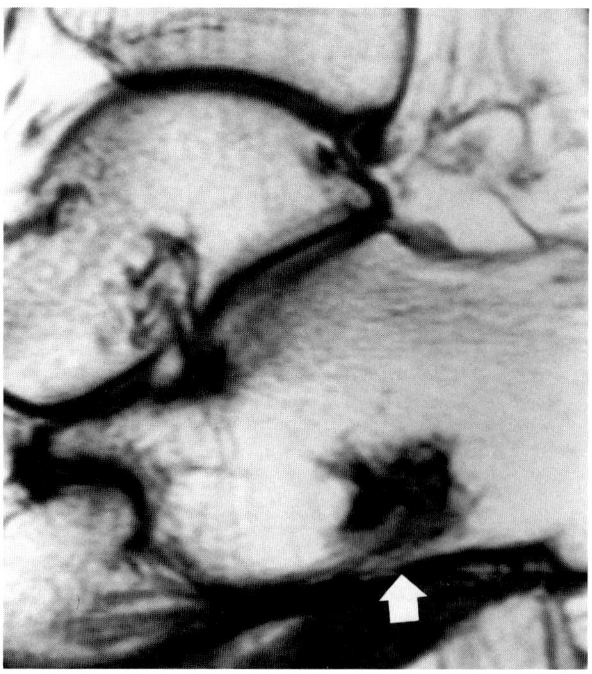

A

FIGURE 14.8 Involuting solitary bone cyst of the calcaneus in a 36-year-old man. Sagittal (A) T1-weighted and (B) FMPIR images reveal an irregular lesion within the mid-calcaneus inferiorly (arrows). The signal characteristics are similar to that of the nearby joint fluid. Irregular margins are consistent with partial healing of the lesion. (C) Additional sagittal T1-weighted image reveals fat deposition (lipidization) within the lesion (thin arrows).

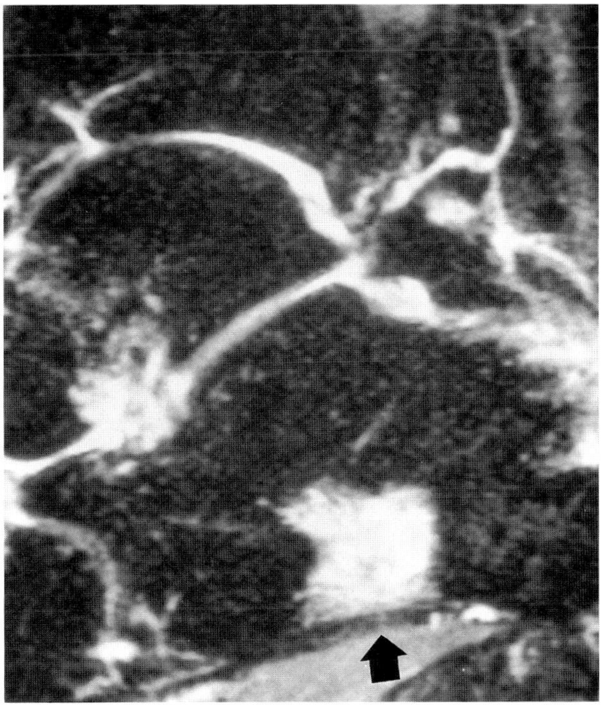

B

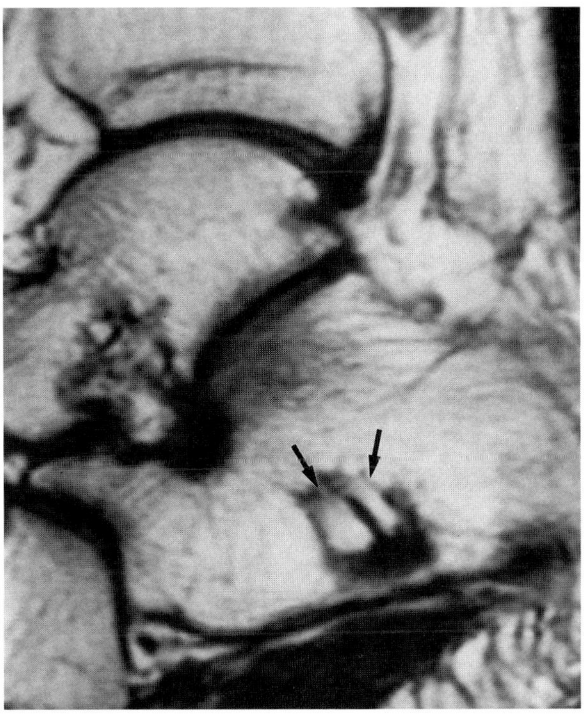

C

Intrasacral Cyst

Definition. An intrasacral cyst results from abnormal dilatation of the dural sac within the confines of the bony canal. This lesion communicates with the subarachnoid space via a thin channel. The sacral nerves often lie outside of the cyst wall pressed against the sacrum, although the sacral nerves may be embedded in the cyst wall or within the cyst itself. The pathogenesis of this lesion may be related to a congenital or acquired dural defect, which allows the herniation of meninges. Similar lesions are identified in patients with dural ectasia (neurofibromatosis, Marfan syndrome, Ehlers-Danlos syndrome).

Clinical Features. Patients usually present in the 3rd–4th decade with a history of chronic pain. Symptoms of bladder or rectal sphincter dysfunction or lower sacral nerve distribution sensory loss may be present.

Location. This lesion occurs within the sacrum in the midline.

Implications. Intrasacral cyst has been previously referred to as an "occult intrasacral meningocele", which is a misnomer. The lesion expands the sacral canal, resulting in erosion of the posterior aspect of the sacral vertebral bodies. A perineural (Tarlov) cyst is a related lesion, but it contains neural tissue and usually does not expand the sacral canal. Asymptomatic lesions should not require treatment.

MRI Findings. A well-marginated midline cystic mass is seen within the sacrum with associated expansion of the sacral canal. There is typically posterior scalloping of the sacral vertebrae. The margins of the lesion may be lobulated. The mass exhibits homogeneously low signal on T1-weighted images and markedly hyperintense and homogeneous signal intensity with T2-weighting. The signal intensity generally parallels the adjacent cerebrospinal fluid, but may also be greater than that of CSF on T2-weighted sequences.

Differential Diagnosis. The differential diagnosis includes other cyst-like masses about the sacrum including perineural (Tarlov) cyst, meningocele, and echinococcal cyst. As described above, a perineural cyst contains neural tissue and does not usually expand the sacral canal. An anterior meningocele would appear as an outpouching of the thecal sac, typically demonstrating a wide connection with the thecal sac. An echinococcal cyst typically appears multiloculated and may contain internal debris. In the appropriate clinical setting, serologic testing should be performed to exclude echinococcus.

References

Mink J. Case report 313. *Skeletal Radiol* 13:314–317, 1985.

Boukobza M, Sichez J, Rolland E, et al. MRI evaluation of sacral cysts. *J Neuroradiologie (Fr)* 20:266–271, 1993.

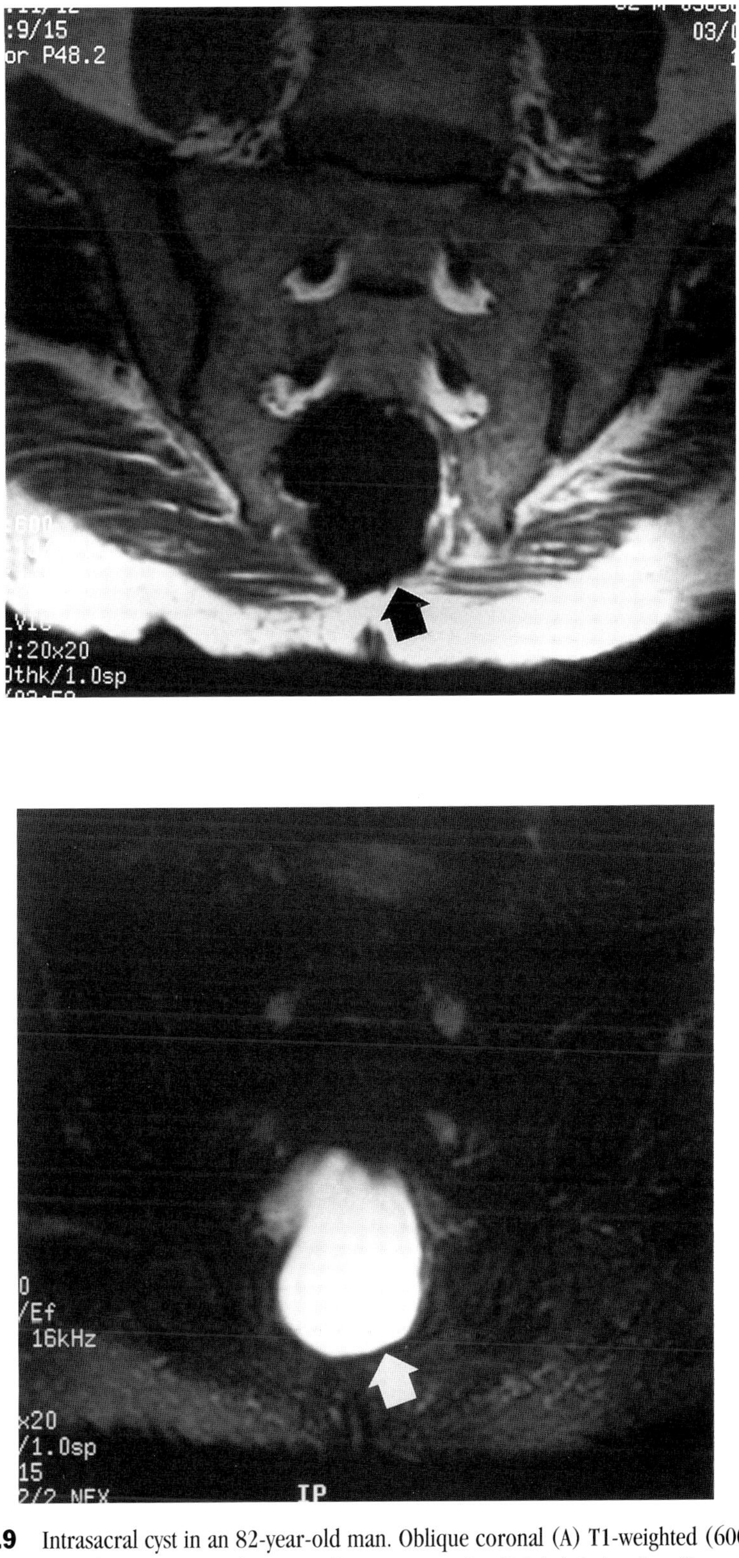

FIGURE 14.9 Intrasacral cyst in an 82-year-old man. Oblique coronal (A) T1-weighted (600/13) and (B) FSE T2-weighted fat suppression (3500/100) images reveal a slightly lobulated, well-marginated mass within the midline of the lower sacrum (arrows). There is homogeneous signal intensity which is low with T1-weighting and very bright with T2-weighting.

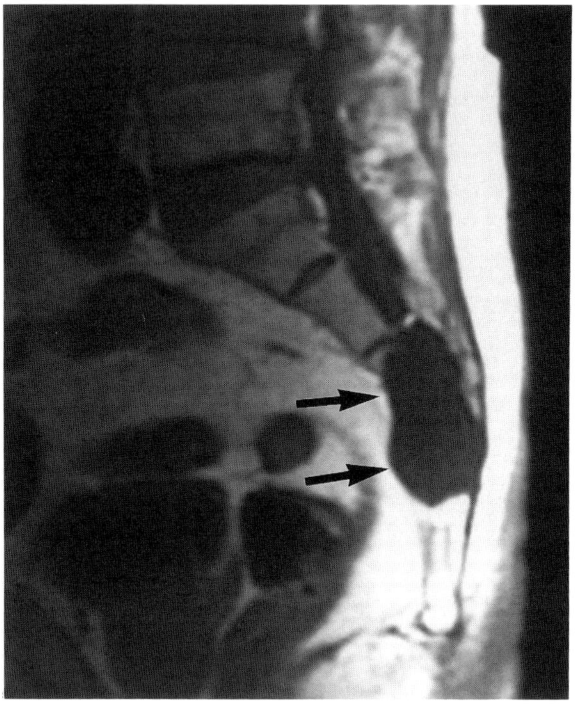

C

FIGURE 14.9 (continued) (C) Sagittal T1-weighted image (500/10) demonstrates the expansile nature of the lesion which has eroded through the S3-S5 vertebrae (thin arrows).

Anterior Sacral Meningocele

Definition. An anterior sacral meningocele is a congenital form of spinal dysraphism in which there is herniation of meninges through a sacral defect, which is typically unilateral and "scimitar-shaped".

Clinical Features. Anterior sacral meningocele is a rare anomaly which may be asymptomatic or present with nonspecific symptoms such as constipation, urinary frequency, or gynecologic abnormalities. Occasionally, headaches may occur (often associated with Valsalva maneuver) as a result of differential cerebrospinal fluid pressures between the meningocele and the subarachnoid space. Rarely, patients will complain of low back pain and radiculopathy secondary to sacral nerve root compression. Symptomatic lesions are usually recognized in the 2nd and 3rd decades of life. Females are more commonly affected. This entity may be sporadic, familial (sex-linked dominant), or may occur in association with anorectal abnormalities. The diagnosis can often be made by rectal or vaginal examination as a fixed or mobile mass.

Location. These lesions arise from the ventral thecal sac and extend through the sacrum (usually through a unilateral defect) into the presacral space.

Implications. The true natural history of anterior sacral meningoceles is unknown since many of these lesions are asymptomatic and remain undetected. However, patients can be at significant risk. Meningitis is the most serious complication and results from erosion of the lesion into the rectum. These lesions are not known to regress spontaneously. Ten to nineteen percent of cases have associated tumors including lipomas, dermoid tumors, and teratomas. Reported mortality rates for patients treated without surgery range from 19 to 30%. Surgery is the treatment of choice and consists of ligation of the communication between the thecal sac and the meningocele. MR imaging is the modality of choice for preoperative planning and provides useful information for deciding upon a surgical approach. An anterior approach should only be used if the communication is large or in the presence of an associated tumor. MRI also provides useful preoperative information regarding the level and size of the lesion.

MRI Findings. Anterior sacral meningoceles appear as well-marginated, variable-sized masses. These lesions communicate with the ventral thecal sac via a neck or stalk. They extend anteriorly through an associated sacral defect (typically unilateral) into the presacral space. These lesions typically demonstrate homogeneous low signal on T1-weighted images and very bright homogeneous signal intensity with T2-weighting. The signal intensity should parallel adjacent cerebrospinal fluid on all pulse sequences. Internal septations may be present.

Differential Diagnosis. Plain radiographs of the sacrum will reveal the pathognomonic "scimitar sacrum sign" in about half of the cases. These lesions have similar signal characteristics to Tarlov (perineural) cysts and intrasacral cysts. Tarlov cysts do not typically extend through the sacrum into the presacral space. Intrasacral cysts should be distinguishable because they are generally midline and connect with the subarachnoid space via a thin channel (versus the typically wide connection of an anterior sacral meningocele). An echinococcal cyst or sacral neoplasms such as giant cell tumor, chordoma, and plasmacytoma could exhibit similar signal characteristics, but would not communicate with the thecal sac.

References

Lee K, Gower D, McWhorter J, et al. The role of MR imaging in the diagnosis and treatment of anterior sacral meningocele. Report of two cases. *J Neurosurg* 69:628–631, 1988.

McGuire R, Metcalf J, Amundson G, et al. Anterior sacral meningocele. Case report and review of the literature. *Spine* 15:612–614, 1990.

Martin B, Boyer de Latour F. Case report. MR imaging of anterior sacral meningocele. *JCAT* 12:166–167, 1988.

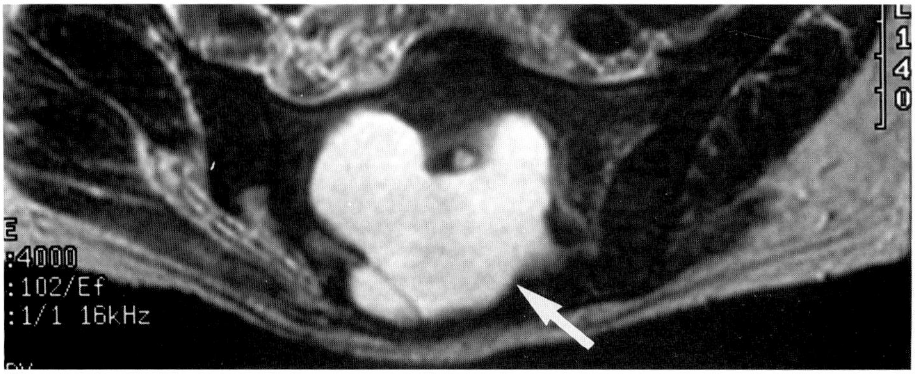

A

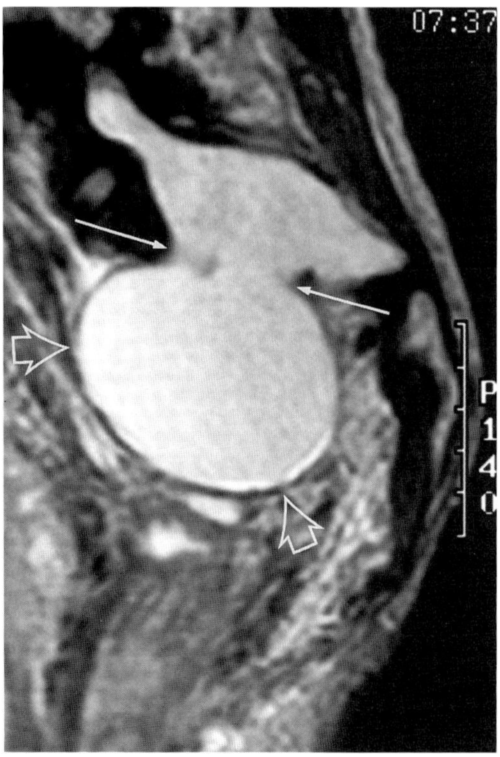

B

FIGURE 14.10 Anterior sacral meningocele in a 25-year-old woman with neurofibromatosis. (A) Axial FSE T2-weighted image (4000/102) reveals a lobulated mass (arrow) within the sacrum which has uniformly bright signal intensity. (B) Sagittal FSE T2-weighted image (3000/102) demonstrates extension of the lesion through the sacrum into the presacral space (open arrows). The lesion communicates with the thecal sac via a large neck (thin arrows). Note that the signal is isointense with cerebrospinal fluid.

15 Miscellaneous Benign Lesions

Aneurysmal Bone Cyst

Definition. Aneurysmal bone cysts (ABCs) are composed of blood-filled, anastomosing, cavernous spaces which are separated by thin cyst-like walls. The etiology is unknown and controversial. Some authors regard ABC as a secondary vascular phenomenon superimposed on a pre-existing lesion. The underlying tumor initiates an intraosseous arteriovenous malformation and creates an ABC via hemodynamic forces. Other investigators prefer classifying the lesions as primary (in which no pre-existing lesion is identified) and secondary (identifiable precursor). Overall, a pre-existing lesion can be identified in approximately 1/3 of cases. The most common precursor is giant cell tumor with additional lesions including osteoblastoma, chondroblastoma, fibrous dysplasia, nonossifying fibroma, chondromyxoid fibroma, solitary bone cyst, eosinophilic granuloma, osteosarcoma, trauma, fibrosarcoma, and metastasis.

Clinical Features. The vast majority of ABCs occur between the ages of 5 and 20. Females are affected slightly more than males. Most patients present with pain and swelling of less than six months duration. Pathologic fracture is not uncommon. Spinal lesions may be associated with scoliosis, kyphosis, or neurologic symptoms.

Location. More than half of aneurysmal bone cysts occur in long bones, where the lesion is usually eccentric and metaphyseal. The lesion may be epiphyseal. Spine involvement accounts for approximately 1/4 of cases. There is a predilection for the posterior vertebral elements, although extension into the vertebral body is common. The lesions may also be cortically or juxtacortically based. Spine lesions may involve contiguous vertebra. The pelvis is the most common flat bone location.

Implications. Treatment is directed at the pre-existing lesion if one is identified. If no precursor lesion is identified, lesions are usually treated with curettage and bone grafting. It is important to remove the entire lesion or as much as possible. Recurrence is seen in 10–44% of cases. Recently, embolotherapy has proven successful in managing these lesions, either alone or in combination with surgery.

MRI Findings. The MR appearance of ABC depends on the stage at which the lesion is imaged. Four radiologic stages have been described: initial, active, stabilization, and healing. Initially, the lesion is not expansile. During the active growth phase, the lesion becomes expansile. This is followed by a period of stabilization. Finally, healing occurs with sclerosis (calcification, ossification) of the lesion. Typically, MRI demonstrates an expansile, lobulated mass surrounded by a thin, well-defined low signal intensity rim, thought to represent fibrous tissue. Internal septa are often seen and adjacent loculations may have markedly differing signal characteristics. Fluid-fluid levels may also be seen within the lesion corresponding to various degraded blood products. Typically, the signal intensity of the fluid increases with T2-weighting. Bright signal on T1-weighted images corresponds to the presence of methemoglobin. Soft tissue extension demonstrates a smooth, sharp, well-defined interface, which is indicative of an intact periosteum.

Differential Diagnosis. For a young patient in the appropriate clinical setting, the identification of an expansile, well-defined, lobulated mass bordered by a thin low signal intensity rim and containing internal septations and fluid-fluid levels is highly suggestive of an aneurysmal bone cyst. The MRI should be correlated with plain films. The identification of fluid-fluid levels is not specific for aneurysmal bone cyst and has been described in numerous other lesions including telangiectatic osteosarcoma, chondroblastoma, giant cell tumor, fibrous dysplasia, simple bone cyst, malignant fibrous histiocytoma, conventional osteosarcoma, and some soft tissue neoplasms.

References

Kransdorf M, Sweet D. Aneurysmal bone cyst: Concept, controversy, clinical presentation, and imaging. *AJR* 164:573–580, 1995.

Munk P, Helms C, Holt RG, et al. MR imaging of aneurysmal bone cyst. *AJR* 153:99–101, 1989.

Tsai J, Dalinka M, Fallon M, et al. Fluid-fluid level: A nonspecific finding in tumors of bone and soft tissue. *Radiology* 175:779–782, 1990.

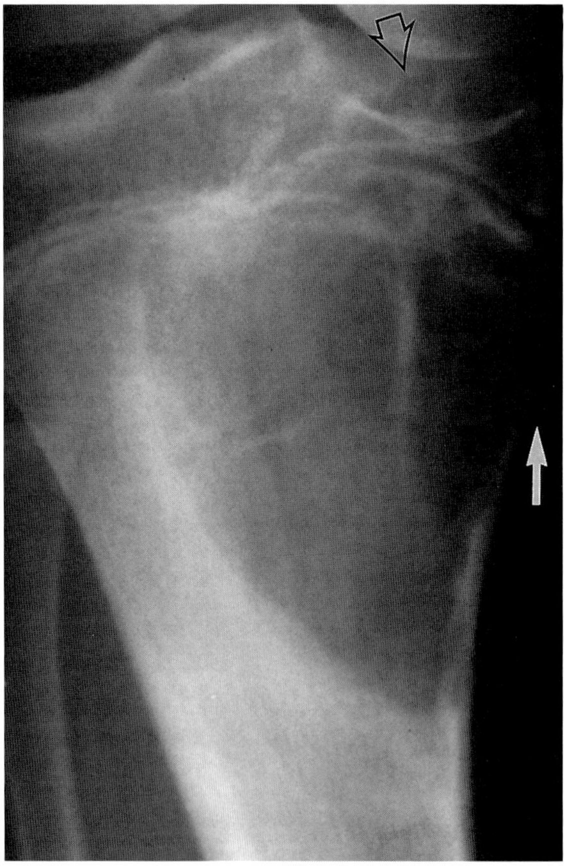

A

Figure 15.1 Aneurysmal bone cyst of the proximal tibia in an 11-year-old girl who presented with a one year history of pain following a minor injury. (A) AP radiograph shows a well-marginated, eccentric, lytic lesion within the medial metaphysis of the proximal tibia. The lesion is minimally expansile (arrow) and appears to extend into the epiphysis (open arrow).

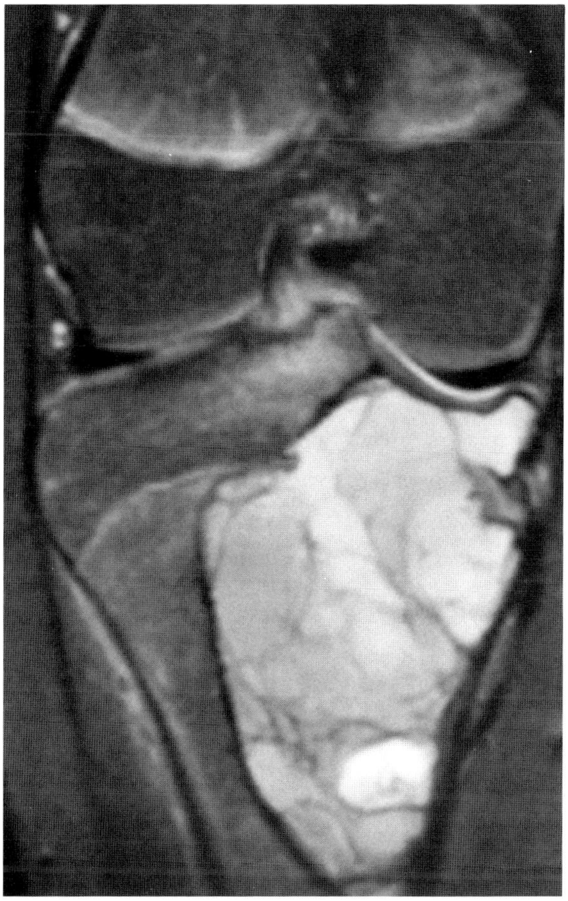

B

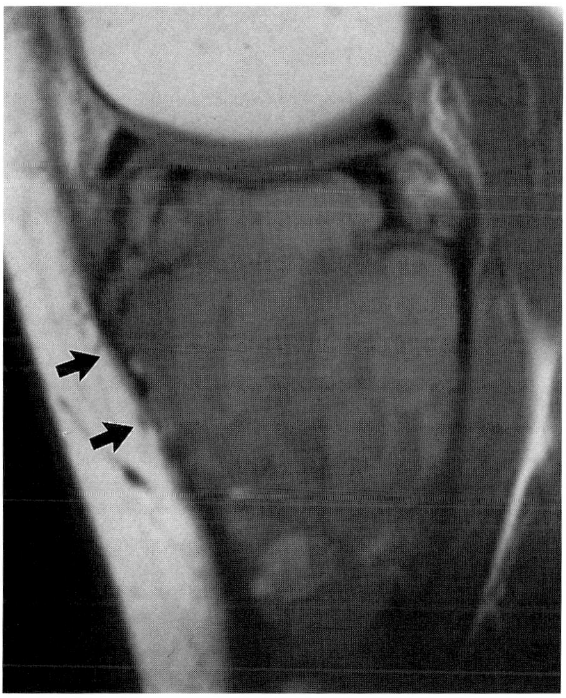

C

FIGURE 15.1 (continued) (B) Coronal FSE T2-weighted fat suppression image gives superior delineation of the epiphyseal extension. The lesion is multiloculated and contains numerous internal septations. There is a peripheral rim of very low signal intensity. Sagittal (C) T1-weighted and

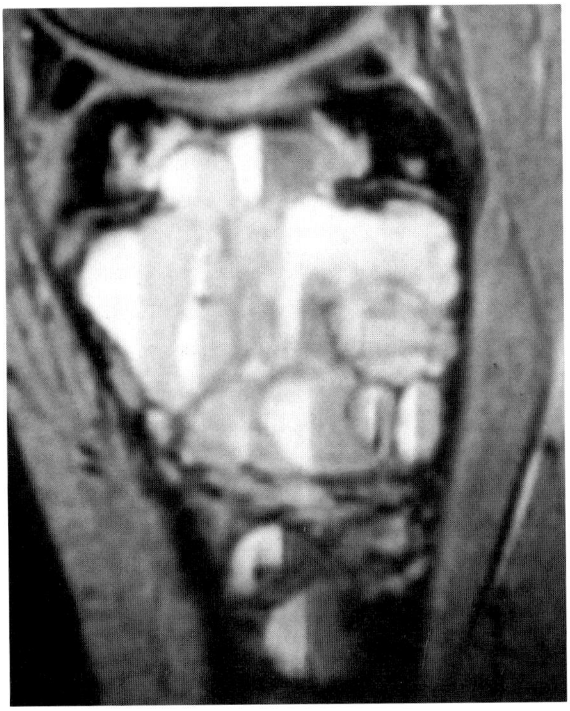

D

FIGURE 15.1 (continued) (D) gradient-recalled echo images reveal numerous fluid-fluid levels and variable signal intensity consistent with various degraded blood products. Note the cortical thinning anteriorly (short arrows).

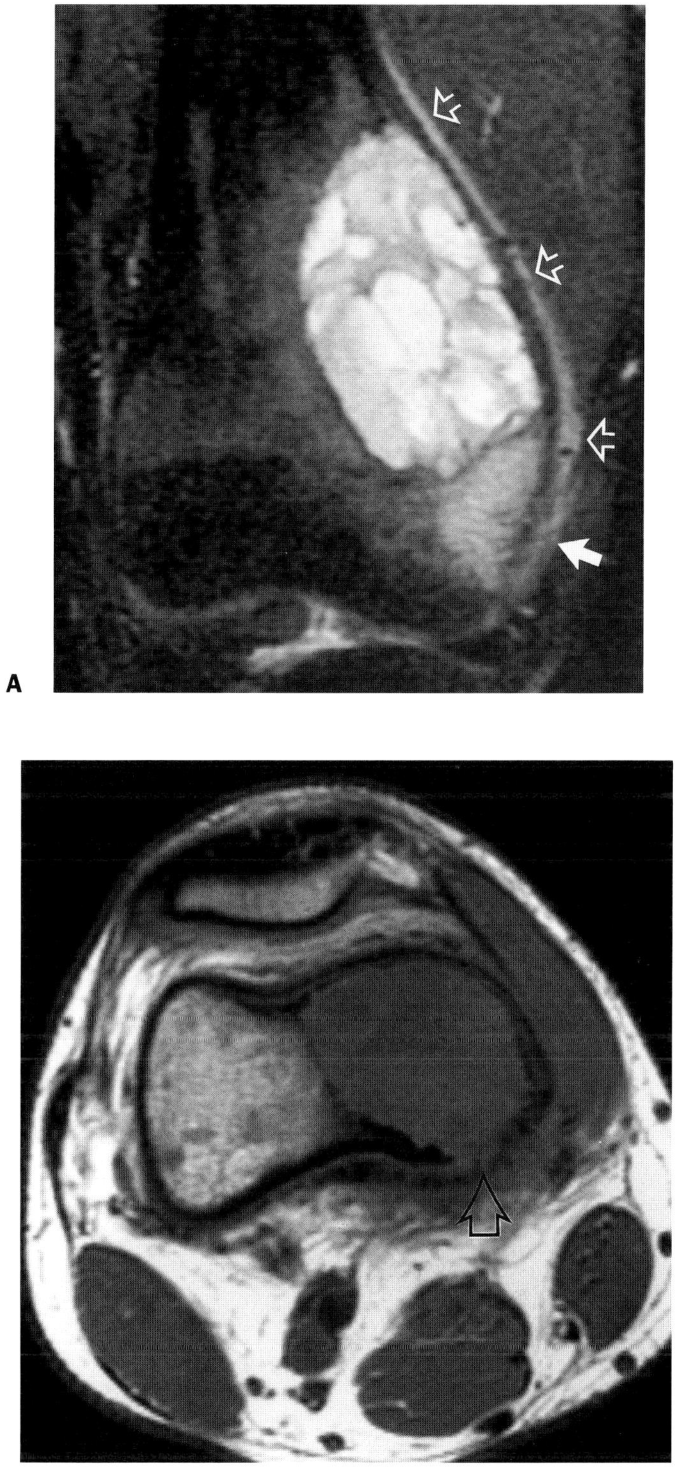

FIGURE 15.2 An 18-year-old male with an aneurysmal bone cyst of the distal femur. (A) Coronal FMPIR image (4000/28, TI-150) reveals a well-marginated, multiloculated lesion within the medial metaphysis of the distal femur. There is associated edema within the epiphysis (arrow) and extending along the periosteal surface (open arrows). Axial (B) T1-weighted (800/13) and

(continued)

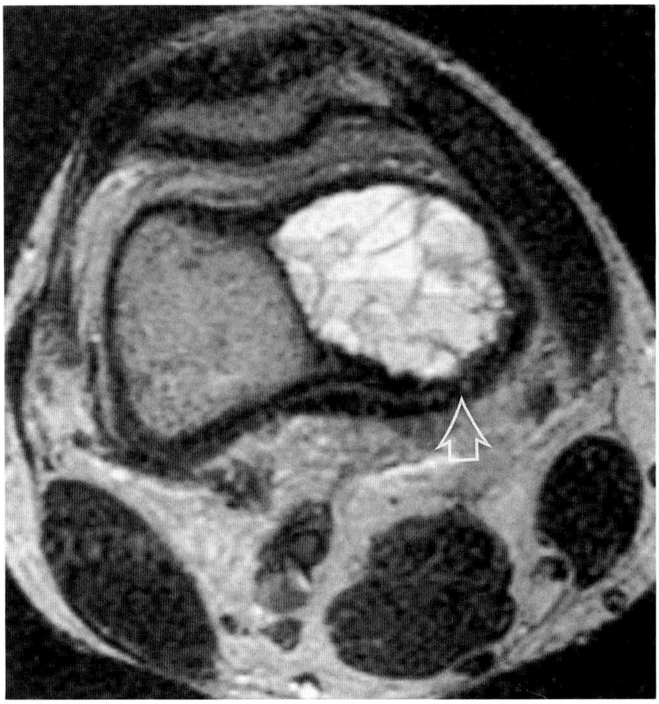

C

Figure 15.2 (continued) (C) T2-weighted (2200/80) images demonstrate numerous fluid-fluid levels. There is a peripheral rim of very low signal intensity. Note extension of the lesion through the cortex (large open arrows).

Giant Cell Tumor

Definition. Giant cell tumors (GCTs) are locally aggressive lesions composed of giant cells, stromal cells, and connective tissue. These lesions often undergo intratumoral hemorrhage and may contain hemosiderin or fluid-filled cyst-like cavities as a result of previous hemorrhage.

Clinical Features. Nearly all GCTs are discovered beyond skeletal maturity, with a peak incidence of 20–40 years of age. The vast majority of lesions present with pain. Pathologic fracture is present in about 10% of cases.

Location. GCTs have a predilection for long tubular bones, especially the distal femur and proximal tibia, followed by the distal radius and proximal humerus ("around the knee, away from the elbow"). The most common flat bone location is the sacrum. In long bones, nearly all lesions abut an articular surface. Typically, the lesion involves both the epiphysis and metaphysis. GCTs are classically eccentrically positioned within a long bone, although this can be difficult to assess with large lesions.

Implications. It is not possible to distinguish between benign and malignant GCTs radiographically or histologically. About 15% of GCTs are considered malignant and may have pulmonary metastasis. Most malignant GCTs occur following radiation therapy, which should be avoided. The recurrence rate following curettage and bone grafting is about 50%, but is much lower following en bloc resection with allograft. If en bloc resection is not preferred, curettage can be combined with cryosurgery to improve the local recurrence rate. There is an association of solitary or multicentric GCTs occurring as an uncommon complication of Paget's disease.

MRI Findings. The MR examination should be interpreted in the presence of corresponding plain films. GCTs exhibit nonspecific signal characteristics. The lesions are often large (greater than 3 cm) at the time of presentation and typically appear well-marginated. On T1-weighted images, these lesions tend to exhibit fairly homogeneous low or intermediate signal intensity. Foci of bright signal intensity on T1-weighted images have also been described and presumably correspond to methemoglobin. GCTs tend to appear heterogeneous with T2-weighting, containing areas of low, intermediate, and high signal intensity. As a result of previous intratumoral hemorrhage, hemosiderin or fluid-filled cyst-like areas may be present within the lesion. The cyst-like areas would exhibit hypointense signal with T1-weighting and bright signal intensity with T2-weighting. Deposits of hemosiderin would exhibit markedly hypointense signal (signal void) on all pulse sequences which would become accentuated on gradient-recalled echo images due to magnetic susceptibility. These tumors may be associated with prominent soft tissue extension and cortical bone destruction. The vast majority of GCTs have a nonsclerotic border on radiographs. A minority of cases may possess a faintly sclerotic border which appears on MRI as a thin peripheral rim of very low signal intensity (similar to cortical bone) on all pulse sequences.

Differential Diagnosis. The MRI findings of GCT are nonspecific. The classic radiographic appearance of GCT is that of a purely lytic, eccentric, expansile, subarticular long bone lesion with a well-defined, nonsclerotic border in a patient with closed epiphyses.

References

Tehranzadeh J, Murphy B, Mnaymneh W. Giant cell tumor of the proximal tibia: MR and CT appearance. *JCAT* 13:282–286, 1989.

Herman S, Mesgarzadeh M, Bonakdarpour A, et al. The role of magnetic resonance imaging in giant cell tumor of bone. *Skeletal Radiol* 16:635–643, 1987.

Aoki J, Tanikawa H, Ishii K, et al. MR findings indicative of hemosiderin in giant-cell tumor of bone: Frequency, cause, and diagnostic significance. *AJR* 166:145–148, 1996.

Aoki J, Moriya K, Yamashita K, et al. Giant cell tumors of bone containing large amounts of hemosiderin: MR-pathologic correlation. *JCAT* 15:1024–1027, 1991.

Potter H, Schneider R, Ghelman B, et al. Multiple giant cell tumors and Paget's disease of bone: Radiographic and clinical correlations. *Radiology* 180:261–264, 1991.

A

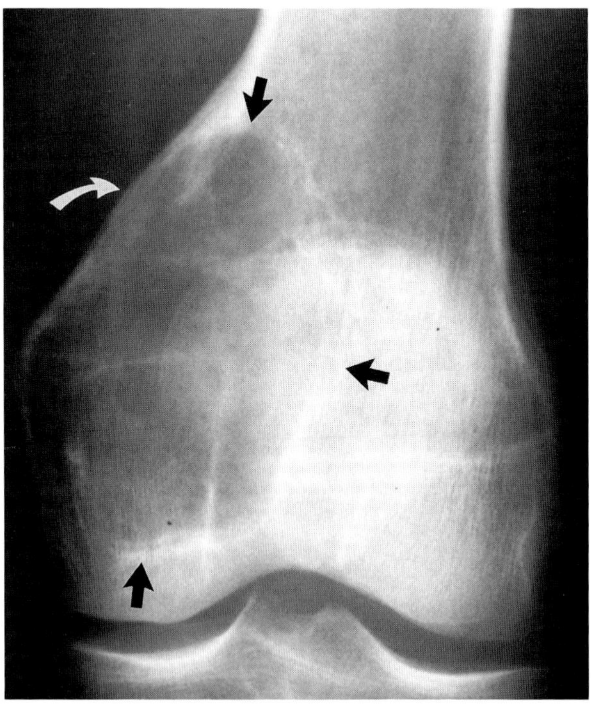

FIGURE 15.3 A 54-year-old male presented with a three-year history of intermittent pain above the knee anteromedially. Histopathologic examination revealed giant cell tumor containing numerous areas of hemosiderin. (A) AP radiograph shows a well-marginated, lytic, slightly expansile lesion involving the medial metaphysis and epiphysis of the distal femur. The lesion is surrounded by a partially nonsclerotic and faintly sclerotic border (arrows). Note the thinned cortex (curved arrow).

B

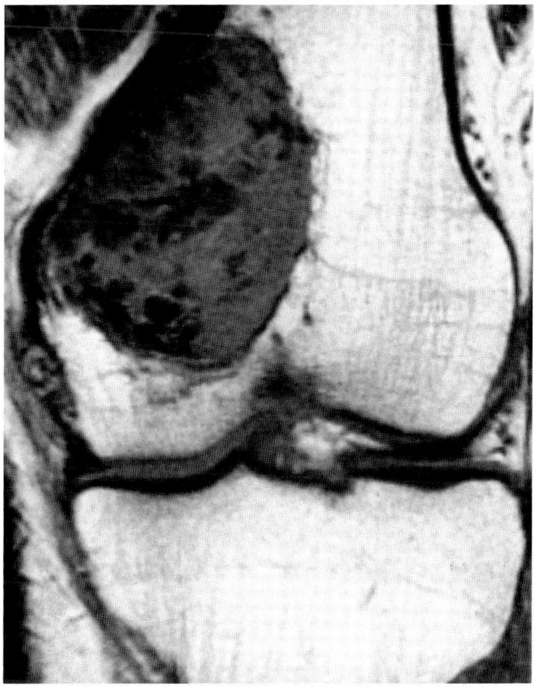

C

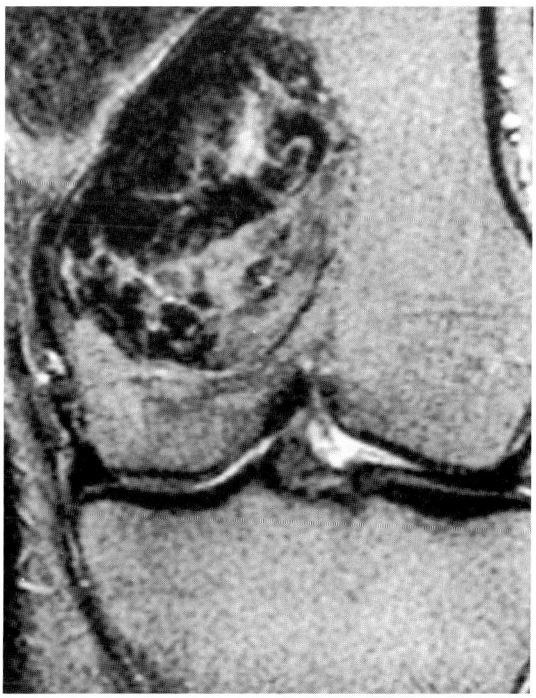

FIGURE 15.3 (continued) Coronal (B) T1-weighted (1000/20) and (C) T2-weighted (2067/70) images reveal that the lesion exhibits heterogeneous, predominantly low signal intensity on both sequences. The areas of markedly low signal intensity likely correspond to the extensive hemosiderin present microscopically.

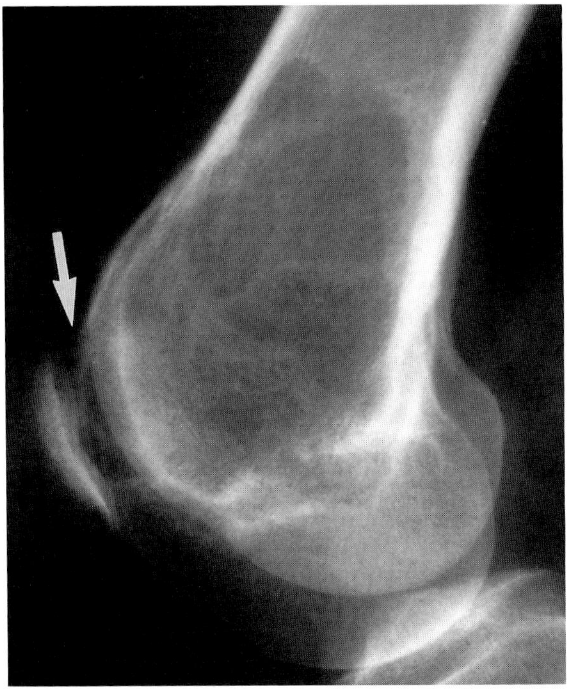

D

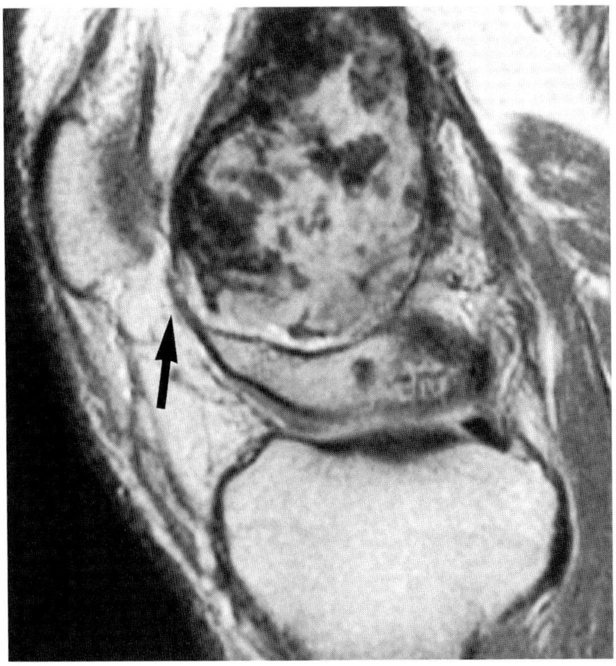

E

FIGURE 15.3 (continued) (D) Lateral radiograph and (E) sagittal proton density image (2367/25) demonstrate that the lesion abuts the patellofemoral articular surface (long arrows).

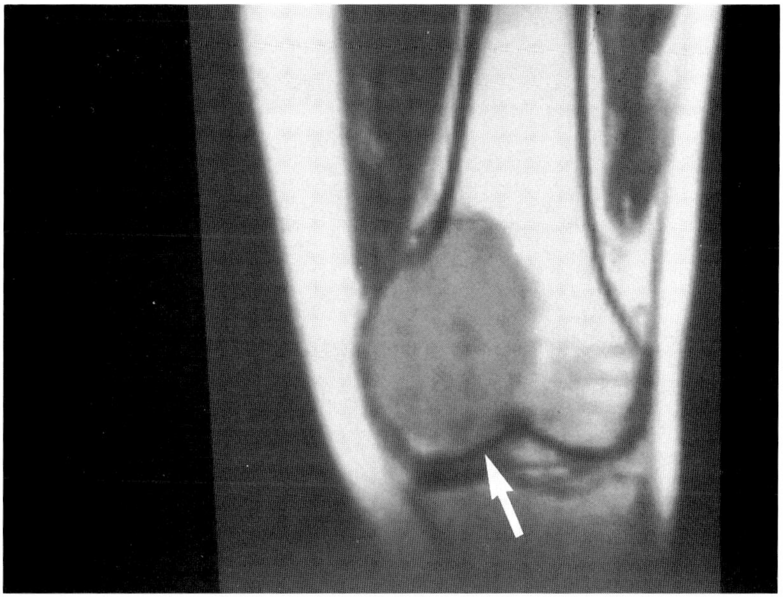

FIGURE 15.4 Giant cell tumor of the distal femur in a 40-year-old male. Coronal T1-weighted image demonstrates an eccentric, expansile lesion within the distal femoral metaphysis and epiphysis with extension into the subarticular region (arrow). Note the intermediate signal intensity of the lesion.

A

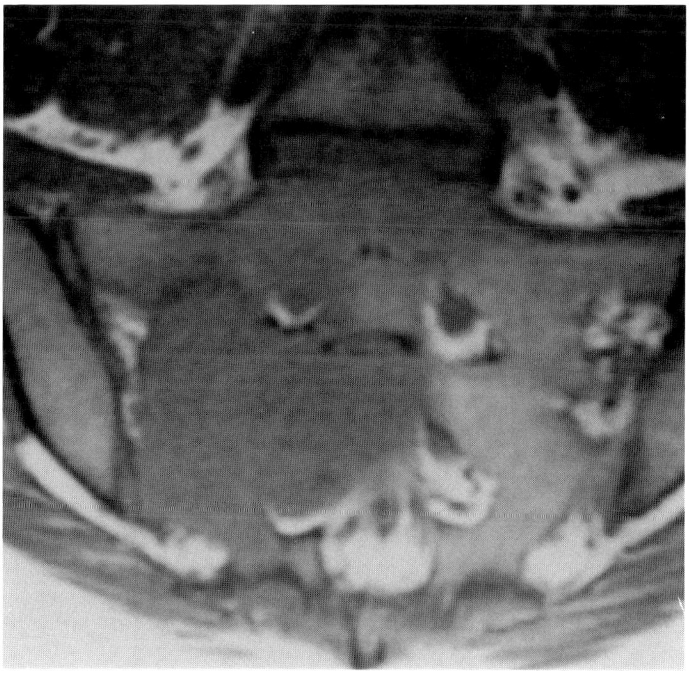

FIGURE 15.5 Giant cell tumor of the sacrum in a 22-year-old woman who presented with low back and right leg pain. (A) Oblique coronal T1-weighted image (600/14) demonstrates a lobulated mass within the right sacrum which exhibits homogeneous intermediate signal intensity. There is involvement of the right S2 nerve.

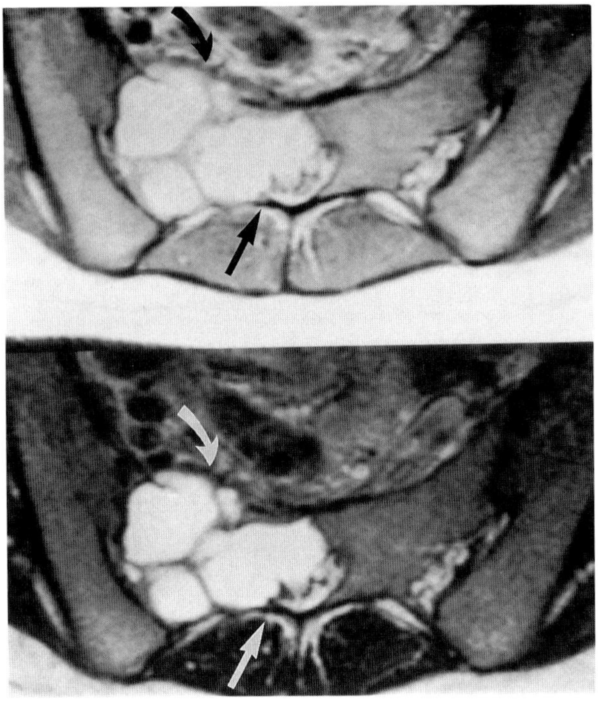

B

C

FIGURE 15.5 (continued) (B), (C) Axial FSE dual-echo T2-weighted images (4600/16, 96) reveal homogeneously bright signal intensity within the multiloculated mass. The lesion is mildly expansile and extends into the spinal canal (arrows). Note extension through the cortex anteriorly (curved arrows).

Eosinophilic Granuloma (Langerhans Cell Histiocytosis)

Definition. Langerhans cell histiocytosis (LCH), previously known as histiocytosis X, is a spectrum of disease characterized by abnormal proliferation of histiocytes and granuloma formation. The distinctive histopathologic feature of the disease is the Langerhans cell, which is a unique histiocyte. The exact cause and pathogenesis of LCH are unknown, but abnormal immune regulation appears to be an important etiologic factor. The histopathologic features of LCH vary with the stage of the disease. In the early phases of the disease, numerous Langerhans and inflammatory cells (eosinophils, lymphocytes, neutrophils) are present, often with associated hemorrhage and necrosis. In later phases, the number of cells progressively decrease and the lesions become more fibrous with increased amounts of collagen. The current classification of LCH encompasses the three diseases formerly known as histiocytosis X, namely eosinophilic granuloma (EG), Hand-Schuller-Christian (HSC), and Letterer-Siwe (LS). EG is the most common of these entities and continues to be a familiar and popular term among radiologists.

Clinical Features. LCH is an uncommon disease occurring almost exclusively in children and young adults with an incidence of 0.5–5 per one million children per year in the United States. There is a slight male predominance (2:1) and non-Caucasians are rarely affected. EG is the localized form of LCH and accounts for 70% of all cases. EG accounts for less than 1% of all biopsied primary osseous lesions. Approximately 90% of patients are 5–15 years old at presentation. EG typically presents with pain, tenderness, and swelling and/or mass lesion. Pathologic fracture may occur. The clinical presentation may mimic osteomyelitis or may be confused with Ewing's sarcoma. EG is limited to bone and/or lung involvement. Solitary or multiple skeletal lesions may be present. The chronic, recurrent form of LCH (20% of cases) is HSC, which is characterized by multifocal osseous lesions and extraskeletal involvement of lymph nodes, skin, and abdominal organs. HSC usually affects children aged 1–5. About 10–15% of patients with HSC have the classic triad of diabetes insipidus, exophthalmos, and destructive bone (skull) lesions. LS is the acute, disseminated form of LCH (10% of cases), usually affecting children less than 2 years of age. It is characterized by rapidly disseminating multisystem involvement.

Location. EG may occur in any bone, although there is a predilection for flat bones. Greater than half of all skeletal lesions occur in the skull (most frequent), ribs, pelvis, and mandible. The clavicle and scapula are occasionally involved. About 30% of lesions occur in long bones, nearly always involving the diaphysis or metaphysis. The most common long bone locations are the femur, humerus, and tibia, in order of decreasing frequency. EG of the spine typically affects the vertebral body, involving the thoracic, lumbar, and cervical regions in order of decreasing incidence. Solitary EG occurs twice as commonly as multifocal EG.

Implications. Treatment options vary with the extent and site of disease and include observation, surgery (curettage, excision), radiation, chemotherapy, intraosseous steroid administration, and a combination of these methods. The prognosis is primarily dependent on the age at presentation and disease extent. Younger patients (less than 2 years old) and those with multiorgan involvement tend to have the poorest prognosis. Patients with EG limited to unifocal or multifocal skeletal involvement generally require minimal therapy and have an excellent prognosis. Lesions may spontaneously heal. Localized lesions have also been managed with excision or curettage with a high degree of success. HSC is usually associated with high morbidity and is fatal in about 15% of those with multiorgan involvement. LS has the poorest prognosis and tends to have a rapidly progressive course resulting in death within 1 to 2 years. The treatment of the acute and chronic disseminated forms of LCH (LS, HSC) remains controversial. It is important to note that the false-negative rate of bone scintigraphy with EG is about 35%. Therefore, a skeletal survey and bone scan should be considered complimentary studies in the evaluation of EG.

MRI Findings. Similar to the histopathologic and radiographic findings, the MRI manifestations vary with the stage of the disease process. Radiographically, early lesions appear lytic and aggressive with permeative destruction, poorly-defined margins, and lamellated periosteal reaction. Accordingly, with MR imaging, early EG lesions typically appear as areas of low to intermediate signal intensity (hypo- to hyperintense to muscle, but hypointense to fat) on T1-weighted images with high signal intensity (iso- or hyperintense to fat) on T2-weighted sequences. The signal intensity tends to be heterogeneous on T2-weighted sequences. Early lesions are typically surrounded by ill-defined areas of hypointensity with T1-weighting and corresponding hyperintensity with T2-weighting in the adjacent bone marrow and soft tissues, corresponding to reactive edema and inflammation. The soft tissue component may be in the form of a focal mass. The size of the soft tissue mass has been shown to be proportional to disease activity. Both intraosseous and extraosseous components exhibit marked enhancement following gadolinium administration. Lesions may be round, oval, multilobular, or dumbbell-shaped. Solitary EG lesions tend to be 1–15 cm in size, but lesions as large as 25 cm may be present in those with disseminated forms of the disease. Endosteal scalloping or cortical expansion may be present. In the later stages of EG, lesions appear more benign with well-defined margins and thick or absent periosteal reaction. On plain films, sclerotic borders may be present. On MRI, a well-defined peripheral rim of low signal (on T1, T2, and STIR sequences), presumably corresponding to sclerosis, has been suggested as a sign of lesion healing. Late stage lesions would tend not to have surrounding edema. EG of the spine classically presents with vertebral collapse (vertebra plana). The collapsed vertebrae exhibit low signal intensity with T1-weighting and high signal intensity with T2-weighting. Associated changes in the paravertebral soft tissues may reflect reactive edema or hematoma.

Differential Diagnosis. The MRI findings of EG are nonspecific and should be interpreted in the presence of corresponding radiographs. The differential diagnosis of EG depends on the stage of the disease as well as the age of the patient. The differential diagnosis of an early, aggressive lesion with soft tissue extension includes osteomyelitis, Ewing's sarcoma, osteosarcoma, and lymphoma. EG may be associated with a bony sequestrum, which is more reliably diagnosed with radiographs or CT than with MRI. Other lesions which may have a sequestrum include osteomyelitis, fibrosarcoma, malignant fibrous histiocytoma, desmoplastic fibroma, lymphoma, and osteoid osteoma (pseudosequestrum).

References

Stull M, Kransdorf M, Devaney K. Langerhans cell histiocytosis of bone. *RadioGraphics* 12:801–823, 1992.

Beltran J, Aparisi F, Bonmati L, et al. Eosinophilic granuloma: MRI manifestations. *Skeletal Radiol* 22:157–161, 1993.

De Schepper A, Ramon F, Van Mark E. MR imaging of eosinophilic granuloma: Report of 11 cases. *Skeletal Radiol* 22:163–166, 1993.

Monroc M, Ducou le Pointe H, Haddad S, et al. Soft tissue signal abnormality associated with eosinophilic granuloma. Correlation of MR imaging with pathologic findings. *Pediat Radiol* 24:328–332, 1994.

Davies A, Pikoulas C, Griffith J. MRI of eosinophilic granuloma. *Eur J Radiol* 18:205–209, 1994.

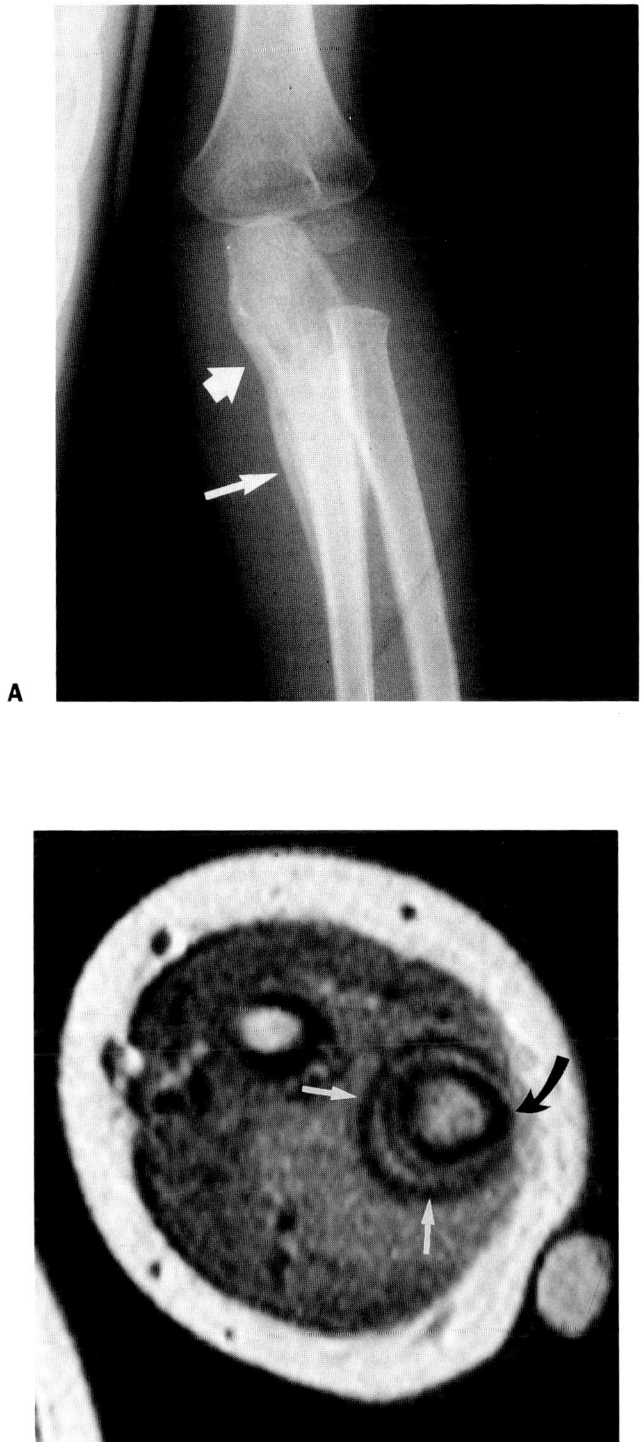

FIGURE 15.6 A 2 1/2-year-old child presented with pain, tenderness, and swelling of the proximal left forearm. (A) AP radiograph reveals a permeative lesion with ill-defined margins involving the metaphysis and proximal diaphysis of the ulna (wide arrow). There is lamellated periosteal reaction (arrow). (B), (C) Axial dual-echo T2-weighted images (1800/20, 80) show heterogeneous,

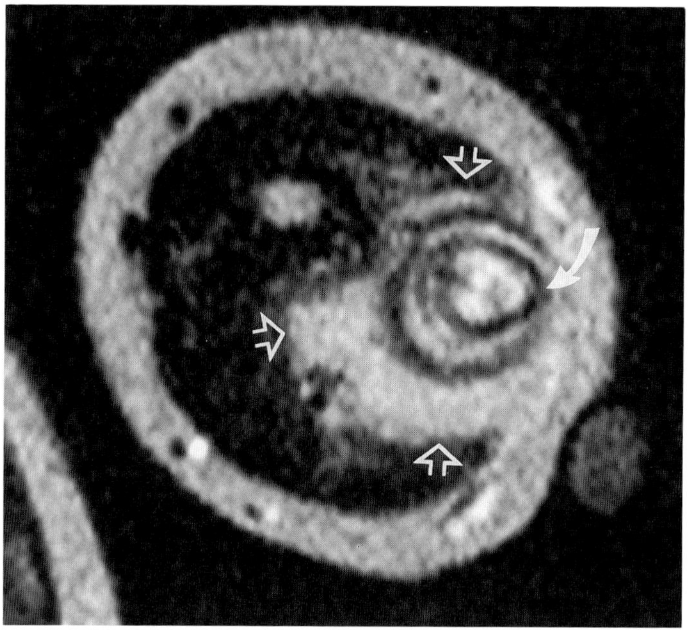

C

FIGURE 15.6 (continued) predominantly increased signal intensity within the lesion (curved arrows). Note the lamellated periosteal reaction (thin arrows) as well as the surrounding soft tissue edema/inflammation (open arrows). Biopsy of the lesion revealed eosinophilic granuloma. (Courtesy of James O. Johnston, MD).

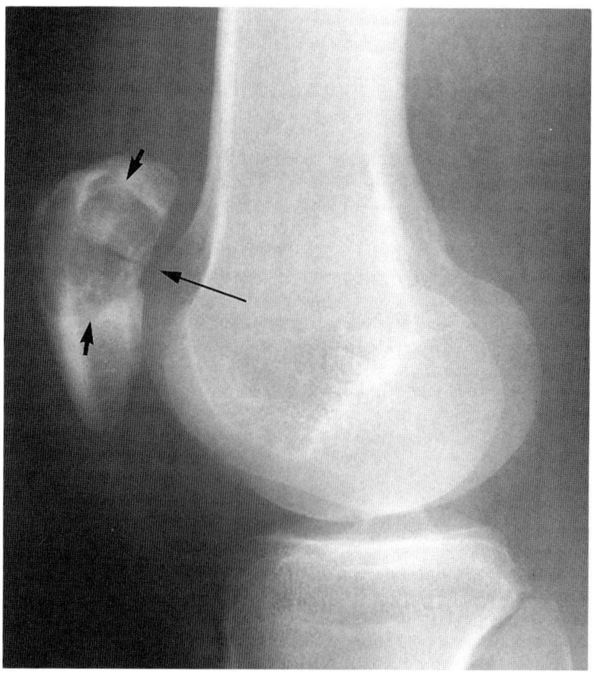

A

FIGURE 15.7 A 28-year-old male presented with a pathologic patella fracture. (A) Lateral radiograph demonstrates a pathologic fracture (thin arrow) through a well-defined lytic patellar lesion (arrows).

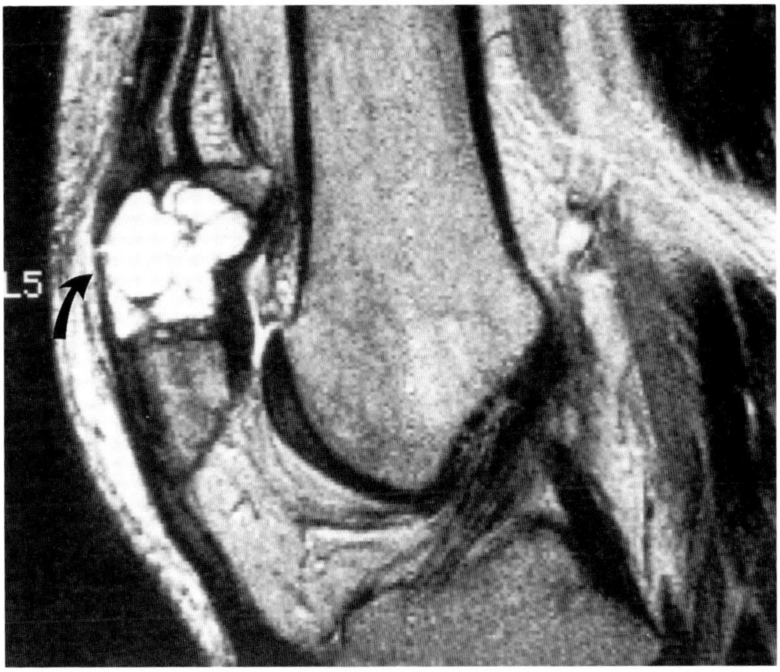

B

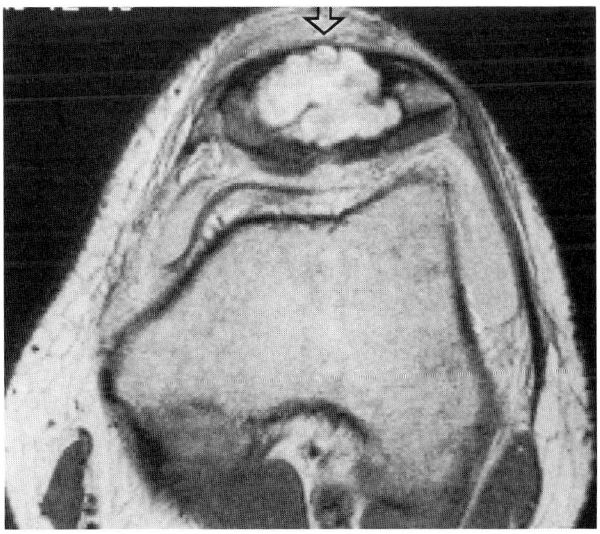

C

Figure 15.7 (continued) (B) Sagittal T2-weighted image (2000/80) reveals a multilobulated mass of very bright signal intensity (curved arrow). A cartilaginous tumor such as chondroblastoma could have this MR appearance. The fracture line is less well visualized than on the corresponding radiograph. (C), (D) Axial dual-echo T2-weighted images (1500/40, 80) delineate the thinned cortex

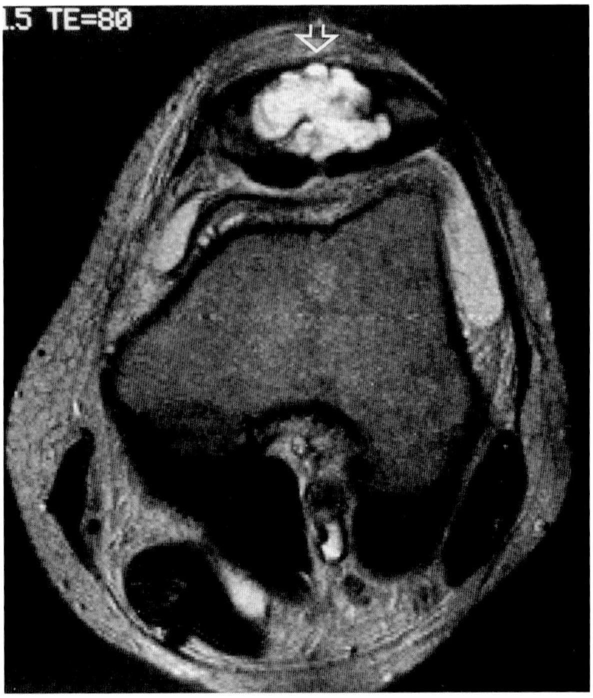

D

FIGURE 15.7 (continued) anteriorly (open arrows). There is an associated joint effusion. Biopsy of the lesion revealed eosinophilic granuloma.

Brodie's Abscess (Bone Abscess)

Definition. Brodie's abscess is a localized form of subacute or chronic hematogenous osteomyelitis. Pathologic examination reveals inflammatory infiltrate, an abscess wall lining of granulation tissue, and surrounding sclerosis. Lesions are of variable size.

Clinical Features. Brodie's abscess usually affects children with an insidious onset. The most common clinical symptom is mild pain. Findings on physical examination may be unremarkable, although local tenderness or swelling are not uncommon. Fever and leukocytosis are usually absent, but the ESR (sedimentation rate) is commonly elevated. The most commonly identified organism is *Staphylococcus aureus*, although cultures are negative in about 20% of cases.

Location. These lesions have a predilection for the metaphysis of long bones, especially the distal and proximal tibia. Rarely, the infection extends across the physis to involve the epiphysis. The lesions may be solitary or multifocal. Occasionally, the lesion is located within the cortex.

Implications. Brodie's abscess is an important entity because it is often misdiagnosed clinically. Biopsy is required for diagnosis and culture. Treatment typically consists of curettage and a six-week course of intravenous antibiotics. Lesions greater than 3 cm in size may require bone grafting. There is usually a rapid response following appropriate therapy.

MRI Findings. A Brodie's abscess may be elongated, oval, or round in shape. In long bone, a distinctive "target" appearance with four layers has been described for Brodie's abscess on MR imaging. This pattern consists of a center, inner ring, outer ring, and peripheral halo. The center abscess cavity exhibits intermediate signal intensity (slightly hyperintense to muscle) on T1-weighted images, corresponding to proteinaceous fluid, leukocytes, and cellular debris. This area appears hyperintense on T2-weighted and STIR sequences. The inner ring appears isointense to muscle on T1-weighted images and hyperintense on T2-weighted and STIR images. This layer represents the pyogen membrane containing granulation tissue and will exhibit marked enhancement following gadolinium administration. The outer ring corresponds to surrounding fibrosis and sclerosis and appears hypointense on all pulse sequences. The peripheral halo appears hypointense on T1-weighted images with variable signal intensity (hypo-, iso-, or hyperintense) on T2-weighted sequences. This layer may represent surrounding edema, sclerosis, or both. Additionally, there may or may not be surrounding bone marrow edema or a soft tissue mass, both exhibiting low signal with T1-weighting and high signal with T2-weighting. A soft tissue mass may represent inflammatory reaction, edema, or purulent material. Occasionally, a tract or channel may be seen extending from the lesion to the growth plate, which could confirm the diagnosis of infection. A sequestrum could be identified, appearing hypointense on all pulse sequences, although sequestra are more confidently identified on plain film or CT.

Differential Diagnosis. The plain film findings of Brodie's abscess are often characteristic and radiographs should be available for comparison. The identification of an elongated or oval metaphyseal lesion in a long bone of a child should suggest Brodie's abscess as a possible diagnosis. The presence of a channel tract extending from the lesion to the physis or the presence of a four-layered "target" MR appearance would confirm the diagnosis. A sequestrum may be present with infection, but can also be seen with eosinophilic granuloma, fibrosarcoma, malignant fibrous histiocytoma, desmoplastic fibroma, osteoid osteoma (pseudosequestrum), and lymphoma. A cortically-based Brodie's abscess is typically associated with prominent surrounding sclerosis and periosteal reaction with an appearance resembling osteoid osteoma or stress fracture, although a linear stress fracture defect is typically seen on MR.

References

Marti-Bonmati L, Aparisi F, Pyatos C, et al. Brodie abscess: MR imaging appearance in 10 patients. *JMRI* 3:543–546, 1993.

Berman A, Levenberg R. Brodie's abscess: A diagnostic dilemma and therapeutic challenge. *Orthopedics* 13:1313–1317, 1990.

Munk P, Vellet A, Hilborn M, et al. Musculoskeletal infection: Findings on magnetic resonance imaging. *Can Assoc Radiol J* 45:355–362, 1994.

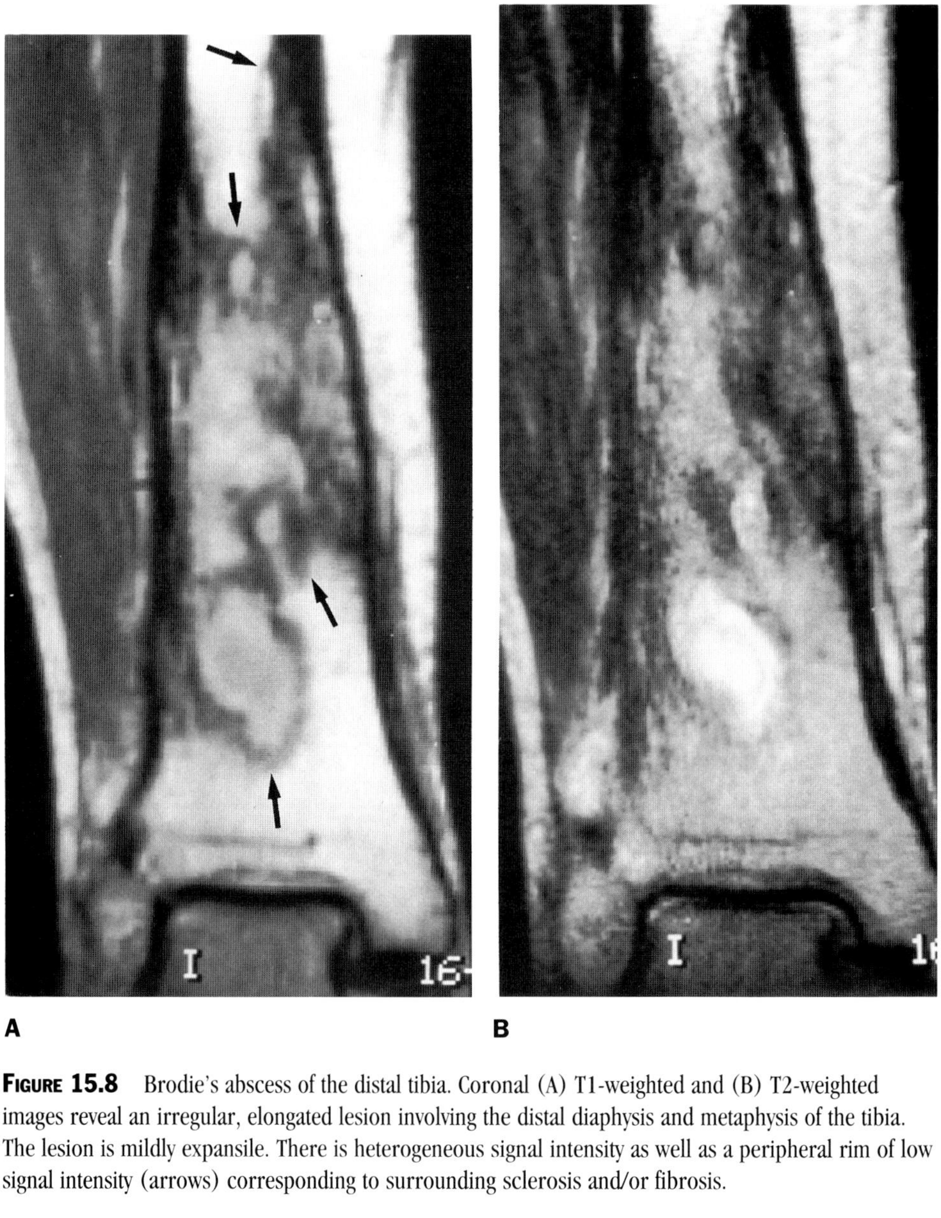

A **B**

Figure 15.8 Brodie's abscess of the distal tibia. Coronal (A) T1-weighted and (B) T2-weighted images reveal an irregular, elongated lesion involving the distal diaphysis and metaphysis of the tibia. The lesion is mildly expansile. There is heterogeneous signal intensity as well as a peripheral rim of low signal intensity (arrows) corresponding to surrounding sclerosis and/or fibrosis.

Hemangioma of Bone

Definition. Osseous hemangiomas are benign vascular tumors which are composed of cavernous, capillary, or venous vascular channels. These lesions are identical histopathologically to soft tissue hemangiomas.

Clinical Features. Osseous hemangiomas are usually identified in middle-aged patients with a peak incidence of 40 to 60 years of age. Females are affected twice as frequently as males. There is an increased incidence with age. These lesions are most often detected as incidental findings. However, some lesions may present with soft tissue swelling, pain, or pathologic fracture. These masses may also result in hemihypertrophy of an extremity. Rarely, vertebral hemangiomas may cause osseous expansion resulting in spinal stenosis, neurologic symptoms, or vertebral compression fracture.

Location. Hemangiomas frequently occur in the vertebrae (especially thoracic and lumbar) and are fairly common in the skull and facial bones. In the spine, hemangiomas typically involve the vertebral body, but may also extend into the posterior elements. Multiple vertebral lesions are not unusual. Hemangiomas of the tubular bones are uncommon, usually affecting the epiphyseal and metaphyseal regions. Intracortical and periosteal lesions are rare, but when present typically occur in the diaphysis of a long tubular bone.

Implications. These benign lesions are often incidental, requiring no further work-up. Intervention should be reserved for those tumors that are symptomatic or at risk for pathologic fracture. These lesions may enlarge slowly over time and may rarely hemorrhage.

MRI Findings. The MR imaging features of osseous hemangiomas are related to the thin-walled vascular channels which contain blood and the presence of fat within these lesions. In the spine, the characteristic imaging features include a coarse vertical trabecular pattern with multiple internal hypointense foci and the presence of fatty signal intensity within the lesion. In extraspinal locations, a slightly expansile lesion with a lattice-like or web-like appearance containing struts that are of marked hypointense signal on all pulse sequences is highly suggestive of the diagnosis.

Differential Diagnosis. In the spine, due to the presence of fatty signal within the hemangioma, the major differential diagnostic consideration is focal fatty replacement within a vertebral body. The MR appearance may also resemble the typical mosaic pattern of Paget's disease.

References

Resnick D, Kyriakos M, Greenway G. Tumors and tumor-like lesions of bone: Imaging and pathology of specific lesions. In: Resnick D (ed), *Bone and Joint Imaging*. Philadelphia, PA, W.B. Saunders Company; 1989, pp 1157–1158.

Melchior B, Bensahel H, Desgrippes Y. Lower limb bone hemangiomas in children: Report of two cases. *J Pediatr Orthop* 11:482–484, 1991.

DelBalso A, Banyas J, Wild L. Hemangioma of the mandibular condyle and ramus. *AJNR* 15:1703–1705, 1994.

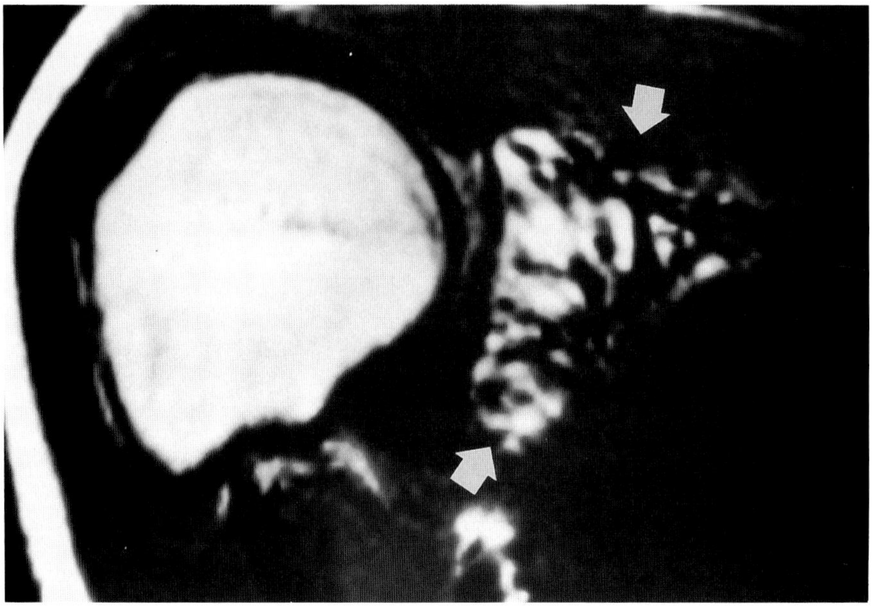

A

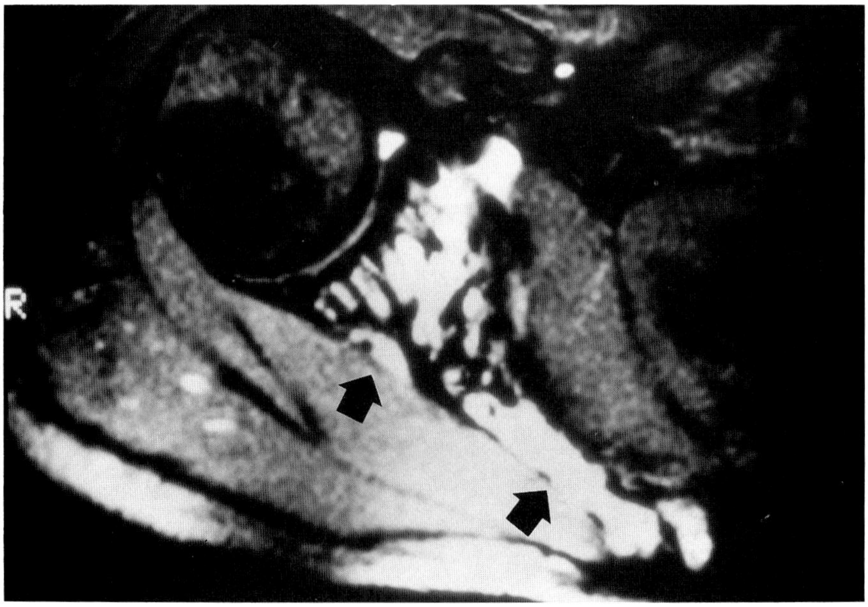

B

FIGURE 15.9 Hemangioma of the scapula in a 17-year-old female. (A) Coronal proton density and (B) axial gradient-recalled echo images reveal extensive involvement of the right scapula (arrows). There are numerous linear struts of signal void surrounding areas of very bright signal intensity corresponding to blood products.

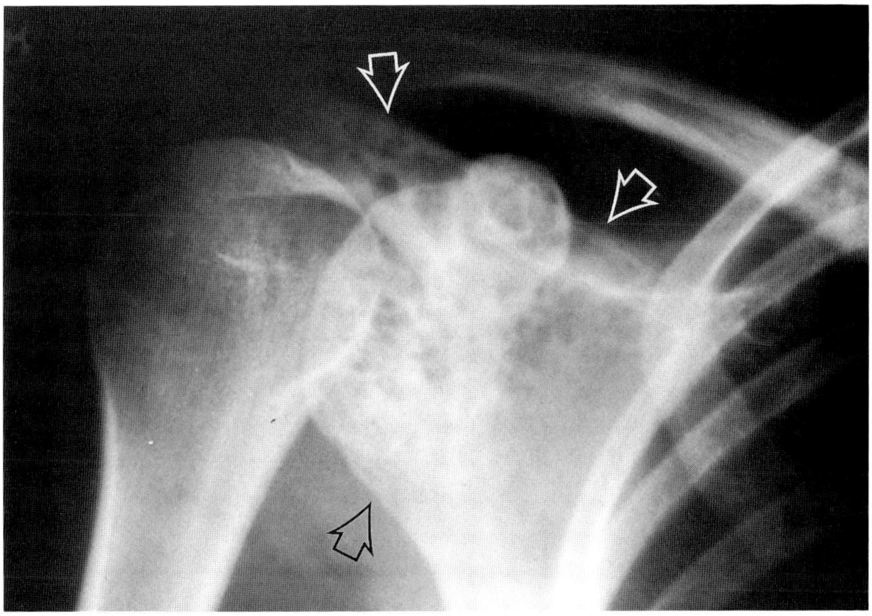

C

FIGURE 15.9 (continued) (C) AP radiograph demonstrates a mixed lytic-sclerotic lesion with a lattice-like trabecular pattern (open arrows). This appearance is highly suggestive of the diagnosis.

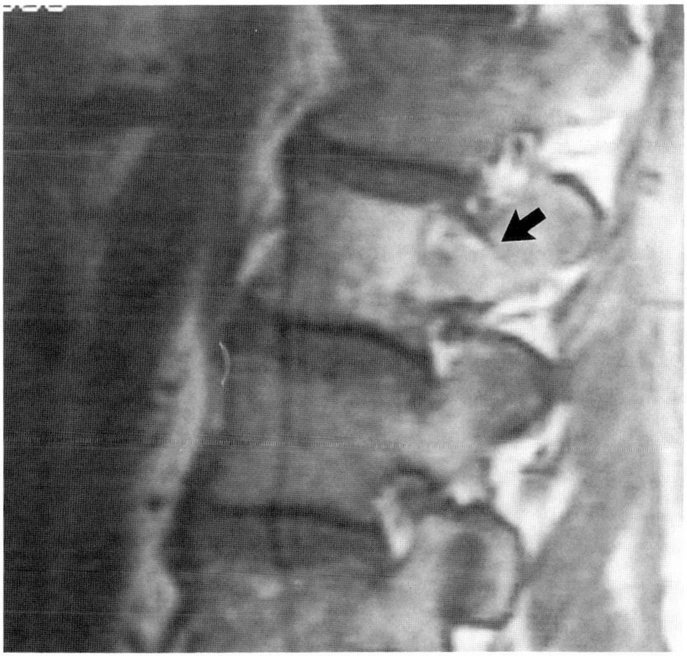

A

FIGURE 15.10 A 77-year-old male with an incidental vertebral hemangioma. Sagittal (A) T1-weighted (600/11) and

(continued)

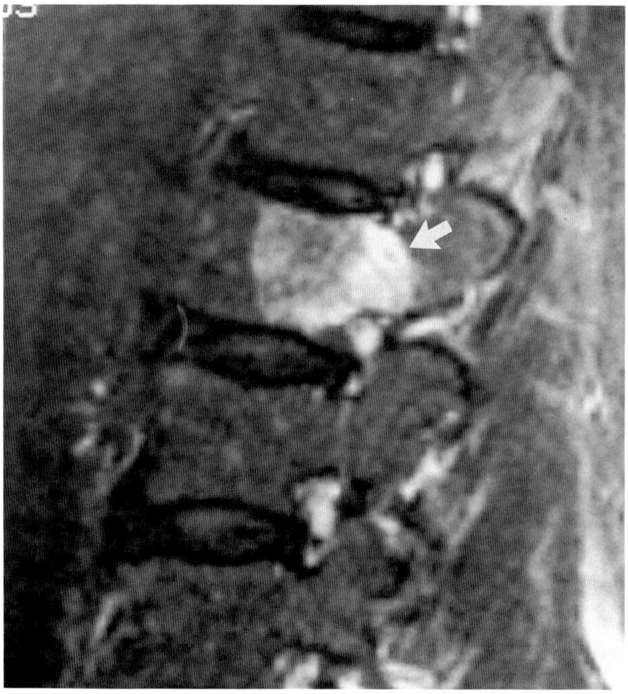

B

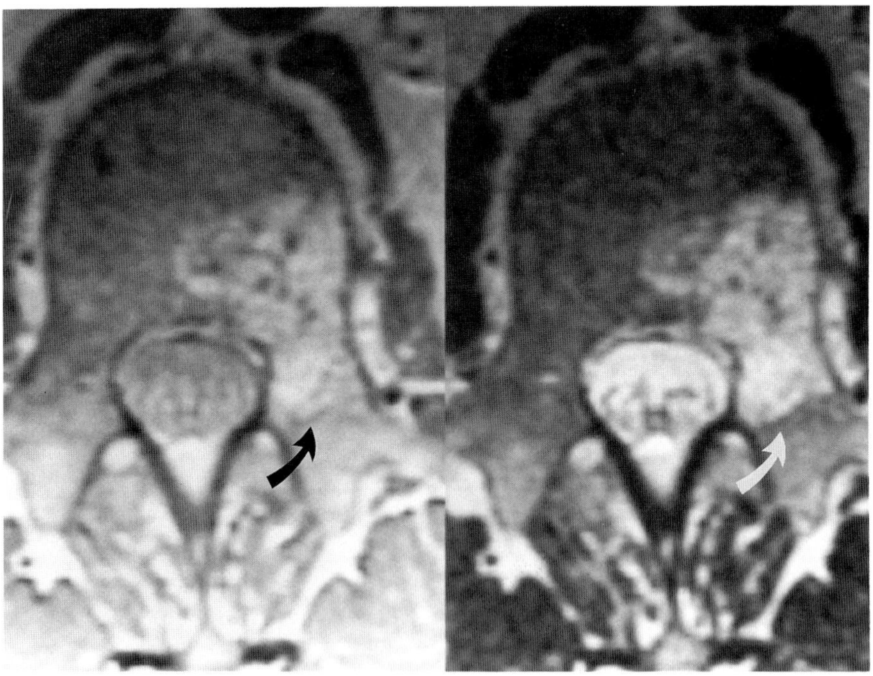

C

FIGURE 15.10 (continued) (B) FSE T2-weighted fat suppression (3800/102) images reveal a hyperintense lesion within the posterior aspect of the L1 vertebral body which extends into the pedicle (arrows). The bright signal with T1-weighting is highly suggestive of the diagnosis and results from the presence of fat and blood within the lesion. (C) Axial FSE dual-echo T2-weighted images (4800/17, 102) further delineate extension of the lesion into the left pedicle (curved arrows). Note the characteristic appearance of internal hypointense foci corresponding to vertical trabeculations.

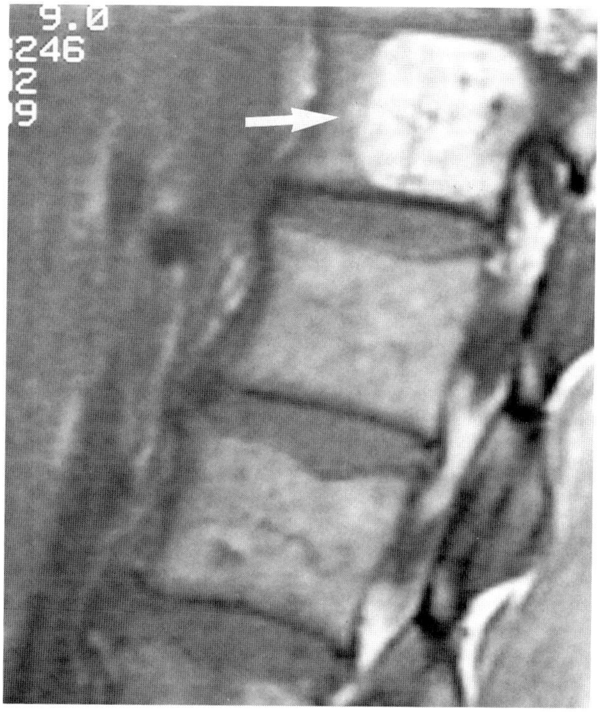

FIGURE 15.11 Incidental L1 vertebral hemangioma in a 49-year-old woman. Sagittal T1-weighted image (500/11) demonstrates a round hyperintense lesion containing numerous internal foci of low signal intensity (arrow). This appearance is characteristic for a vertebral hemangioma.

Paget's Disease

Definition. Paget's disease, also known as osteitis deformans, is a disorder of abnormal and excessive bone remodeling which may affect one or more bones. The exact etiology is unknown, although many authors favor a viral cause. Paget's disease can be divided into three phases: initial (active), middle (intermediate), and late (inactive). Each phase is associated with distinctive pathologic, radiologic, and clinical features. The initial phase is characterized by markedly increased osteoclastic activity with an advancing wedge of osteolysis. Normal marrow is replaced by fibrovascular tissue. The middle phase is characterized by the presence of both osteoclastic resorption and osteoblastic repair. The intense osteoblastic activity is stimulated by the bone loss resulting from unopposed resorption in the initial phase. The new bone formation tends to predominate, resulting in trabecular and cortical thickening and areas of sclerosis. Bone widening also occurs in this phase. Thickened and disorganized trabeculae along with irregular bone fragments result in the classic mosaic pattern seen pathologically. During the late phase, there is gradual diminution of osteoclastic and osteoblastic activity. A prominent mosaic pattern is seen histologically. Cortical and trabecular thickening are present as well as enlargement/widening of bone, which may also become bowed. In long bones, Paget's disease typically starts at one end of a bone and advances toward the other. Therefore, there are commonly different phases coexisting within the same bone. Also, additional bones may become affected throughout the course of the disease and the phase and extent of disease may vary considerably from one bone to another.

Clinical Features. Paget's disease is a relatively common disorder affecting about 3% of individuals over the age of 40 and 10% of the population greater than 85 years of age. The disease is rare in Asians and African-Americans. There is a slight male predominance (3:2). Patients with a positive family history have an incidence of disease seven times higher than the normal population. The vast majority of patients with Paget's disease (up to 90%) are asymptomatic at all stages. Paget's disease is commonly detected incidentally on imaging studies. Most patients with symptomatic Paget's disease present in the middle phase and a majority of the symptoms are related to weakened and thickened bone. The most common presenting complaint is pain. Additional clinical features include insufficiency and pathologic fracture, bone enlargement and deformity, bone bowing, and numerous neurologic symptoms related to spine and/or skull involvement. Increased vascularity with Paget's disease can be so extensive as to result in bruit, warmth, and high output cardiac failure. Abnormal laboratory values include elevated serum alkaline phosphatase and urinary hydroxyproline.

Location. Although any bone may be involved with Paget's disease, the most common sites are the pelvis, spine, femur, and skull, followed by the tibia, humerus, scapula, and clavicle. One or multiple (two-thirds of cases) bones may be affected. In long bones, Paget's disease typically begins in one subarticular region and advances toward the other. The most common exception to this general rule is the tibia.

Implications. Paget's disease can be treated with calcitonin and diphosphonates which reverse bone loss by depressing osteoclastic resorption and stimulating osteoblastic activity. The dread complication of Paget's disease is malignant transformation, which occurs in about 1% of all patients and approximately 10% of those with extensive polyostotic disease. Malignant conversion typically occurs in patients who have had symptomatic Paget's disease with moderate to severe morbidity for 15–25 years. These patients most commonly present with unrelenting pain and/or a mass. The most frequent histologic types of Paget's sarcoma are osteosarcoma, malignant fibrous histiocytoma, fibrosarcoma, and chondrosarcoma, respectively. These patients have an extremely poor prognosis, with a mortality rate of greater than 90% within three years of diagnosis. Giant cell tumor may occur as a very rare complication of Paget's disease and even less commonly, multicentric giant cell tumors may occur in association with familial Paget's disease.

MRI Findings. The MRI findings of Paget's disease are highly variable depending on the phase, histologic composition, and extent of involvement. In later stages, bone enlargement and cortical thickening are identified. The thickened cortex appears as a peripheral rim of signal void on all pulse sequences. Coarsened trabeculae appear as thick linear areas of signal void. There may also be round or oval foci of signal void corresponding to sclerosis. Signal void (on all pulse sequences) in the medullary space may be focal, heterogeneous, or diffuse depending on the extent of sclerosis present. There are typically focal or large areas of normal yellow marrow signal consistent with residual or repopulated fatty marrow tissue. Cyst-like areas of fat-filled marrow cavities may also be present. Foci which are hypointense with T1-weighting and hyperintense with T2-weighting may be identified and correspond to fibrovascular/granulation tissue. Areas of hemorrhage with variable signal intensity may also be present. A soft tissue mass may be seen in association with pathologic fracture with hematoma, Paget's sarcoma, or rarely giant cell tumor.

Differential Diagnosis. Although the signal characteristics are variable, the MR findings of Paget's disease are often diagnostic. The presence of an enlarged bone with cortical and trabecular thickening and containing focal areas of signal corresponding to sclerosis, fat, and granulation tissue strongly suggests the diagnosis. Nevertheless, corresponding radiographs should be obtained for comparison. The radiographic hallmarks of Paget's disease include an advancing wedge of resorption, coarsened and thickened trabeculae, cortical thickening, and bone enlargement. Occasionally, the radiographic findings are not pathognomonic and additional possibilities such as fibrous dysplasia, chronic infection, and blastic metastasis are considered. Paget's disease should be readily distinguishable from these entities with measurement of serum alkaline phosphatase and urinary hydroxyproline levels.

References

Mirra J, Brien E, Tehranzadeh J. Paget's disease of bone: Review with emphasis on radiologic features, Part I. *Skeletal Radiol* 23:163–171, 1995.

Mirra J, Brien E, Tehranzadeh J. Paget's disease of bone: Review with emphasis on radiologic features, Part II. *Skeletal Radiol* 23:173–184, 1995.

Roberts M, Kressel H, Fallon M, et al. Paget disease: MR imaging findings. *Radiology* 173:341–345, 1989.

Kaufmann G, Sundaram M, McDonald D. Magnetic resonance imaging in symptomatic Paget's disease. *Skeletal Radiol* 20;413–418, 1991.

Griffiths H. Radiology of Paget's disease. *Curr Opinion Radiol* 4:124–128, 1992.

Potter H, Schneider R, Ghelman B, et al. Multiple giant cell tumors and Paget disease of bone: Radiographic and clinical correlations. *Radiology* 180:261–264, 1991.

A

B

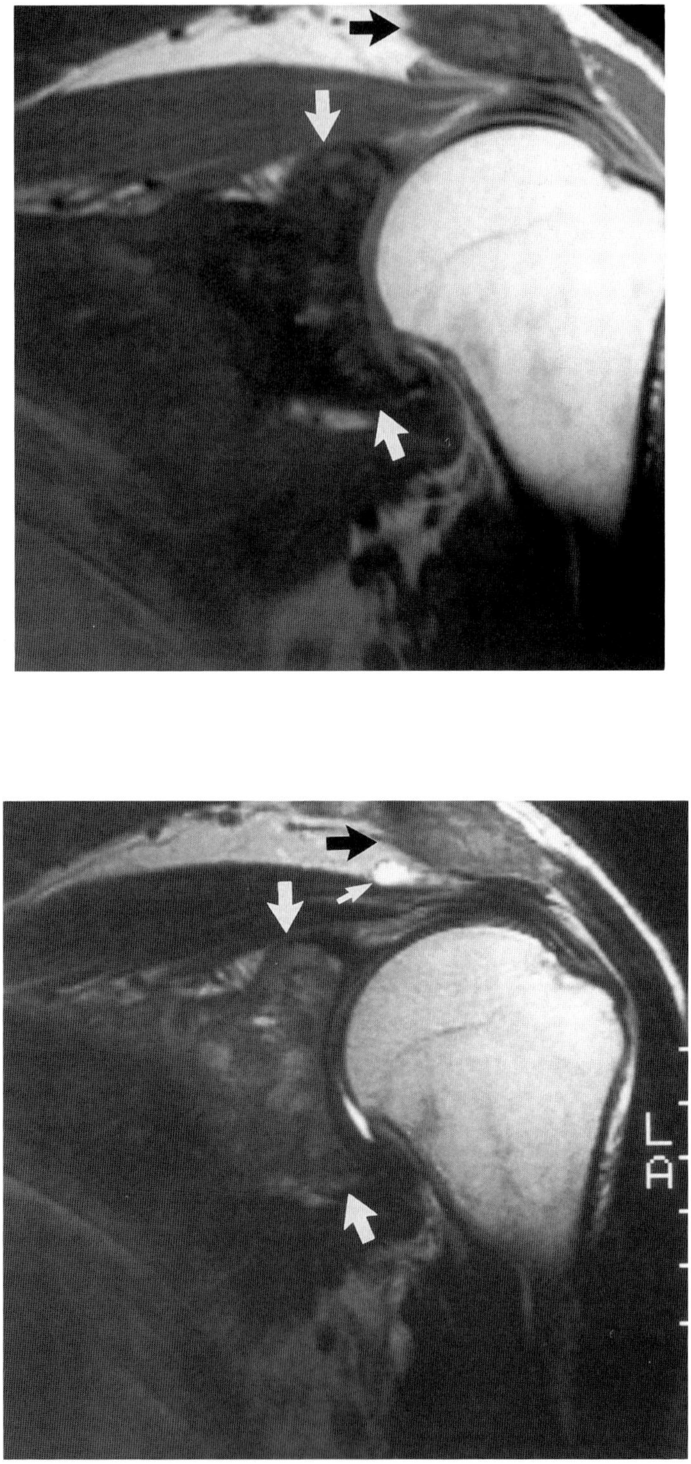

FIGURE 15.12 A 62-year-old male with left shoulder pain and clinical suspicion for rotator cuff pathology. Coronal (A) T1-weighted (683/18) and (B) FSE T2-weighted (3600/126) images reveal replacement of the normal marrow of the glenoid and acromion with a heterogeneous, predominantly low signal intensity process (arrows). Enlargement and lateral downsloping of the acromion is present. There is associated fluid within the subacromial-subdeltoid bursa (small arrow).

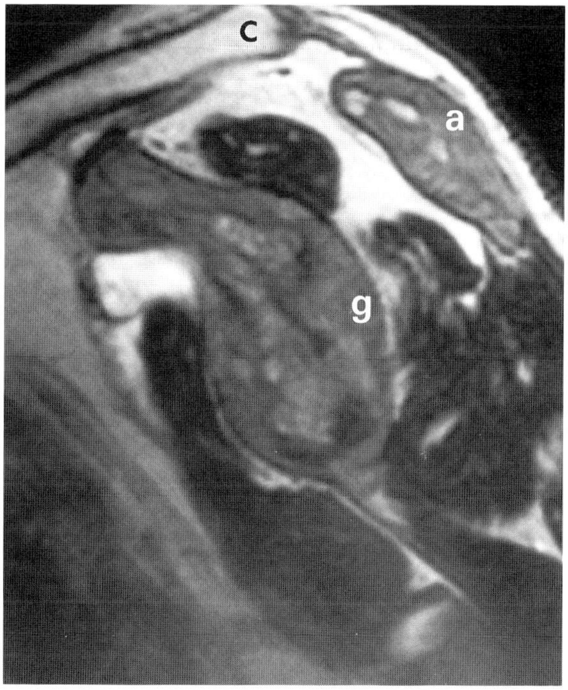

C

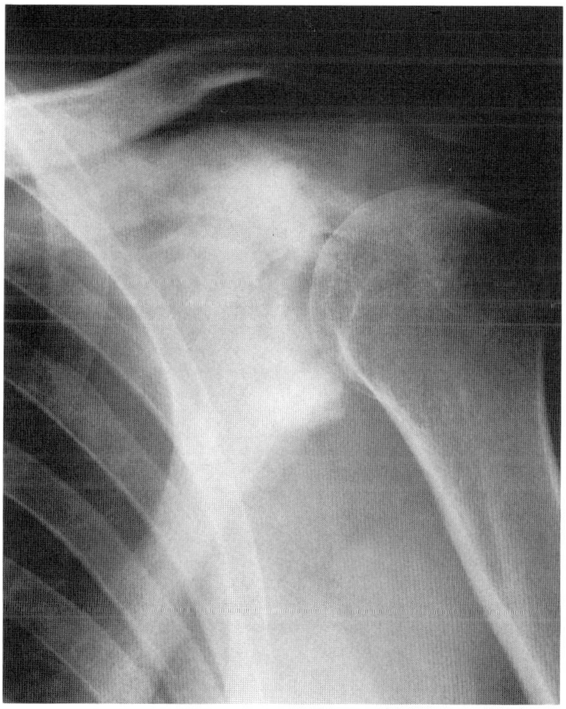

D

FIGURE 15.12 (continued) (C) Sagittal FSE T2-weighted image (3000/119) again demonstrates heterogeneous signal intensity involving the scapula and enlargement of the acromion. The MR appearance is strongly suggestive of Paget's disease. In contrast, note the normal appearance of the uninvolved clavicle (c). Glenoid (g), acromion (a). (D) AP radiograph of the left shoulder is characteristic for Paget's disease, revealing trabecular thickening and sclerosis throughout the left scapula with some associated bone enlargement.

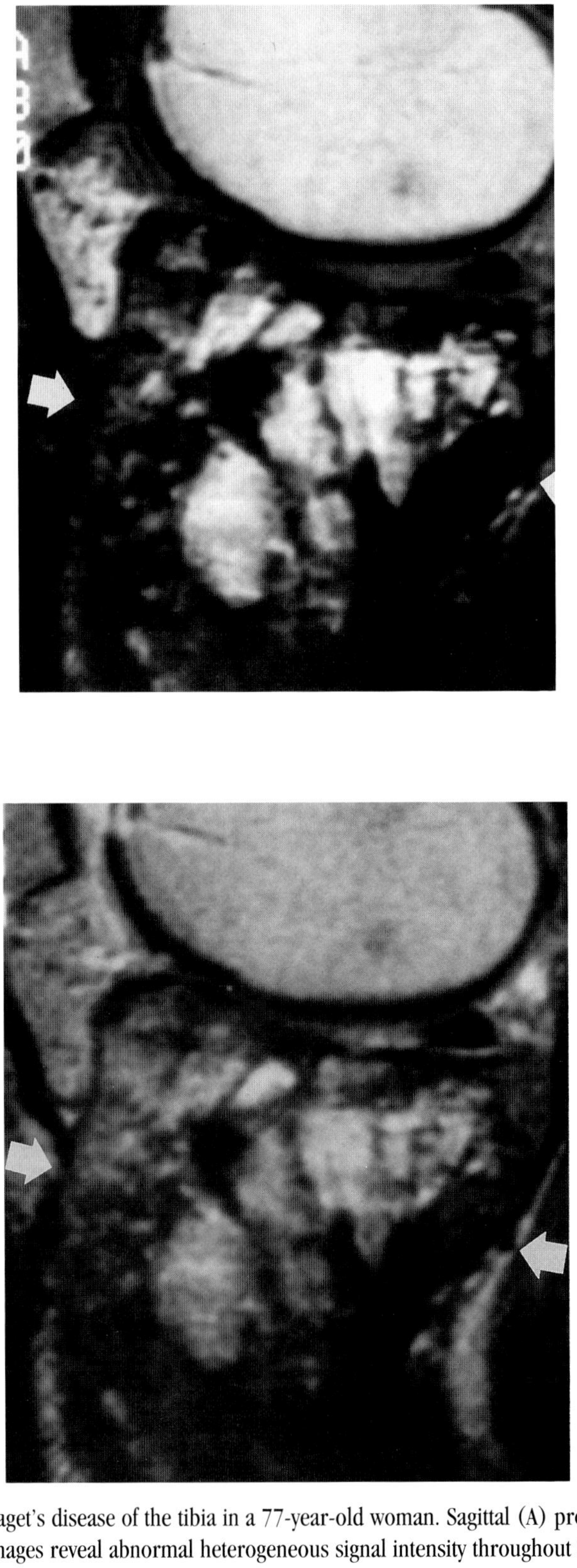

A

B

FIGURE 15.13 Paget's disease of the tibia in a 77-year-old woman. Sagittal (A) proton density and (B) T2-weighted images reveal abnormal heterogeneous signal intensity throughout the proximal tibia with numerous linear and rounded areas of signal void corresponding to thickened trabeculae and sclerosis (arrows).

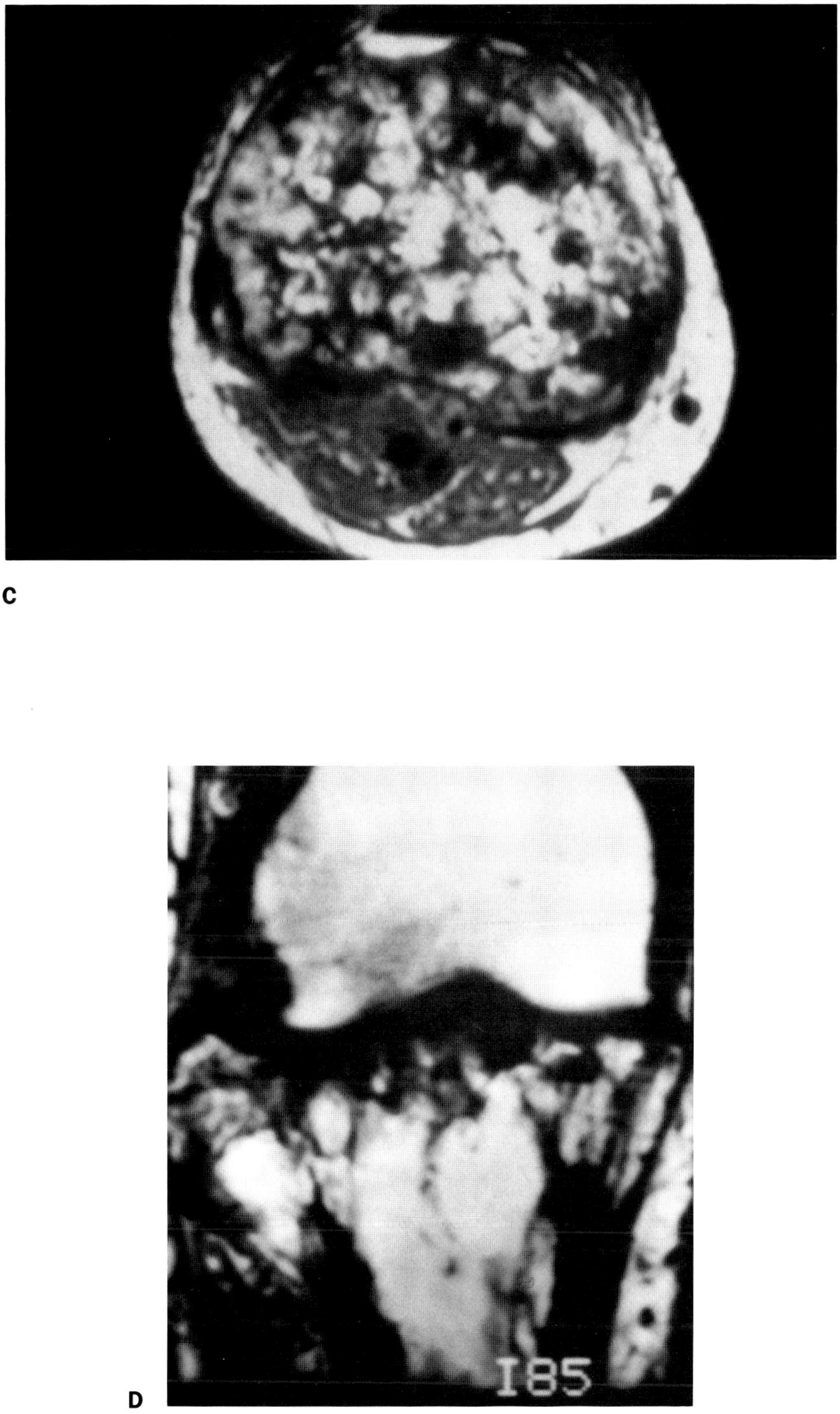

C

D

FIGURE 15.13 (continued) T1-weighted (C) axial and (D) coronal images demonstrate numerous areas of fatty marrow, which appear hyperintense. Areas of signal void again represent coarsened trabeculae and sclerosis. Note the marked osseous enlargement.

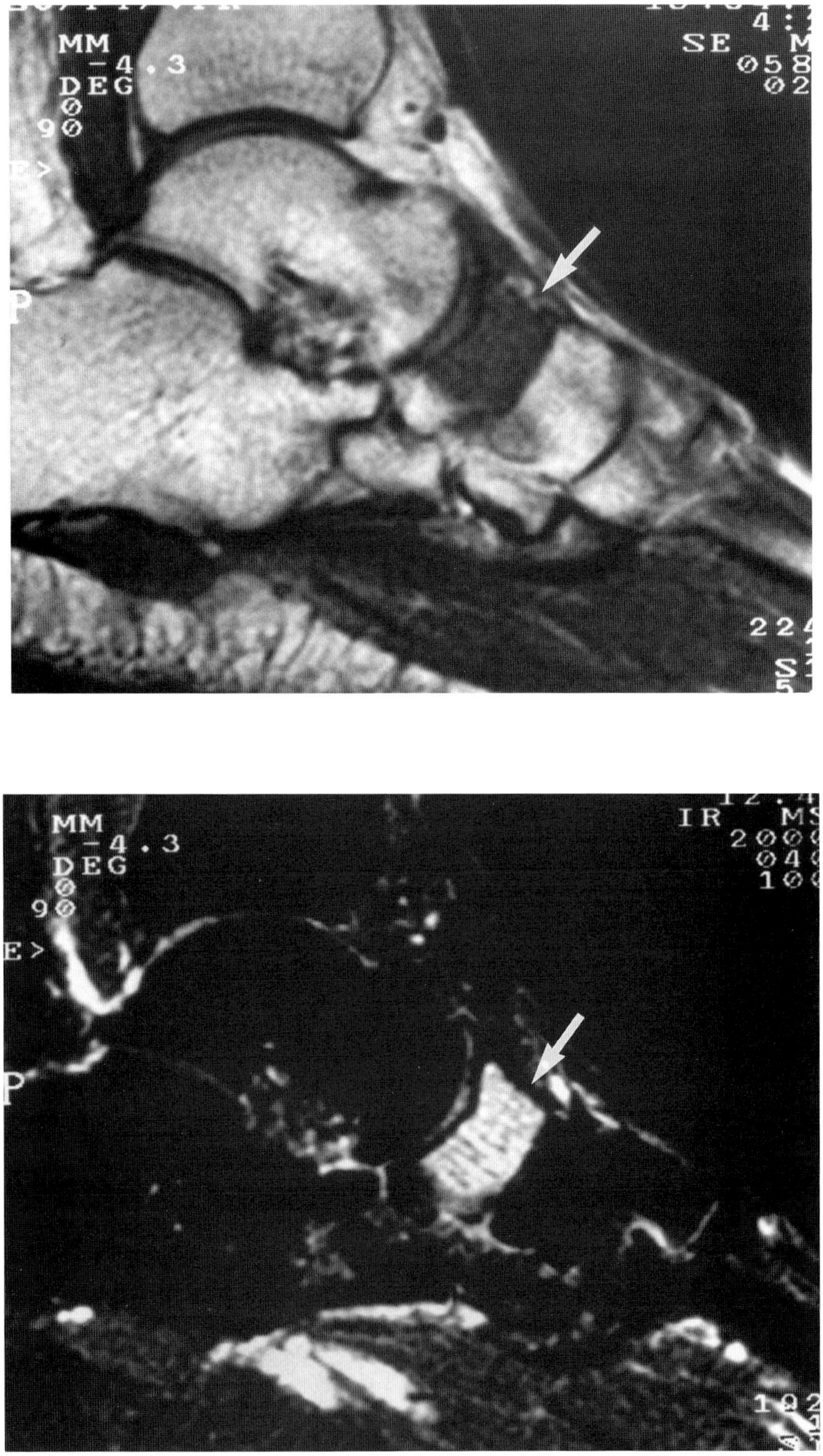

A

B

FIGURE 15.14 Biopsy-proven Paget's disease of the tarsal navicular in a 30-year-old male who presented with chronic pain exacerbated with exercise. Sagittal (A) T1-weighted (580/25) and (B) inversion recovery (2000/40, TI-100) images demonstrate abnormal signal within the navicular bone (arrows). Note the thin linear areas of very low signal corresponding to thickened trabeculae. (Courtesy of Quentin Reeves, MD).

Intraosseous Lipoma

Definition. Intraosseous lipomas are histopathologically identical to soft tissue lipomas, consisting of lobular collections of adipose tissue separated by thin fibrous septa. With involution, these lesions may contain areas of fat necrosis and calcification with eventual development of myxoid degeneration, cyst formation, and reactive ossification.

Clinical Features. Intraosseous lipomas are among the rarest of all benign bone tumors. They may occur at nearly any age and have no sex predilection. Although the lesions may be asymptomatic, the majority present with localized pain and/or swelling.

Location. Although nearly any bone may be involved, the most common sites of intraosseous lipomas include the intertrochanteric and subtrochanteric regions of the femur, ilium, calcaneus, proximal tibia, and fibula. The true incidence of lesions involving the calcaneus is unknown, since some authors believe that many of the lesions reported to occur in the calcaneus may actually represent solitary bone cysts that have undergone lipidization. Those lesions reported in the calcaneus occur in the same classic location as solitary bone cysts, namely the antero-middle region of normal rarefaction.

Implications. Treatment should be directed by the individual clinical setting. Surgery may be indicated for painful lesions. Rare cases of malignant transformation have been reported.

MRI Findings. Since these lesions are composed predominantly of fat, the signal intensity will be isointense with the surrounding yellow marrow and subcutaneous fat on all pulse sequences. Therefore, intraosseous lipomas typically blend in with the surrounding yellow marrow and have ill-defined margins on MRI, as opposed to the well-defined lytic appearance on radiographs. Corresponding radiographs are helpful in delineating the tumor margin and in the presence of plain films, the MR findings should be diagnostic. The signal intensity should be homogeneous unless the lesion has undergone involution. If calcification is present, it is typically located centrally within the lesion and appears as signal void on all pulse sequences. With progressive involution, areas of very bright signal may be seen within the lesion on T2-weighted sequences, corresponding to cystic or myxomatous degeneration.

Differential Diagnosis. In general, correlation of the MR imaging and radiographic findings should allow the correct diagnosis. The diagnosis may not be straightforward in the presence of extensive cystic or myxomatous degeneration, which may result in prominent areas of hypointense signal with T1-weighting and corresponding bright signal with T2-weighting. The latter signal characteristics are very nonspecific. The key to establishing the diagnosis is the identification of fat within the lesion. A hemorrhagic lesion containing methemoglobin could be mistaken for a fat-containing mass on T1-weighted sequences, but the signal from methemoglobin should not parallel yellow marrow and subcutaneous fat on all pulse sequences.

Reference

Blacksin M, Ende N, Benevenia J. Magnetic resonance imaging of intraosseous lipomas: A radiologic-pathologic correlation. *Skeletal Radiol* 24:37–41, 1995.

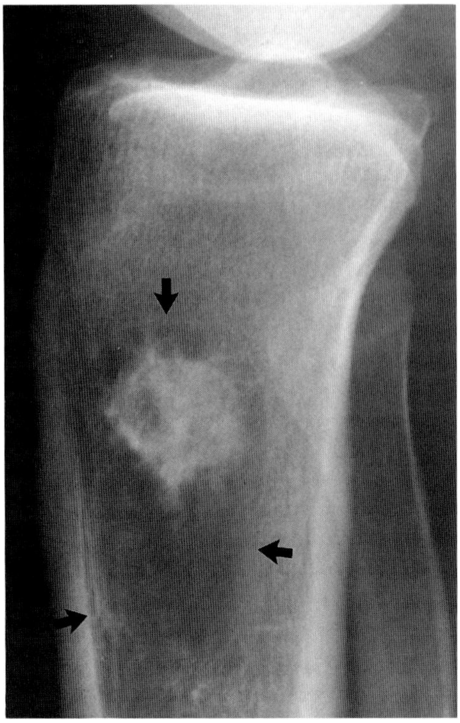

A

B

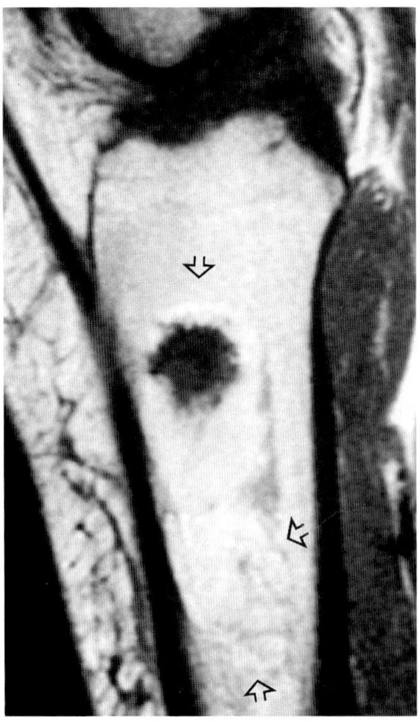

FIGURE 15.15 A 33-year-old woman presented with anteromedial pain below the knee. (A) Lateral radiograph demonstrates a well-marginated lytic lesion within the metadiaphyseal region of the proximal tibia (arrows). The mass contains a prominent area of calcification/ossification superiorly. (B) Sagittal T1-weighted image (600/16) reveals very bright signal intensity corresponding to the radiographically-lytic component. Note that the margin of the mass is difficult to distinguish from the surrounding fatty marrow (open arrows). (C), (D) Coronal dual-echo T2-weighted images (2000/19, 70) show that the predominant component of the lesion remains isointense to the subcutaneous fat and very similar in intensity to the adjacent fatty marrow. Portions of a thin fibrous capsule are identified (curved open arrows). These findings are diagnostic of an intraosseous lipoma. The superior focus of signal abnormality contains areas of signal void representing calcification/ossification, but also contains bright signal likely corresponding to cystic or myxomatous degeneration (thin arrow).

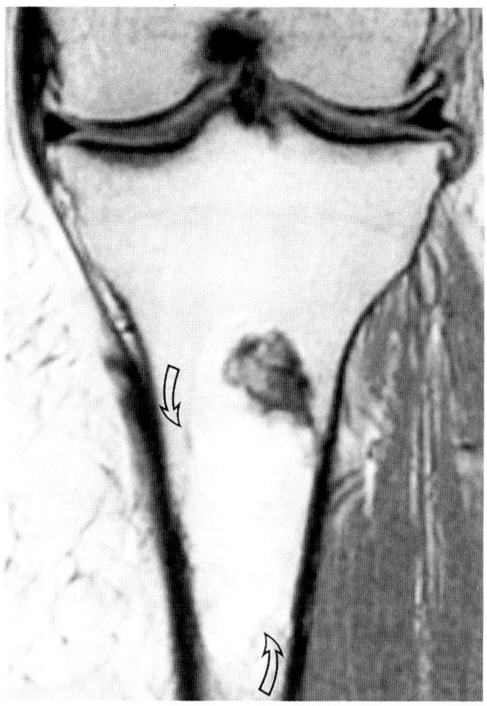

C

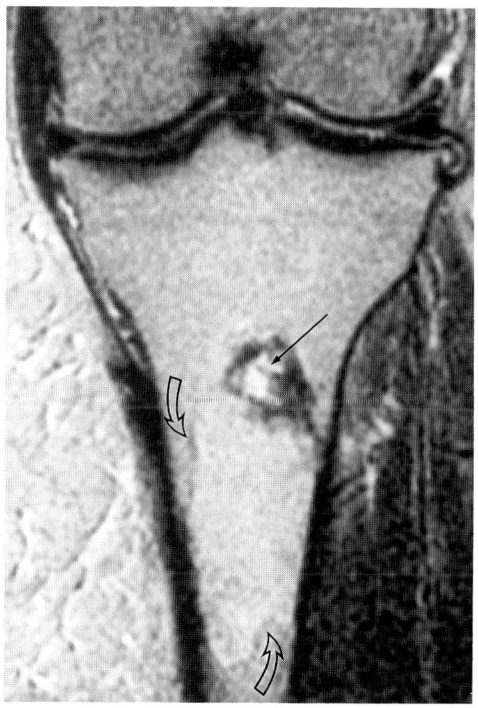

D

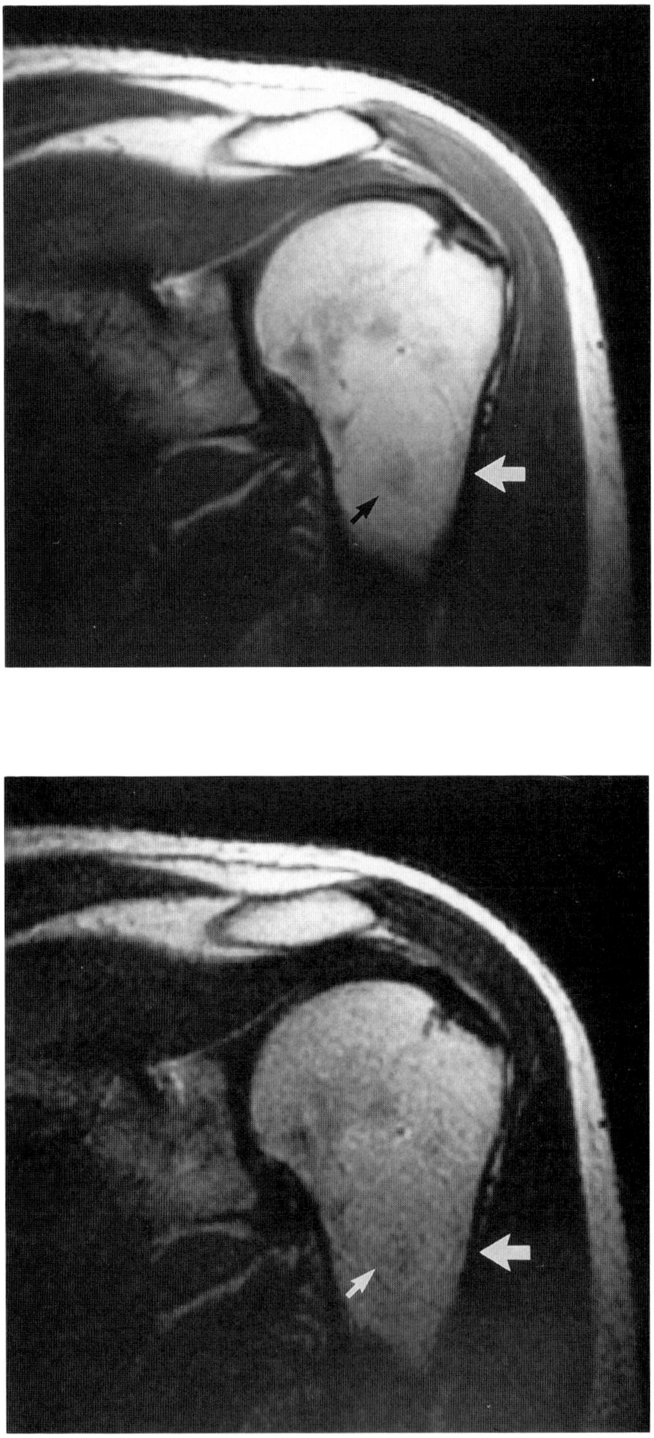

A

B

FIGURE 15.16 Intraosseous lipoma of the proximal humerus in a 49-year-old male. (A), (B) Coronal dual-echo T2-weighted images (2000/20, 80) reveal a barely-perceptible lesion within the metadiaphyseal region of the proximal left humerus (arrows). The margins of the mass are difficult to distinguish from the surrounding yellow marrow. The predominant signal intensity is isointense to subcutaneous fat. There is a central focus of hypointensity corresponding to calcification/ossification (small arrows).

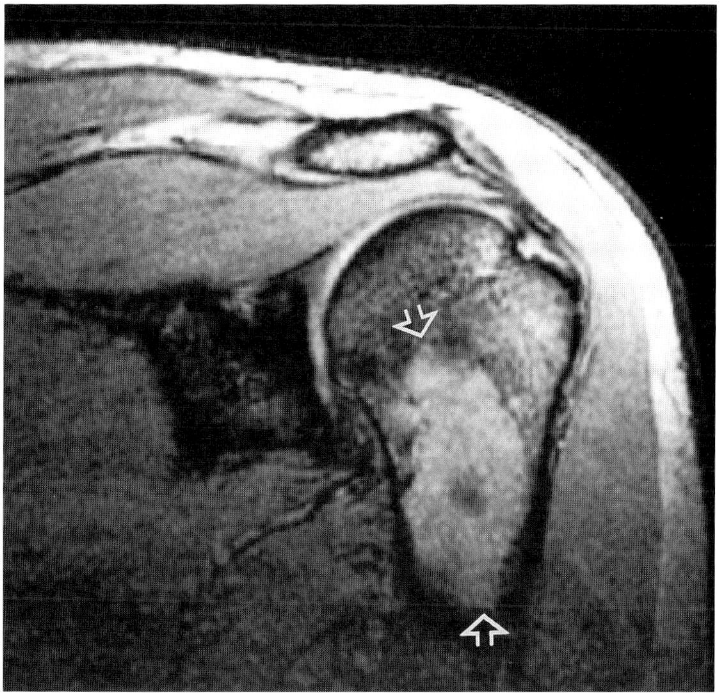

C

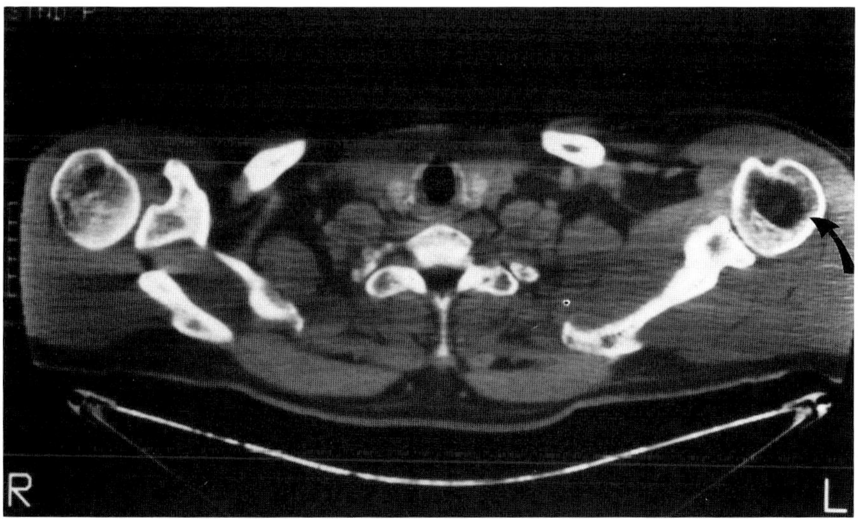

D

Figure 15.16 (continued) (C) Coronal MPGR image (600/20, 30 degrees) demonstrates increased conspicuity of the lesion due to magnetic susceptibility artifact of the surrounding trabeculae. The margins of the lesion are much better delineated (open arrows). Magnetic susceptibility also causes the central focus of calcification/ossification to become more prominent. Note that the signal intensity of the lesion remains isointense to subcutaneous fat. (D) Axial CT image also confirms the fatty nature of the mass (curved arrow) by revealing its very low density, equal to that of the subcutaneous fat.

Medullary Bone Infarct

Definition. Medullary bone infarction results from a decrease in blood supply to the affected area. One or more of three general mechanisms may occur: (1) intravascular occlusion (thromboembolic phenomenon, sludging, stasis); (2) intraosseous vascular compression (increased marrow contents and/or pressure); (3) physical alteration of the vessel wall (trauma, vasculitis). Some common causes of bone infarction are steroids, collagen vascular disease, sickle cell anemia, radiation, and alcohol.

Clinical Features. Medullary bone infarcts are commonly encountered on imaging studies. A known risk factor can often be established by clinical history. Early/immature infarcts may be painful and may clinically mimic infection, neoplasm, or joint space pathology. Old/mature infarcts are typically asymptomatic.

Location. Medullary bone infarcts typically occur in the metadiaphyseal portion of long bones, partly because of a poorer collateral blood supply. The distal femur and proximal tibia are classic sites of involvement. Involvement is often bilateral and symmetrical.

Implications. In the vast majority of cases, the diagnosis of medullary bone infarct can be established on imaging studies and biopsy should not be performed. Malignant transformation is a rare complication of bone infarction, occurring with long-standing lesions. Secondary malignancies include fibrosarcoma, malignant fibrous histiocytoma, and osteosarcoma. The prognosis in these cases is poor.

MRI Findings. The MRI findings are often pathognomonic. An oblong medullary lesion with a thin serpiginous peripheral rim that is hypointense on T1- and T2-weighted sequences is characteristic. On T1-weighted images, the center of the lesion tends to exhibit signal intensity that is isointense or hyperintense in relation to the adjacent marrow. On T2-weighted sequences, the central region tends to be isointense to the surrounding marrow or hyperintense if there is associated edema. Old infarcts which contain prominent calcification or fibrosis may exhibit predominantly hypointense signal on both T1- and T2-weighted sequences. Very early infarcts may have a nonspecific MR appearance, exhibiting decreased signal intensity with T1-weighting and hyperintense signal with T2-weighting without the presence of a serpiginous border.

Differential Diagnosis. In the vast majority of cases, the MR findings are characteristic and a confident diagnosis of medullary bone infarct can be made. There are cases of very early infarction in which the MR features are nonspecific and can be seen with various other conditions including infection, trauma, and numerous benign and malignant neoplastic processes.

References

Munk P, Helms C, Holt R. Immature bone infarcts: Findings on plain radiographs and MR scans. *AJR* 152:547–549, 1989.

Gillespy T, Genant H, Helms C. Magnetic resonance imaging of osteonecrosis. *Radiol Clin North Am* 24:193–208, 1986.

Gaucher A, Regent D, Gillet P, et al. Case report 656. *Skeletal Radiol* 20;137–140, 1991.

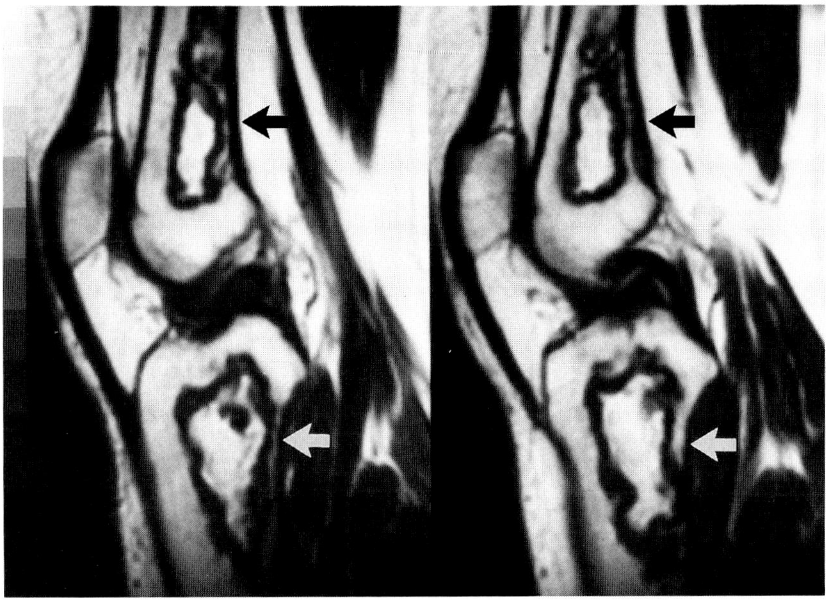

FIGURE 15.17 A 35-year-old woman status post knee injury. MRI was obtained to rule out internal derangement. Sagittal T1-weighted images (600/15) reveal elongated medullary lesions (arrows) within the metadiaphyseal portions of the distal femur and proximal tibia. Note the serpiginous peripheral rims of very low signal intensity as well as the presence of high signal intensity centrally. This appearance is characteristic for medullary bone infarcts.

16 Miscellaneous Malignant Masses

Ewing's Sarcoma

Definition. Ewing's sarcoma is a highly malignant primary bone tumor of uncertain origin. Histologically, it is characterized by sheets of small round cells with frequent areas of hemorrhage and necrosis.

Clinical Features. Ewing's sarcoma is the sixth most common malignant bone neoplasm. Ninety percent of patients are less than 30 years of age at the time of diagnosis. Patients typically present with pain and swelling of relatively long duration (weeks to months). There may also be erythema and warmth in the involved area, which can be clinically confused for infection. Ewing's sarcoma has a predilection for Caucasians, with African-Americans and Asians infrequently affected.

Location. Any bone may be involved. Over half of the cases occur in the long bones of the extremities (lower extremity greater than upper extremity). Long bone lesions most often involve the metadiaphyseal and diaphyseal regions. The most common flat bone sites are the ribs and ilium. Rarely, Ewing's sarcoma may be purely extraosseous.

Implications. Approximately 30% of patients have metastatic disease at the time of presentation. Those without distant metastasis at presentation have five-year survival rates between 55% and 75%. Preoperative multiagent chemotherapy is typically used to reduce the size of the tumor. Surgery following chemotherapy offers the best chance of a cure. Radiation therapy may also be utilized. Ewing's sarcoma has a tendency to recur locally, sometimes after periods as long as five years of apparent remission. The initial response of the tumor to chemotherapy is a prognostic indicator. Nonresectable central lesions (especially those occurring in the pelvis) are associated with a poorer prognosis. Additional poor prognostic indicators include diameter greater than 8 cm, older age, elevated sedimentation rate, and increased white blood cell count at the time of presentation.

MRI Findings. MR is the imaging modality of choice for defining the intraosseous and extraosseous extent of the tumor, which are important in preoperative planning. Ewing's sarcoma is frequently associated with a soft tissue mass and flat bone lesions characteristically have a larger extraosseous component relative to the amount of intraosseous disease. Both the marrow and soft tissue components typically exhibit hypointense signal on T1-weighted images and intermediate to high signal intensity on T2-weighted sequences. The signal intensity is frequently heterogeneous. Associated periosteal reaction and cortical thickening are commonly seen, which appear very low in signal intensity on all pulse sequences. Following chemotherapy, there are frequently areas of high signal intensity on T2-weighted sequences which correspond histologically to tumor necrosis, cystic hemorrhagic areas, and highly vascular fibroblastic repair tissue. In addition, there may be areas of signal void on all pulse sequences corresponding to dense cortical bone or hemosiderin. It has been shown that following chemotherapy, there are commonly microscopic areas of viable tumor present in regions of both low and high signal intensity on T2-weighted sequences. MRI cannot reliably exclude the presence of residual/active disease following chemotherapy.

Differential Diagnosis. Plain films are the standard modality for diagnosing Ewing's sarcoma and the MR images should be interpreted in the presence of recent radiographs. In a younger age group, a symptomatic mass with both intraosseous and extraosseous components on MRI could represent various lesions including Ewing's sarcoma, osteosarcoma, infection, and eosinophilic granuloma.

References

Eggli K, Quiogue T, Moser R. Ewing's sarcoma. *Radiol Clin of North Am* 31:325–337, 1993.

MacVicar A, Olliff J, Pringle J, et al. Ewing sarcoma: MR imaging of chemotherapy-induced changes with histologic correlation. *Radiology* 184:859–864, 1992.

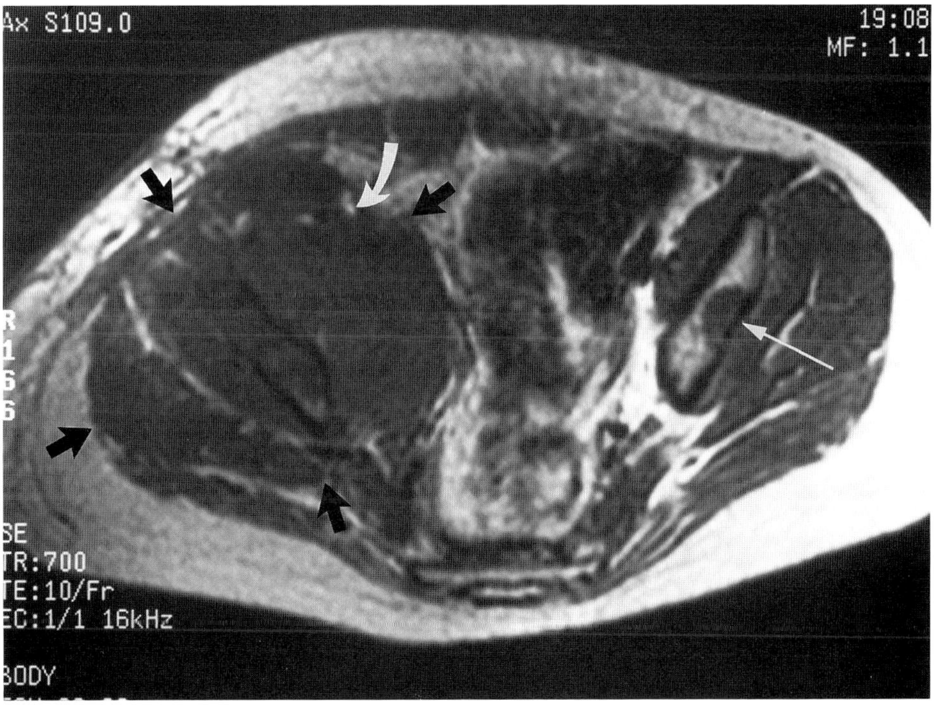

A

Figure 16.1 A 15-year-old male with Ewing's sarcoma of the right ilium. Axial (A) T1-weighted (700/10) and

(continued)

B 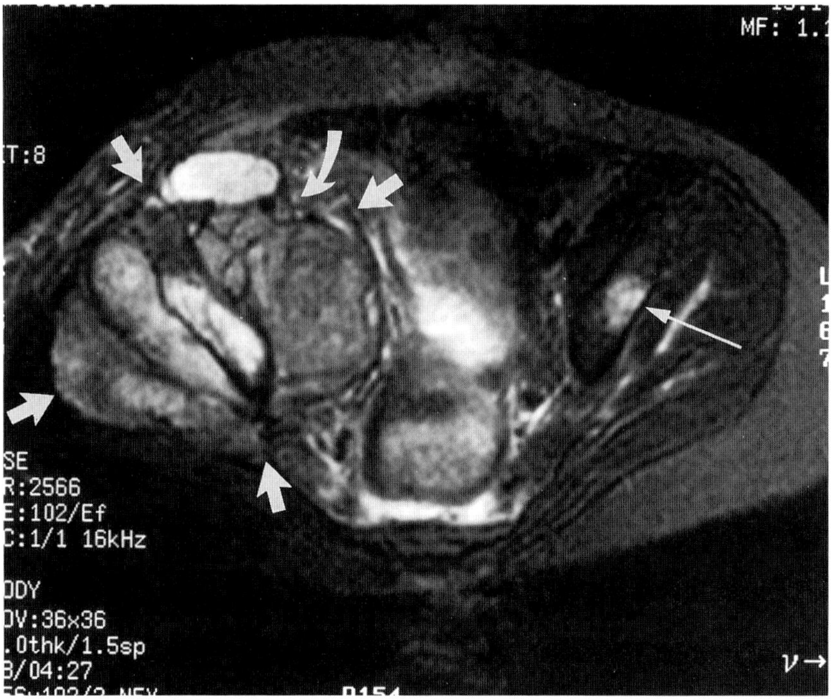

FIGURE 16.1 (continued) (B) FSE T2-weighted fat suppression (2566/102) images reveal a very large mass arising from the right ilium. The extraosseous component (arrows) predominates over the intraosseous component. The signal is isointense to muscle with T1-weighting, but heterogeneous on the T2-weighted image with areas of low, intermediate, and high signal intensity. There is mass effect on the right iliac vessels (curved arrows). Note the presence of a metastatic lesion within the left ilium (thin arrows).

Chordoma

Definition. Chordoma is a malignant osseous neoplasm which arises from rests of the primitive notochord. Chordomas are classified into two pathologic types, typical chordomas and chondroid chordomas. Typical chordomas consist of physaliphorous (vacuolated) cells arranged in sheets and cords. The tumor mass may consist of fairly compact tissue, but is frequently gelatinous or semiliquid in nature. Chondroid chordomas contain multiple areas of cartilaginous tissue interspersed in the tumor matrix. Chordomas are associated with calcification and significant bone destruction.

Clinical Features. Chordoma is an uncommon entity, accounting for 3–4% of all primary malignant bone neoplasms. It is the most common primary tumor of the sacrum. The lesions are often large at presentation. They are typically associated with localized pain and there may be symptoms related to mass effect on adjacent structures. Chordomas may occur at any age, but most commonly affect patients in the fourth through seventh decades of life.

Location. Chordomas may arise anywhere along the distribution of the primitive notochord, i.e., in the midline from the spheno-occipital region to the coccyx. Approximately 50% of chordomas are sacrococcygeal, 35% are spheno-occipital (especially involving the clivus), and 15% arise from a vertebral body (especially C2).

Implications. The prognosis is variable. Many lesions are very large at the time of presentation with invasion into the adjacent structures. Hematogenous metastasis have been reported to occur in 10–48% of cases and are much more common with lesions involving the sacrococcygeal region or vertebrae. Radiation therapy is often used in conjunction with surgery in treating these lesions. Chondroid chordomas have a significantly better prognosis than typical chordomas and the prognosis improves with increasing cartilaginous content.

MRI Findings. Chordomas generally appear as lobulated masses surrounded by a low signal intensity fibrous pseudocapsule. Typically, the signal is hypointense on T1-weighted sequences and markedly hyperintense (similar to cerebrospinal fluid) on T2-weighted sequences. They are usually associated with a large soft tissue mass. Calcification is usually present within the lesion and appears as foci of signal void on all pulse sequences. Chondroid chordomas have shorter T1 and T2 relaxation times compared with typical chordomas due to the presence of cartilaginous tissue. MRI may be helpful in distinguishing between chondroid and typical chordomas.

Differential Diagnosis. The MR findings are not diagnostic, but the presence of a highly destructive mass in a typical location which exhibits very bright signal intensity on T2-weighted images and contains areas of signal void consistent with calcification is suggestive of the diagnosis. Tarlov cysts, intrasacral cysts, and anterior sacral meningoceles may exhibit similar signal characteristics, but these lesions are connected with the thecal sac and are not associated with local destruction or soft tissue extension. An echinococcal cyst would not be associated with local destruction or a soft tissue mass. Giant cell tumor and plasmacytoma may have a similar appearance in the sacrum, but these lesions are generally not as bright as chordomas on T2-weighted sequences.

References

Sze G, Uichanco L, Brant-Zawadzki M, et al. Chordomas: MR imaging. *Radiology* 166:187–191, 1988.

Rosenthal D, Scott J, Mankin H, et al. Sacrococcygeal chordoma: Magnetic resonance imaging and computed tomography. *AJR* 145:143–147, 1985.

Yuh W, Flickinger F, Barloon T, et al. MR imaging of unusual chordomas. *JCAT* 12:30–35, 1988.

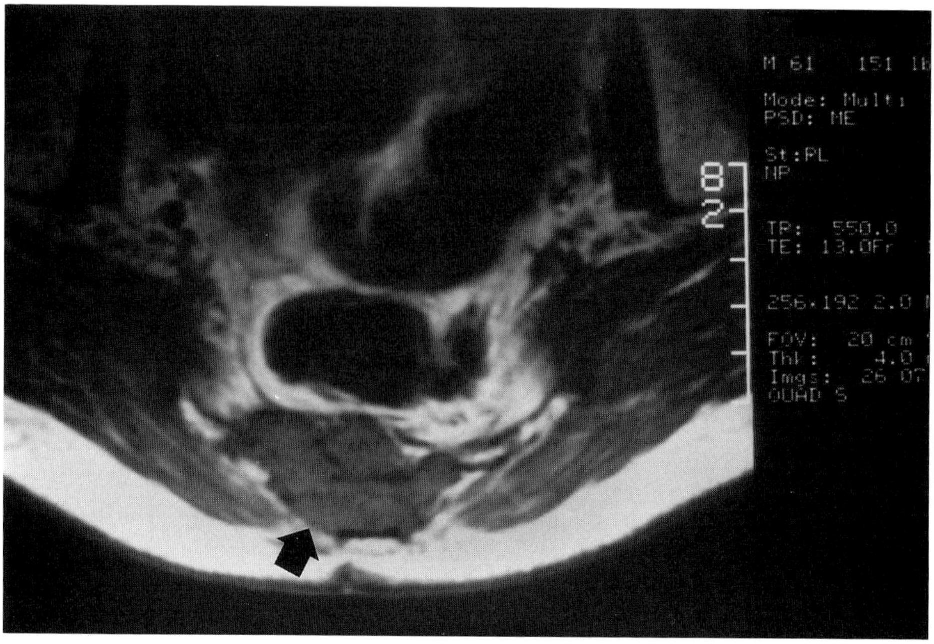

A

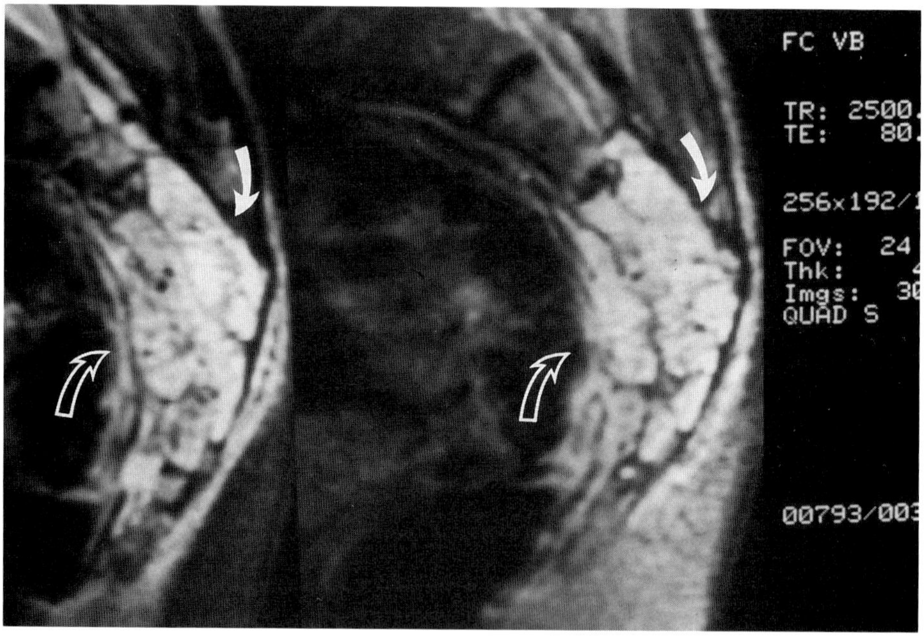

B

Figure 16.2 A 61-year-old male with a sacrococcygeal chordoma. (A) Axial T1-weighted image (550/13) demonstrates a sacral mass (arrow) which is isointense to muscle. (B) Sagittal T2-weighted images (2500/80) reveal that the lesion is lobulated and exhibits very bright signal intensity. There is soft tissue extension of the mass anteriorly into the presacral space (curved open arrows) as well as posteriorly into the spinal canal (curved arrows). Internal foci of signal void may well represent calcification.

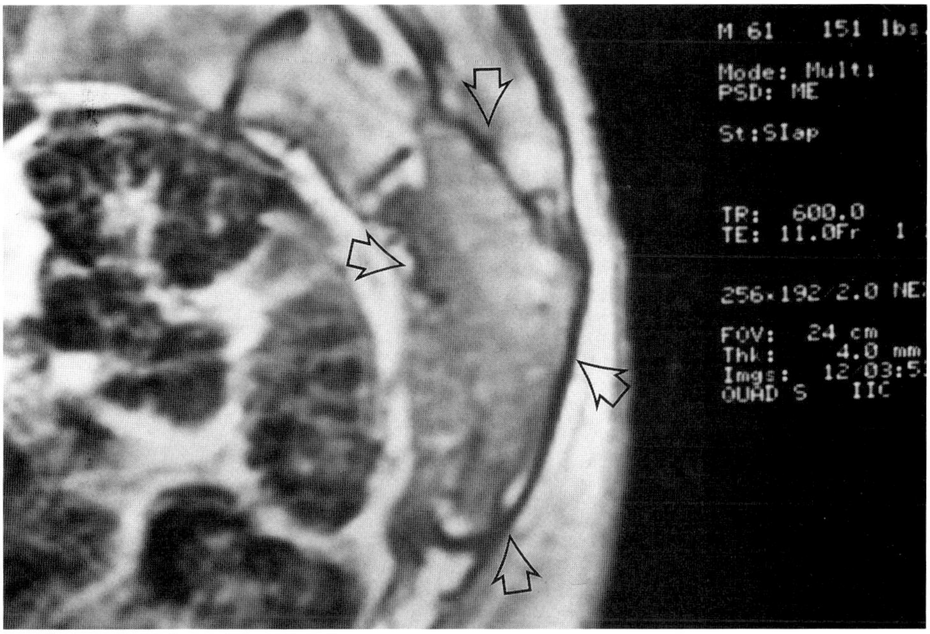

C

Figure 16.2 (continued) (C) Gadolinium-enhanced sagittal T1-weighted image (600/11) reveals uniform enhancement of the mass (open arrows). (Courtesy of James O. Johnston, MD).

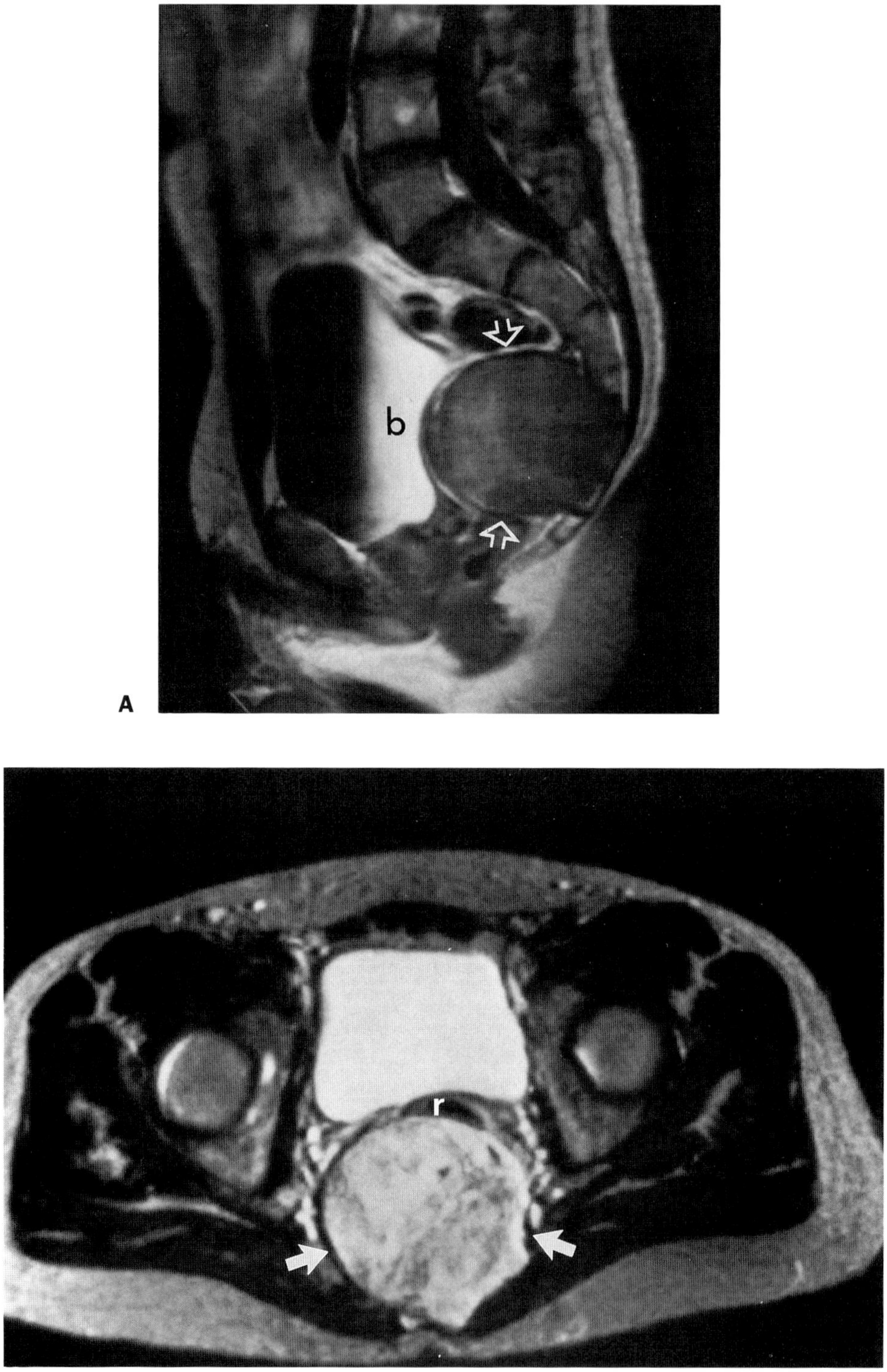

B

FIGURE 16.3 Sacrococcygeal chordoma in a 48-year-old male. (A) Sagittal T1-weighted image following gadolinium administration depicts a large soft tissue component extending into the presacral space with mass effect on the bladder (b). There is inhomogeneous contrast enhancement. Note the thin low signal fibrous pseudocapsule (open arrows). (B) Axial T2-weighted image reveals that the mass exhibits heterogeneous, predominantly bright signal intensity (arrows). Internal foci of signal void may represent calcification. Mass effect on the rectum (r) is present. (Courtesy of James O. Johnston, MD).

Primary Lymphoma of Bone

Definition. Primary lymphoma of bone is defined as lymphomatous involvement of a single bone without involvement of other tissues at presentation. The vast majority of cases are non-Hodgkin's lymphoma, which are of B-cell morphology. Primary lymphoma of bone only rarely consists of Hodgkin's lymphoma. Histologically, the lesions typically contain a dense network of reticulin and collagen fibers. Areas of intratumoral necrosis are generally present and there may be cyst formation as well. Previous terms used to define this entity include reticulum cell sarcoma and lymphosarcoma.

Clinical Features. Primary lymphoma of bone is an uncommon tumor accounting for 3–5% of all primary malignant bone neoplasms. These lesions may occur at any age with a mean age of approximately 45 years old. There is a slight male predominance. Patients typically present with localized pain and swelling, often without associated constitutional symptoms. Pathologic fracture may occur.

Location. These lesions most commonly involve the metaphysis or diaphysis of long bones, especially around the knee. The pelvis is also a relatively frequent location. Any bone may be affected.

Implications. Primary lymphoma of bone has a better prognosis than most primary malignant osseous tumors. The presence of periostitis, soft tissue extension, and pathologic fracture are associated with a poorer prognosis. These lesions are generally treated with radiation therapy and/or chemotherapy.

MRI Findings. On T1-weighted images, these lesions typically appear as homogeneous hypointense (isointense to muscle) masses. On T2-weighted sequences, they generally appear as heterogeneous lesions with signal that is isointense or hyperintense to fat, but hypointense to fluid. Small foci of bright signal intensity are typically seen as well. The dominant signal intensity has been reported to be less than that of many primary bone malignancies, which is probably due to the high fibrous tissue content of primary lymphoma of bone. There is commonly an associated soft tissue mass. Joint effusion and intra-articular extension may also be present.

Differential Diagnosis. The MR signal characteristics of primary lymphoma of bone may be seen with numerous other aggressive/malignant osseous lesions. It has been recently reported that bone sequestra (detached or dead pieces of separated bone) are present in 11% of cases of primary lymphoma of bone on plain films. If a sequestrum is identified, entities such as fibrosarcoma, malignant fibrous histiocytoma, desmoplastic fibroma, osteomyelitis, and eosinophilic granuloma should also be considered.

References

Stiglbauer R, Augustin I, Kramer J, et al. MRI in the diagnosis of primary lymphoma of bone: Correlation with histopathology. *JCAT* 16:248–253, 1992.

Mulligan M, Kransdorf M. Sequestra in primary lymphoma of bone: Prevalence and radiologic features. *AJR* 160:1245–1248, 1993.

Vincent J, Ng Y, Norton A, et al. Case report: Primary lymphoma of bone—MRI appearance with pathologic correlation. *Clin Radiol* 45:407–409, 1992.

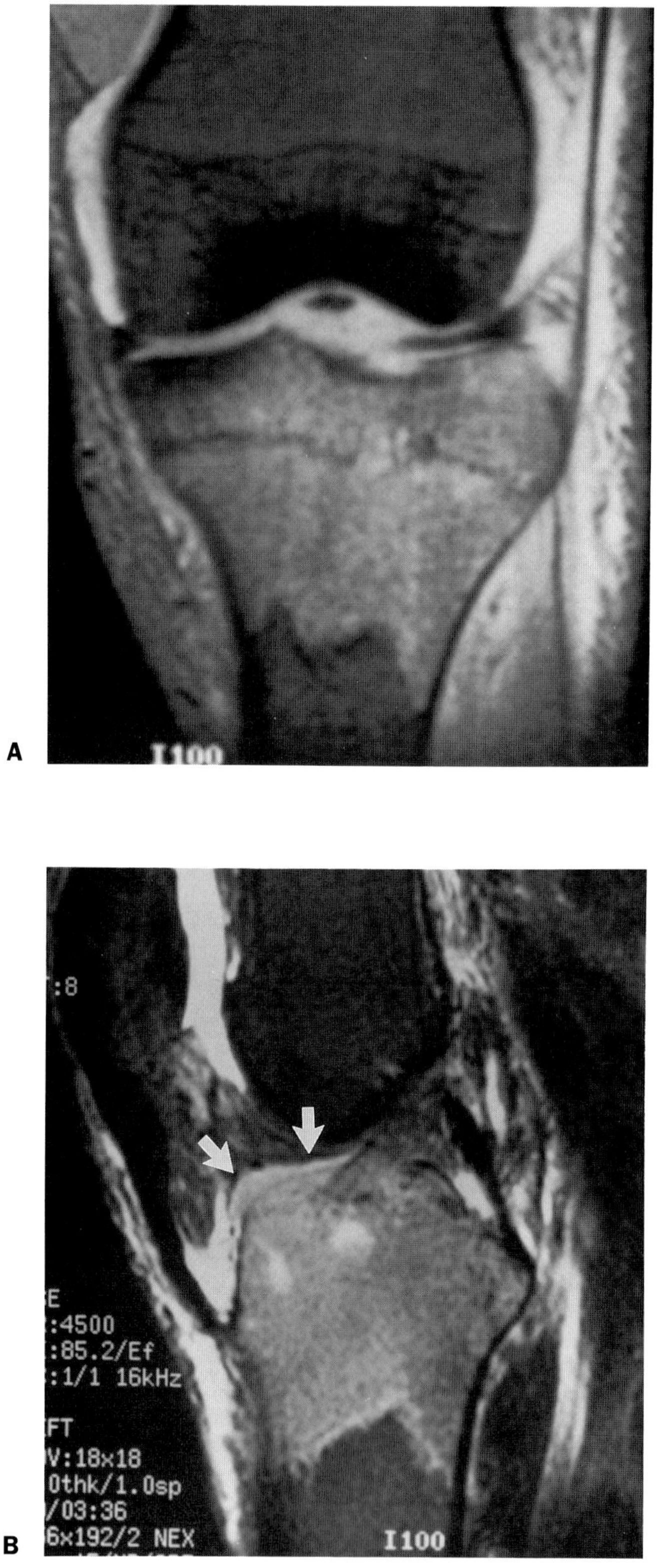

Figure 16.4 A 37-year-old male with a three-week history of severe knee pain. (A) Coronal MPGR (833/10, 25 degrees) and (B) sagittal FSE T2-weighted fat suppression (4500/85) images show an infiltrative lesion within the proximal tibia. The mass extends through the cortex into the intercondylar notch and Hoffa's fat pad (arrows). There is an associated joint effusion and surrounding soft tissue edema.

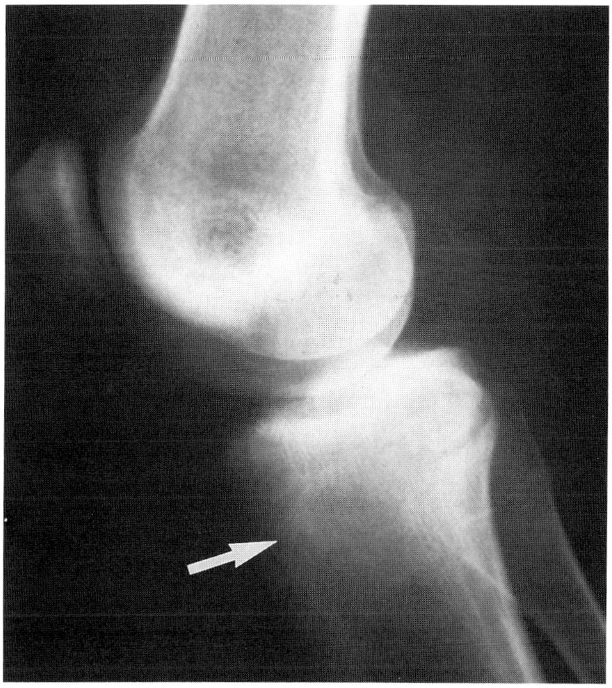

C

FIGURE 16.4 (continued) (C) Lateral radiograph demonstrates very subtle ill-defined sclerosis within the proximal tibia (long arrow). Biopsy of the lesion revealed primary lymphoma of bone. (Courtesy of Alan Massengill, MD).

Osseous Metastasis

Definition. Metastasis to bone may result from various mechanisms of tumor spread including hematogenous dissemination and direct extension, and less commonly via lymphatic and intraspinal pathways. Hematogenous (arterial and venous) routes are the predominant mechanism by which primary malignant tumors spread to osseous structures. Batson's plexus is a particularly important venous route by which tumors spread to the vertebrae.

Clinical Features. The skeletal system is a common site of tumor metastasis. The most common sources of osseous metastases (in decreasing frequency) are carcinomas of the breast, prostate, lung, and kidney. The vast majority of bone metastases occur in middle-aged or older patients. Common sources in the pediatric population include neuroblastoma, Ewing's sarcoma, and osteosarcoma. Common presenting symptoms include pain and pathologic fracture.

Location. Bones that are rich in hematopoietic marrow are the most common sites for osseous metastasis and are (in order of decreasing frequency) the spine, pelvis, ribs, sternum, proximal femoral and humeral shafts, and skull. Within the spine, the lumbar region is most frequently affected. Spinal metastases are most frequently located in the vertebral bodies, although the pedicles are not uncommonly involved. In tubular bones, hematogenous metastases generally begin in the cancellous bone of the medullary cavity and with growth, involve the cortex. Infrequent locations for osseous metastases include the mandible, patella, and bones distal to the elbow and knee. In cases involving metastasis to the hands or feet, bronchogenic carcinoma is the most frequent source. Metastases to the external cortical bone surface (cookie-bite lesions) and intracortical metastases are also most often secondary to bronchogenic carcinoma. Although multiplicity is the general rule regarding skeletal metastases, approximately 15% of cases present with a single metastatic focus.

Implications. The presence of a metastatic lesion weakens the underlying bone and not infrequently leads to pathologic fracture, which occurs most commonly in the spine and proximal femur. The amount of cortical destruction in a tubular bone is an important predictor for the development of a pathologic fracture. Large lesions are often treated with radiation therapy in hopes of preventing this complication. Destruction of greater than half of the underlying cortex is associated with a high risk of pathologic fracture.

MRI Findings. MR is the most sensitive imaging modality for the detection of osseous metastasis, in addition to providing the best depiction of tumor localization and extent. MR imaging has proven helpful in the planning of palliative surgery or radiation therapy for these lesions. On T1-weighted sequences, osseous metastases exhibit hypointense signal (hypointense to isointense in relation to muscle). On T2-weighted sequences, the signal intensity of metastases depends on numerous factors including tissue type, cellularity, water content, and the amount of any possibly associated fibrosis, necrosis, hemorrhage, calcification, and inflammatory cells. However, metastases generally demonstrate increased signal intensity with T2-weighting. The most sensitive pulse sequences in detecting skeletal metastases are STIR, T2-weighted with fat suppression, and T1-weighted.

Differential Diagnosis. Although the MR signal characteristics of skeletal metastases are nonspecific, there are some differential generalizations that can be made. Multiplicity is clearly one of the best signs that can be used to suggest metastases versus primary neoplastic processes. Notable exceptions include multiple myeloma, multifocal infection, eosinophilic granuloma, multiple brown tumors associated with hyperparathyroidism, polyostotic fibrous dysplasia, and enchondromatosis. Large soft tissue masses are infrequent with osseous metastases and favor primary aggressive bone lesions. There are several general rules which can be used in trying to distinguish between metastasis and multiple myeloma. These include:

(1) involvement of a pedicle is seen more frequently with metastasis; (2) myelomatous lesions tend to be fairly uniform in size, whereas metastases are often more variable in size; (3) scintigraphy is much more likely to be falsely negative in multiple myeloma than metastasis; and (4) mandibular involvement is more frequent with multiple myeloma than metastasis. A common dilemma is trying to distinguish between osteoporotic vertebral compression fractures and pathologic fractures from vertebral metastases. In our experience, we have found that the use of a single general rule has been most helpful and practical in distinguishing the vast majority of osteoporotic compression fractures from pathologic compression fractures: there must be complete replacement of the fatty marrow within a vertebral body by a metastatic lesion before a pathologic fracture will occur; on the contrary, osteoporotic compression fractures typically have preservation of at least a portion of yellow marrow. It is important to note that this generalization does not apply to primary bone marrow processes such as multiple myeloma. Additional signs suggesting pathologic compression fracture include the presence of an associated soft tissue mass and distortion of the vertebral endplates.

References

Gold R, Seeger L, Bassett L, et al. An integrated approach to the evaluation of metastatic bone disease. *Radiol Clin North Am* 28:471–483, 1990.

Schweitzer M, Levine C, Mitchell D, et al. Bulls-eyes and halos: Useful MR discriminators of osseous metastases. *Radiology* 188:249–252, 1993.

Yuh W, Zachar C, Barloon T, et al. Vertebral compression fractures: Distinction between benign and malignant causes with MR imaging. *Radiology* 172:215–218, 1989.

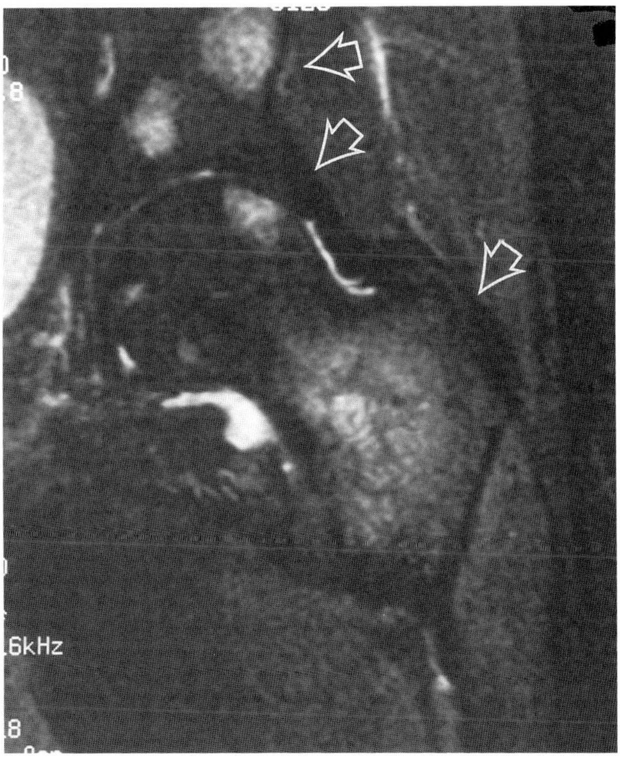

FIGURE 16.5 Numerous bone metastases from Ewing's sarcoma. Coronal FMPIR image (3050/51, TI-150) of the left hip reveals multiple foci of increased signal within the proximal left femur and acetabulum (arrows). A small joint effusion is present.

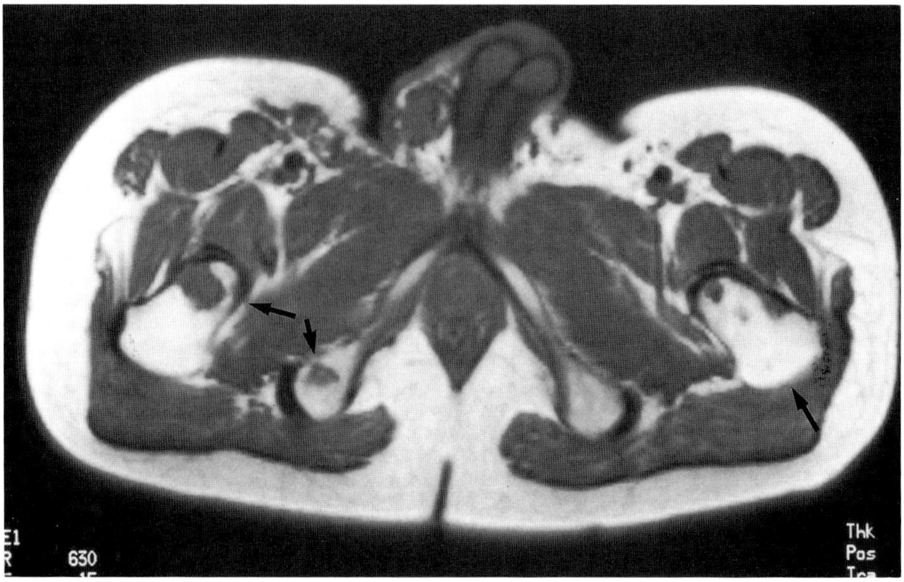

A

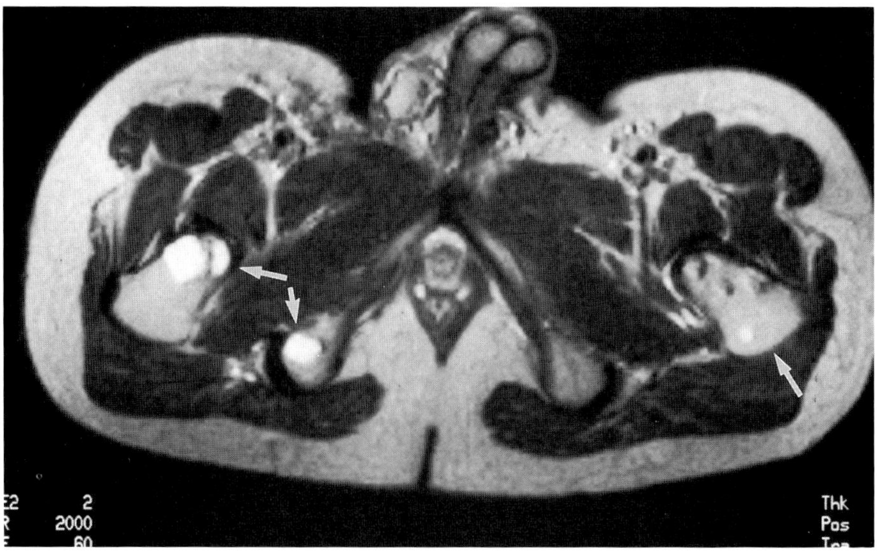

B

FIGURE 16.6 Extensive bone metastasis. Axial (A) T1-weighted (630/15) and (B) T2-weighted (2000/60) images reveal lesions within both proximal femora and the right ischial tuberosity (arrows).

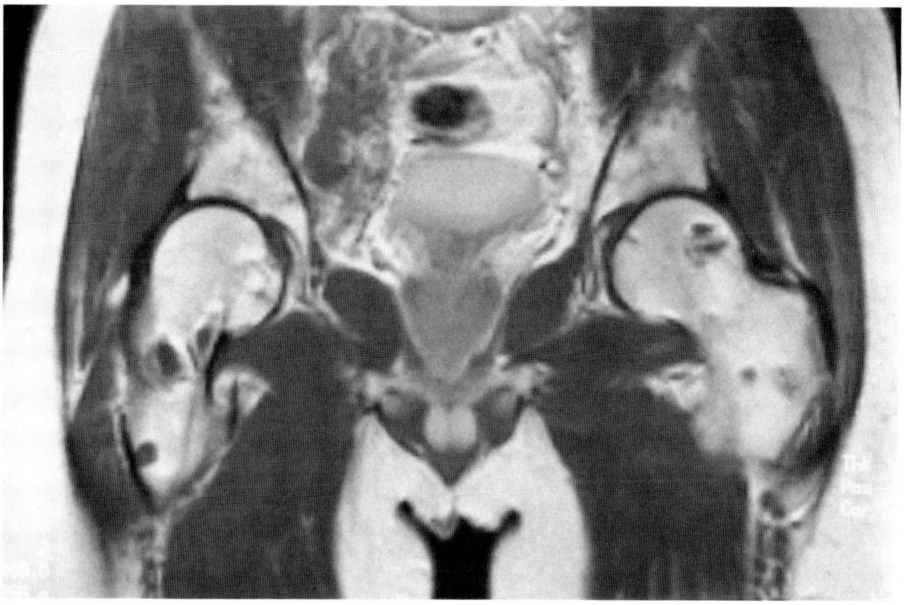

C

FIGURE 16.6 (continued) (C) Gadolinium-enhanced coronal T1-weighted image (500/15) demonstrates peripheral enhancement of multiple necrotic metastases within the right and left proximal femora.

Multiple Myeloma (Plasma Cell Myeloma, Plasmacytoma)

Definition. Multiple myeloma (MM) is a malignant disorder of bone marrow in which there is monoclonal proliferation of plasma cells. Plasma cell infiltration of the bone marrow may occur in a diffuse or nodular fashion. Solitary lesions are known as plasmacytomas.

Clinical Features. MM is the most common primary malignant bone lesion, occurring with a yearly incidence of about 3 per 100,000 persons. The disease typically occurs between 40 and 80 years of age. Patients with plasmacytoma tend to be about 10 years younger than those with multifocal disease. There is a slight male predominance. The most common symptom is bone pain which is present in about 75% of cases. In most patients, a monoclonal protein band is present on urine or serum electrophoresis, but there is a form of the disease in which no abnormal protein can be demonstrated in urine or serum (nonsecretory MM). Patients may present with pathologic fracture. Vertebral lesions may lead to kyphosis or neurologic symptoms. Infection and renal insufficiency are common in patients with MM. Amyloidosis occurs in about 15% of those with MM. There is a rare sclerotic form of MM which occurs in less than 2% of cases. This form may occur in conjunction with other clinical abnormalities, known as POEMS syndrome (polyneuropathy, organomegaly, endocrinopathy, M protein, and skin changes).

Location. The axial skeleton is the predominant site of involvement. MM most commonly affects the vertebrae, ribs, skull, pelvis, and long bones (especially femur), in order of decreasing frequency. At the time of diagnosis, the disease is often widely disseminated throughout the axial skeleton.

Implications. The prognosis of MM is poor with an average survival time of approximately three years. The prognosis is poorer with increased tumor cell mass, decreased renal function, and increased serum beta 2-microglobulin levels. The primary treatment is chemotherapy. Radiation therapy may be used for lesions that are progressive, symptomatic, or associated with pathologic or compression fracture. Bone marrow transplantation can also be performed. Response to therapy is typically assessed by serial monitoring of myeloma protein levels. Some authors have suggested that MR may prove useful for following disease status in patients with nonsecretory MM or equivocal protein findings.

MRI Findings. On T1-weighted sequences, MM lesions typically appear hypointense, but may appear of intermediate intensity (slightly hyperintense to muscle). On T2-weighted and STIR images, the lesions typically exhibit hyperintense signal. MR patterns of spinal MM include diffuse, focal, and numerous small scattered foci. Vertebral compression fractures may occur without complete myelomatous replacement of marrow. Extension into the soft tissues or epidural space may be present. In long bones, endosteal scalloping is a characteristic finding. Lesions may be expansile and fluid-fluid levels have been reported.

Differential Diagnosis. The MRI signal characteristics of MM are nonspecific. Corresponding plain films should be obtained. Plasmacytomas or individual MM lesions may have a benign appearance radiographically. Lesion multiplicity is clearly one of the best signs in distinguishing MM from other entities. In these cases, the principle differential consideration is metastasis. In the spine, multiple vertebral hemangiomas are also common. Vertebral hemangiomas characteristically appear hyperintense on T1-weighted sequences due to the presence of fat within the lesions. However, vertebral hemangiomas may also appear hyperintense on T2-weighted sequences. A characteristic imaging feature of vertebral hemangiomas is a coarse vertical trabecular pattern resembling corduroy or honeycomb. On individual MR slices, this would appear as a speckled appearance of multiple small round foci of hypointense signal on all pulse sequences. Several general rules can be applied when trying to distinguish between MM and skeletal metastasis. These include: (1) pedicle involvement is more common with metastasis; (2) MM lesions tend to be fairly uniform in size, whereas metastases are often variably sized; (3) scintigraphy is much more likely to be falsely negative in MM than metastasis; and (4) mandibular involvement is more frequent with MM than with metastasis. In addition, if a lesion causes a pathologic vertebral compression fracture and there is some preservation of yellow marrow on MR images, the lesion is much more likely to be MM than metastasis. Another general rule can be applied when attempting to distinguish between extensive hematopoietic marrow throughout the spine and diffuse MM. Hematopoietic marrow should be at least slightly hyperintense in relation to normal disc or muscle on T1-weighted sequences. Therefore, if the marrow signal appears hypointense or isointense to normal disc or muscle, diffuse MM or other infiltrative marrow process cannot be excluded. It is important to note that this rule serves only as a general guideline, since MM lesions can occasionally appear slightly hyperintense to muscle on T1-weighted images.

References

Moulopoulos L, Varma D, Dimopoulos M, et al. Multiple myeloma: Spinal MR imaging in patients with untreated newly diagnosed disease. *Radiology* 185:833–840, 1992.

Moulopoulos L, Dimopoulos M, Alexanian R, et al. Multiple myeloma: MR patterns of response to treatment. *Radiology* 193:441–446, 1994.

Rahmouni A, Divine M, Mathieu D, et al. MR appearance of multiple myeloma of the spine before and after treatment. *AJR* 160:1053–1057, 1993.

Rahmouni A, Divine M, Mathieu D, et al. Detection of multiple myeloma involving the spine: Efficacy of fat-suppression and contrast-enhanced MR imaging. *AJR* 160:1049–1052, 1993.

Libshitz H, Malthouse S, Cunningham D, et al. Multiple myeloma: Appearance at MR imaging. *Radiology* 182:833–837, 1992.

Carlson K, Astrom G, Nyman R, et al. MR imaging of multiple myeloma in tumour mass measurement at diagnosis and during treatment. *Acta Radiologica* 36:9–14, 1995.

Carroll K, Feller J. Useful internal standard for distinguishing infiltrative marrow pathology from hematopoietic marrow at MR imaging. *Radiology* 193(P):237, 1994.

Harter S, Nokes S. Plasmacytoma of the sacrum: Fluid-fluid levels on MR images. *AJR* 165:741–742, 1995.

A

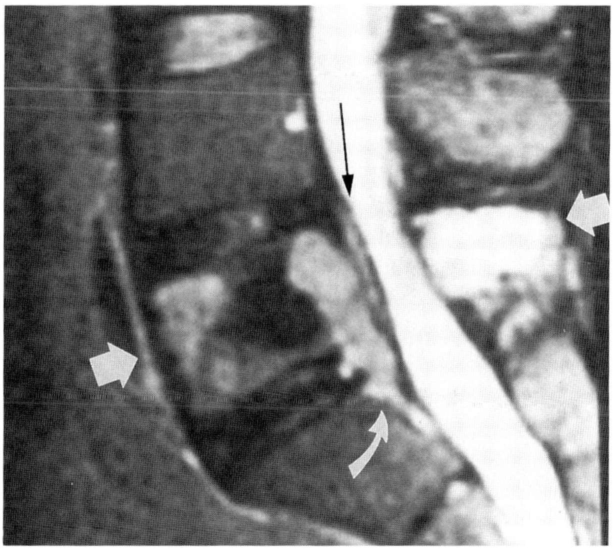

FIGURE 16.7 Plasmacytoma of the lumbar spine in a 33-year-old male. (A) Sagittal T2-weighted image (2500/90) demonstrates an extensive mass involving the L5 vertebral body and spinous process (arrows). There is extension of the lesion into the anterior epidural space (thin arrow) and extension across the L5-S1 disc space posteriorly (curved arrow). Incidental note of disc dessication at L4-5 and L5-S1.

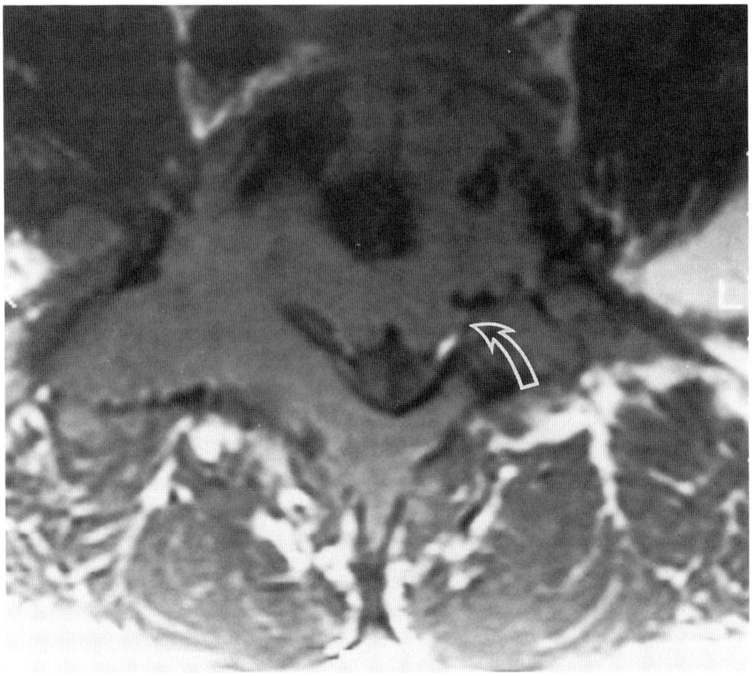

B

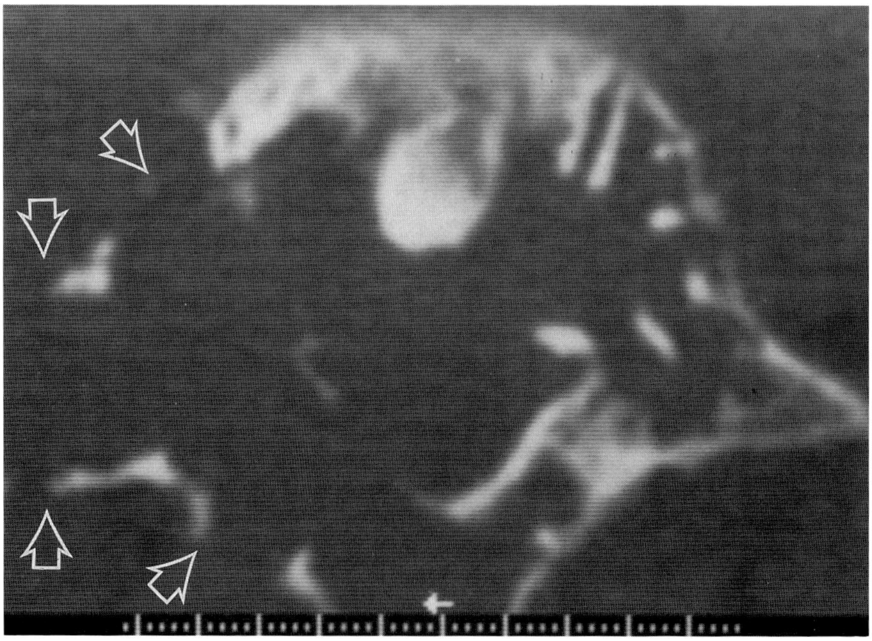

C

FIGURE 16.7 (continued) (B) Axial T1-weighted image (650/14) and (C) corresponding axial CT image further depict extensive involvement of the L5 vertebral body and posterior elements including multiple areas of cortical destruction as well as osseous expansion (open arrows). Extension of disease into the anterior epidural space is again seen (curved open arrow). Note that the lesion is of intermediate signal intensity with T1-weighting.

Leukemia

Definition. Leukemia refers to a malignant condition of the bone marrow in which there is proliferation of lymphocytes or granulocytes. Leukemia is divided into acute and chronic forms. A chloroma (also known as myeloblastoma or granulocytic sarcoma) is a solid mass of leukemic cells which may occur in soft tissue or bone.

Clinical Features. Adults may have acute or chronic forms, whereas children nearly always have the acute form of the disease. Acute leukemia affecting children occurs with a peak incidence between ages 2 and 5. Chronic leukemia has a peak frequency in middle age. Patients may present with fever, constitutional symptoms, arthralgia, bone pain or tenderness, infection, splenomegaly, or lymphadenopathy. Chloromas may occur in about 5% of leukemic patients.

Location. Leukemic infiltrates may be seen throughout the bone marrow and have a predilection for the metaphysis of long bones.

Implications. These patients are treated with chemotherapy and possibly bone marrow transplantation. Chloromas may require additional therapy with radiation or even surgical resection.

MRI Findings. Leukemic infiltrates typically appear hypointense on T1-weighted sequences and hyperintense with T2-weighting. The distribution may be diffuse or patchy.

Differential Diagnosis. The MR appearance of leukemia can resemble other infiltrative malignancies including metastasis and multiple myeloma. In patients with a known history of leukemia, the differential diagnosis of leukemic infiltrates may include hematopoietic marrow, osteomyelitis, and bone infarction. Hematopoietic marrow typically exhibits signal intensity that is slightly greater than muscle on T1-weighted sequences, whereas leukemic infiltrate typically demonstrates signal that is hypointense or isointense to muscle. Medullary bone infarcts are typically surrounded by a serpiginous peripheral rim of low signal intensity on all pulse sequences, which should allow distinction from leukemic infiltration. However, very early bone infarction may not have a serpiginous border and may be indistinguishable from leukemic infiltrate on MRI. In addition, it may not be possible to differentiate osteomyelitis from leukemic infiltrate based upon the MRI findings.

References

Bohndorf K, Benz-Bohm G, Gross-Fengels W, et al. MRI of the knee region in leukemic children. Part I. Initial pattern in patients with untreated disease. *Pediat Radiol* 20:179–183, 1990.

Benz-Bohm G, Gross-Fengels W, Bohndorf K, et al. MRI of the knee region in leukemic children. Part II. Followup: Responder, non-responder, relapse. *Pediat Radiol* 20:272–276, 1990.

Ruzal-Shapiro C, Berdon W, Cohen M, et al. MR imaging of diffuse bone marrow replacement in pediatric patients with cancer. *Radiology* 181:587–589, 1991.

Pui M, Fletcher B, Langston J. Granulocytic sarcoma in childhood leukemia: Imaging features. *Radiology* 190:698–702, 1994.

Resnick D, Haghighi P. Myeloproliferative disorders: In Resnick D: *Bone and Joint Imaging*. Philadelphia, PA, W.B. Saunders Company; 1989, pp 703–707.

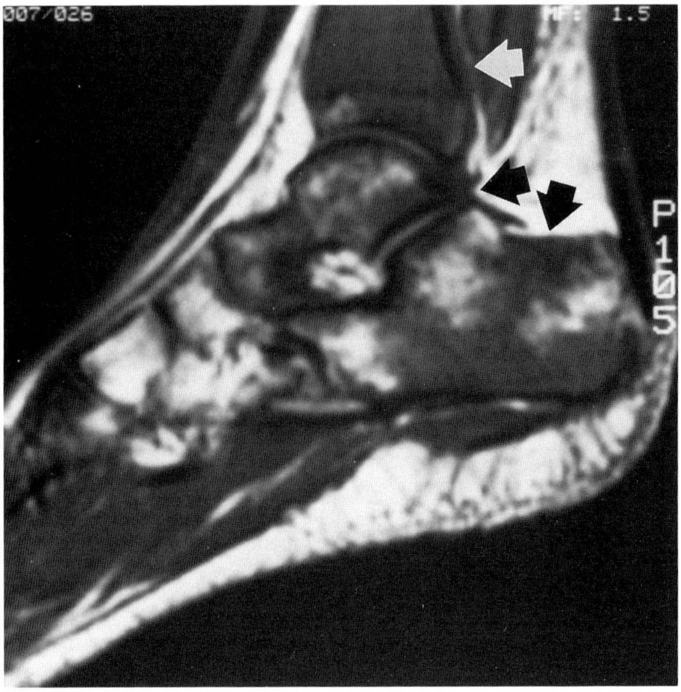

A

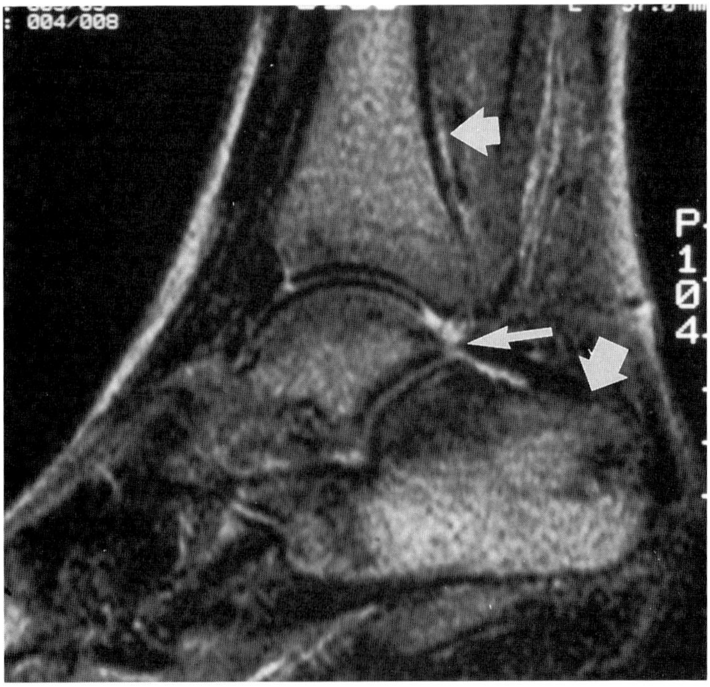

B

FIGURE 16.8 A 45-year-old male with leukemia. Sagittal (A) T1-weighted (550/11) and (B) inversion recovery (1800/30, TI-160) images reveal extensive leukemic infiltrates involving the distal tibia, talus, and calcaneus (arrows). The signal is isointense to muscle with T1-weighting and mildly hyperintense with inversion recovery technique.

SECTION III

JOINT SPACE

17 Intra-articular Masses

Pigmented Villonodular Synovitis

Definition. Pigmented villonodular synovitis (PVNS) is an idiopathic monoarticular arthropathy characterized histologically by hyperplastic synovium (in the form of villous projections and nodules) containing lipid-laden foam cells, histiocytes, giant cells, and hemosiderin. PVNS can be diffuse or less commonly localized. The erosive changes of PVNS are due to a pressure phenomenon resulting from entrapment of soft tissue masses between articulating surfaces.

Clinical Features. PVNS is an uncommon disorder with an estimated incidence of 2 cases per one million persons annually. It occurs most commonly between the ages of 20 and 50, but may be seen in teens and the elderly. The clinical presentation consists of an insidious onset and progression of joint swelling, stiffness, and discomfort, but without isolated pain. Joint effusions are the rule. The clinical picture of a marked joint effusion and swelling, which are out of proportion to the amount of accompanying discomfort, with no history of trauma, is reported to be unique for diffuse PVNS. There may be a diffuse palpable synovial mass, particularly in the suprapatellar region. Mild to moderate tenderness and a slight flexion posture are present in the vast majority of cases. Due to chronic distension, symptoms of extensor mechanism dysfunction are often present and frequently lead to misdiagnosis. There seems to be a predilection for Caucasian, sedentary individuals. Although aspiration of xanthochromic or serosanginous joint fluid is often present, performance of an aspiration to detect a bloody effusion has been shown to be an unreliable diagnostic tool.

Location. Monoarticular involvement is the rule. Polyarticular involvement has only rarely been reported. Most cases affect the knee, with less common locations including the hip, ankle, shoulder, and elbow. Involvement of numerous other joints has been described. In the knee, there is a predilection for involvement posterior to the posterior cruciate ligament. Associated subchondral cystic lesions are more commonly identified in joints with tight capsules such as the hip and elbow. These lesions are usually nonmarginal in location and may be multiple.

Implications. Total synovectomy is the treatment of choice for diffuse PVNS. There is a high local recurrence rate (approaching 50%) following surgical treatment. This high recurrence rate is probably secondary to a persistence of disease resulting from the technical difficulty of performing a total synovectomy. Arthrodesis or arthroplasty is often performed in cases where the disease is extensive. Low-dose radiation therapy or radiation synovectomy is sometimes used to provide palliation or control of the disease in poor surgical candidates or in those with recurrence following synovectomy. In addition to providing a diagnosis of PVNS, MRI is useful in delineating the full extent of the disease for treatment planning as well as in assessing the disease status following surgery or radiation therapy.

MRI Findings. The MRI findings of PVNS include hemosiderin deposition, joint effusion, hyperplastic synovium in the form of frond-like villous masses, subchondral cystic lesions, marginal pressure erosions, occasional lipid production, and the absence of significant cartilage loss and joint destruction. Due to the presence of hemosiderin and its unique signal characteristics, MRI allows a highly confident diagnosis of PVNS in the appropriate clinical setting. Hyperplastic, hemosiderin-laden synovium appears hypointense on all pulse sequences. The signal is hypointense or isointense to muscle on T1-weighted images and hypointense to muscle with T2-weighting. On gradient-echo images, due to magnetic susceptibility, the hypointense signal of hemosiderin becomes more prominent resulting in improved detection. Hemosiderin may be identified within associated subchondral cystic lesions or popliteal cysts. A lipid component may also be identified, appearing hyperintense on T1-weighted images and of intermediate signal intensity on T2-weighted images.

Differential Diagnosis. The MRI differential diagnosis of PVNS includes other causes of hemosiderotic synovitis such as trauma, hemophilia, and rheumatoid arthritis. Post-traumatic hemorrhage can usually be distinguished on the basis of clinical history. Hemophilia and rheumatoid arthritis are usually associated with marked cartilage loss and should also be readily distinguished on clinical grounds. Synovial osteochondromatosis may simulate PVNS on MRI. Calcification within these loose bodies results in hypointense signal on all pulse sequences. Plain films would easily identify these calcified loose bodies and distinguish this condition from PVNS. In synovial chondromatosis, in which plain films will not reveal calcification, the appearance of the loose bodies as discrete, well-circumscribed masses should allow differentiation from PVNS. A fibrous tumor, such as a desmoid, may demonstrate hypointense signal on all pulse sequences due to the fibrous content. However, the location outside of the joint space and absence of the characteristic intra-articular changes of PVNS should allow differentiation.

References

Steinbach L, Neumann C, Stoller D, et al. MRI of the knee in diffuse pigmented villonodular synovitis. *Clin Imag* 13:305–316, 1989.

Flandry F, Hughston J, McCann S, et al. Diagnostic features of diffuse pigmented villonodular synovitis of the knee. *Clin Ortho* 298:212–220, 1994.

Jelinek J, Kransdorf M, Utz J, et al. Imaging of pigmented villonodular synovitis with emphasis on MR imaging. *AJR* 152:337–342, 1989.

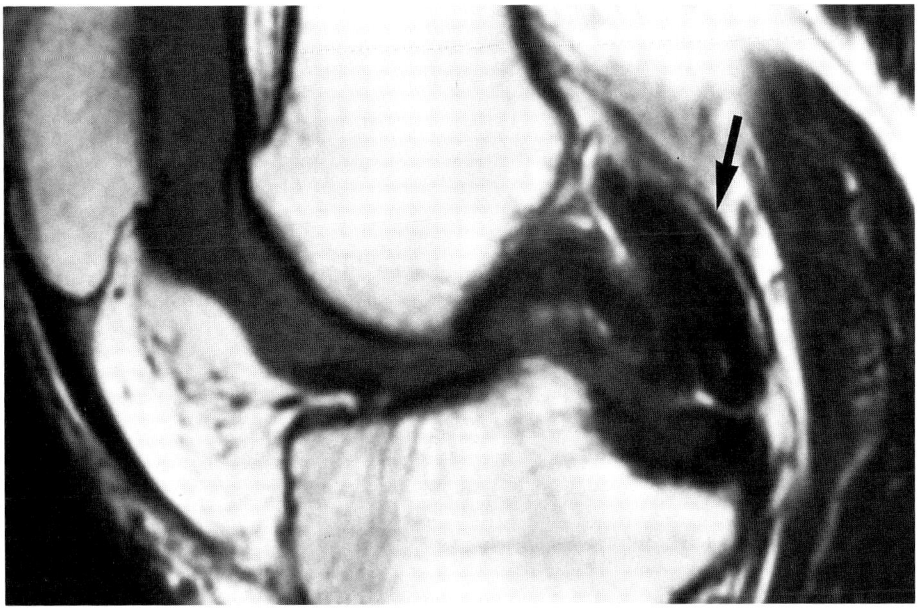

A

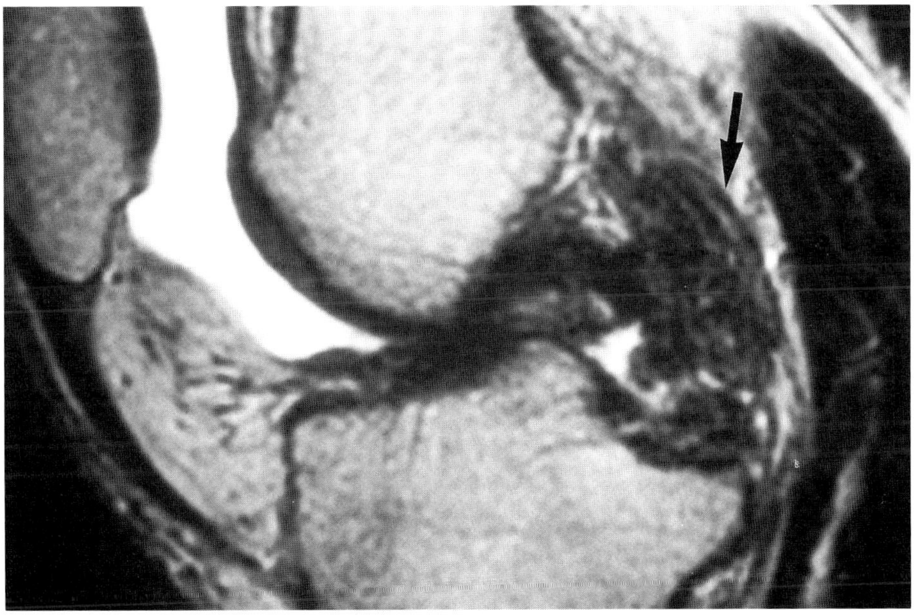

B

FIGURE 17.1 A 62-year-old woman with knee discomfort and swelling. Sagittal (A) T1-weighted (600/20) and (B) FSE T2-weighted (4000/135) images demonstrate a prominent joint effusion and lobulated hypointense soft tissue (arrows) centered posterior to the posterior cruciate ligament. This appearance is characteristic of pigmented villonodular synovitis. The hypointense signal results from the presence of hemosiderin. Gradient-recalled echo imaging can be used to improve detection of the hemosiderin present with PVNS. This technique will result in "blooming" of the signal void due to magnetic susceptibility artifact.

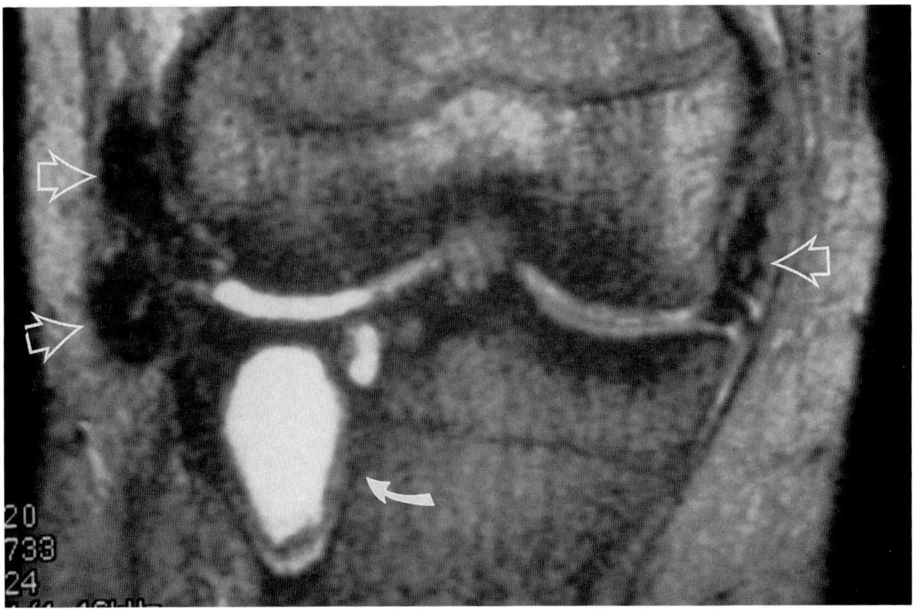

C

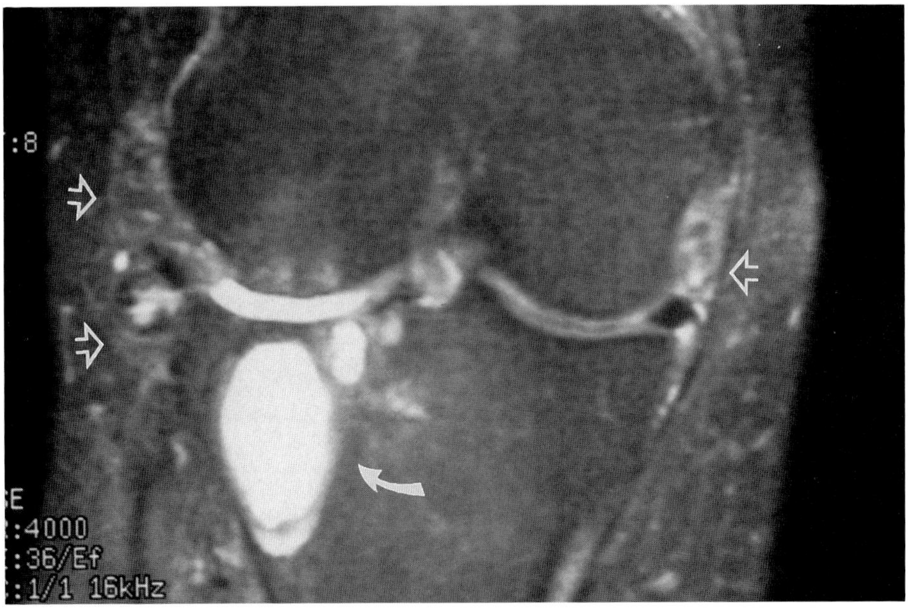

D

FIGURE 17.1 (continued) Coronal (C) MPGR (733/24, 20 degrees) and (D) FSE T2-weighted fat suppression (4000/36) images illustrate this point. The signal void related to hemosiderin is accentuated on the gradient-recalled echo image (large open arrows), but is difficult to identify on the fast spin-echo image (open arrows). Fast spin-echo imaging is known to minimize magnetic susceptibility artifact. Note the prominent subchondral cystic change within the lateral tibial plateau (curved arrows) as well as lateral compartment chondromalacia.

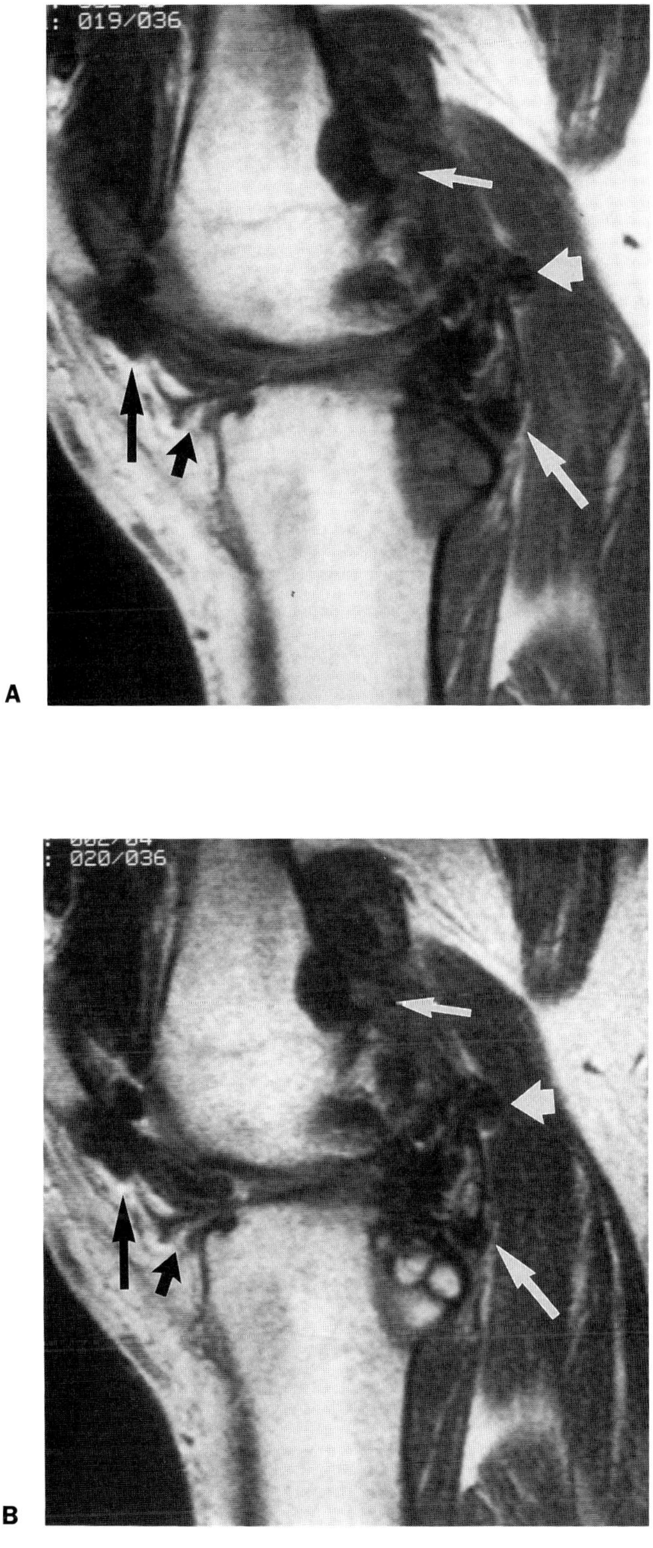

FIGURE 17.2 PVNS of the knee in a 37-year-old woman. (A), (B) Sagittal dual-echo T2-weighted images (1500/20, 60) reveal numerous nodular areas of very low signal (arrows). This appearance is characteristic of PVNS.

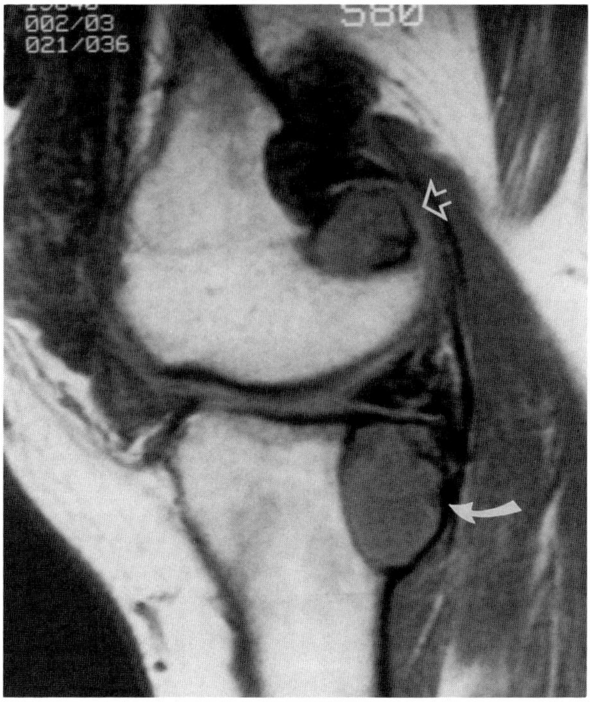

C

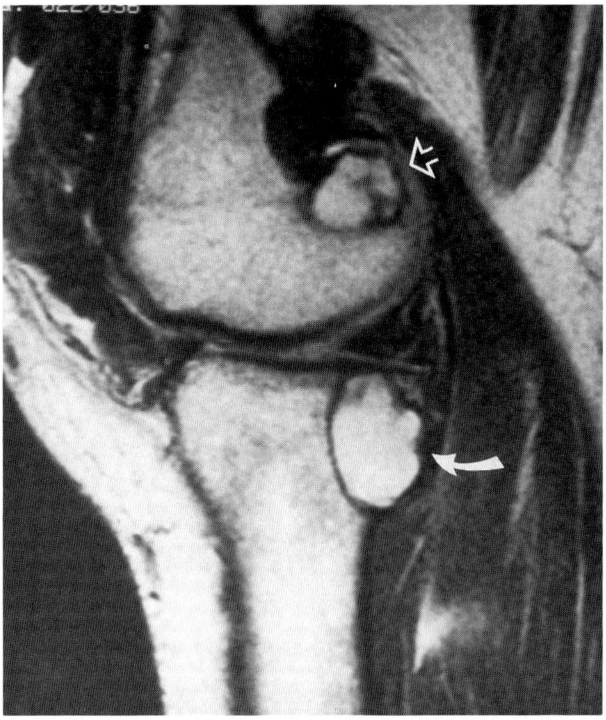

D

FIGURE 17.2 (continued) (C), (D) More medial sagittal dual-echo T2-weighted images demonstrate a marginal erosion (open arrows) and subchondral cystic lesion (curved arrows). A tear of the posterior horn of the medial meniscus is also present. (Courtesy of Chuck Fiske, MD).

Synovial (Osteo) Chondromatosis

Definition. Idiopathic synovial chondromatosis represents chondroid metaplasia of the synovium resulting in cartilaginous masses within a joint, bursa, or tendon sheath. Histologically, this entity consists of nodules of proliferating hyaline cartilage formed by synovial metaplasia. This disorder is nearly always monoarticular. The chondroid bodies may detach from the synovium and grow, receiving nourishment from the synovial fluid. They may subsequently reattach to the synovium, become vascularized and eventually calcify or ossify (hence the term synovial osteochondromatosis).

Clinical Features. Synovial chondromatosis is twice as common in men as in women and usually occurs in the third to fifth decades of life. Patients tend to present with a several-year history of joint pain and limited range of motion. A palpable soft tissue mass may be identified.

Location. The knee is the most commonly involved joint, followed by the hip and elbow. This entity may occur in bursae or tendon sheaths.

Implications. This benign disorder is associated with a chronic progressive course. Synovectomy is the treatment of choice. Focal recurrence following surgery is not uncommon.

MRI Findings. A joint effusion is usually present, which may be hemorrhagic. The MRI appearance of the chondroid bodies depends on their size, age, and attachment. Immature lesions (without calcification or ossification) appear as intermediate signal intensity masses on T1-weighted images and as intermediate to high signal intensity lesions on T2-weighted sequences. The lesions typically appear around the periphery of the joint space. With calcification and ossification, the osteochondromata appear as hypointense structures on T1- and T2-weighted sequences. Occasionally, these lesions may contain marrow fat which appears as hyperintense on T1-weighted images. This condition is typically associated with a large number of cartilaginous or osteocartilaginous bodies which are discrete and fairly uniform in size. The hypointense signal of osteocartilaginous bodies becomes more prominent on gradient-echo images due to magnetic susceptibility. A variable amount of nodular synovial thickening is identified. The nodules may cause erosions of the adjacent bone.

Differential Diagnosis. Idiopathic synovial osteochondromatosis may be distinguished from secondary synovial chondromatosis (from degenerative joint disease) by the absence of osteoarthritic changes. In addition, secondary synovial osteochondromatosis is generally associated with fewer bodies (usually less than 10) which are of variable size. The signal intensity of synovial osteochondromatosis may resemble that of pigmented villonodular synovitis. However, the presence of well-marginated, discrete masses which are of uniform size should allow differentiation from PVNS. Plain radiographs should also allow distinction because calcification is not seen with PVNS.

References

Munk P, Helms C. *MRI of the Knee*. Gaithersburg, MD: Aspen Publishers; 1992; p 174.

Resnick D. *Bone and Joint Imaging*. Philadelphia, PA; W.B. Saunders Company; 1989; pp 390, 1186.

Janzen D, Peterfy C, Forbes J, et al. Cystic Lesions around the knee joint: MR imaging findings. *AJR* 163:155–161, 1994.

Dahlin D, Unni K. *Bone Tumors*. 4th ed, Springfield, Il: Charles C. Thomas Publisher; 1986; pp 462–465.

A

B

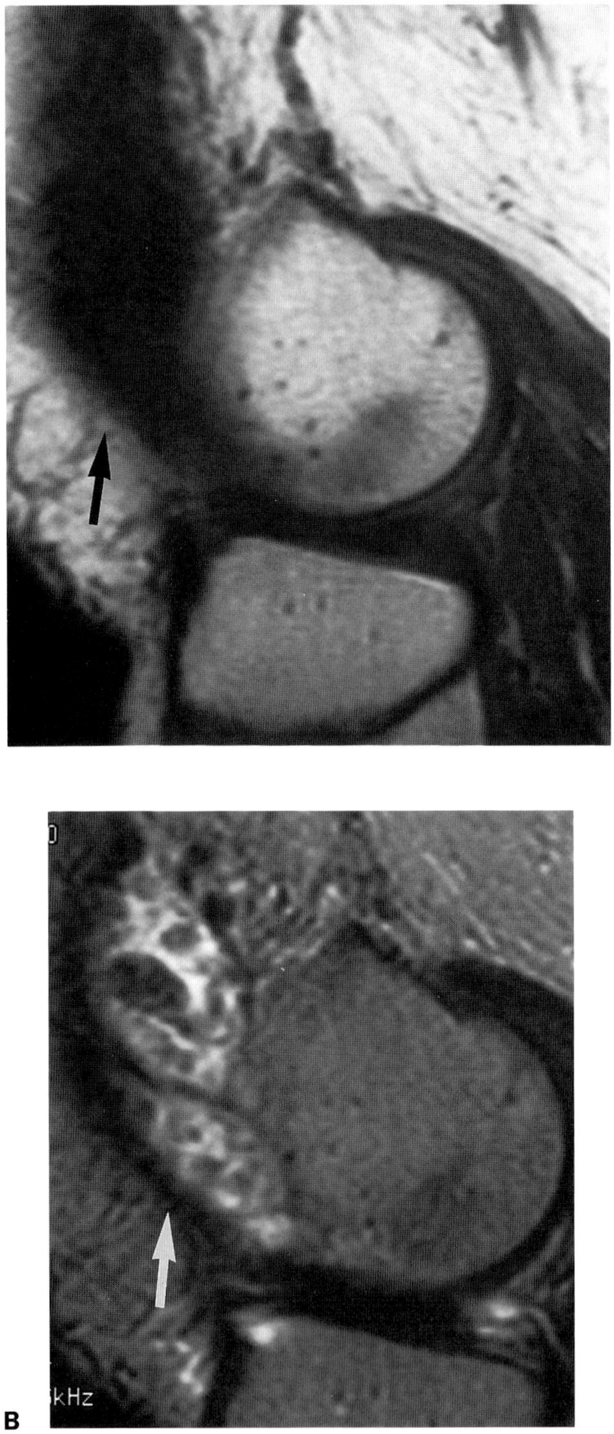

FIGURE 17.3 Synovial chondromatosis in a 64-year-old woman who presented with knee pain and swelling. Radiographs were negative except for the presence of a joint effusion. Sagittal (A) T1-weighted (600/16) and (B) FSE T2-weighted (4000/144) images reveal numerous round and oval intra-articular bodies (arrows) which are isointense to joint fluid with T1-weighting and of intermediate signal intensity with T2-weighting. (C) Axial FSE T2-weighted fat suppression image (3500/51) shows that the chondral bodies are of fairly uniform size (open arrows). There is an associated joint effusion.

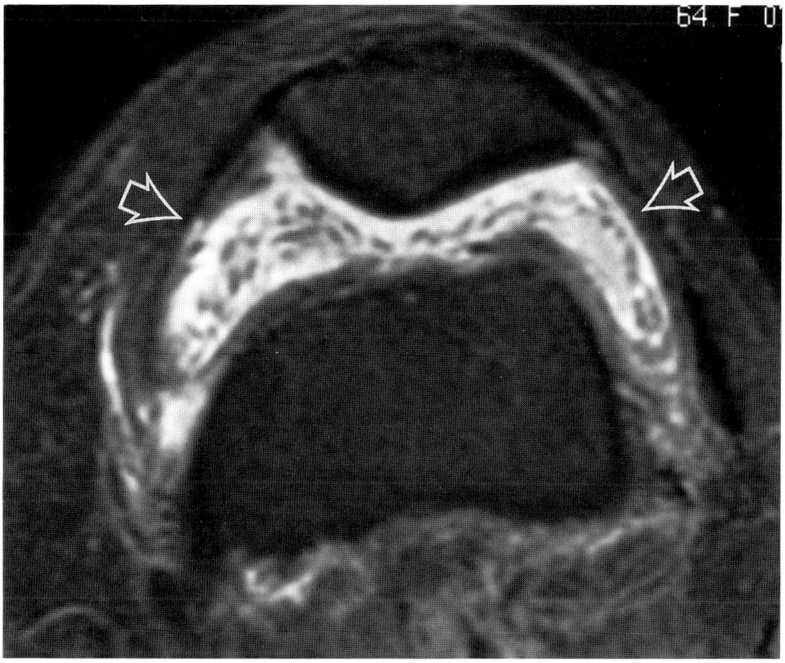

C

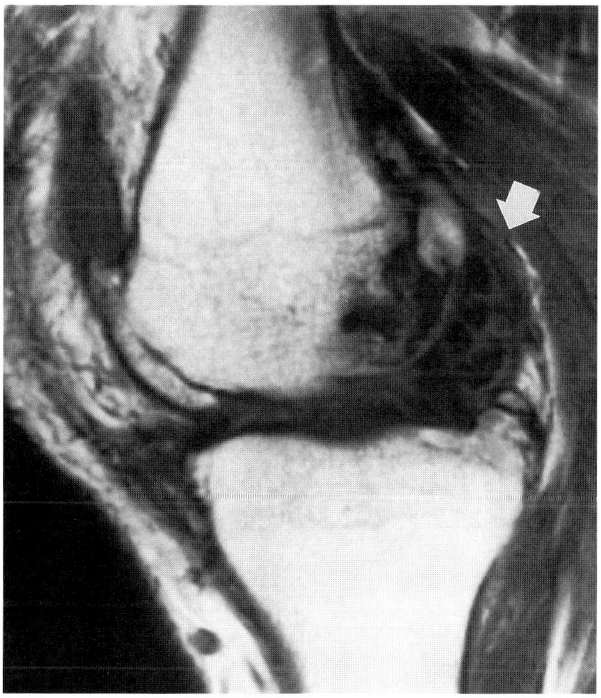

A

FIGURE 17.4 A 47-year-old male with synovial osteochondromatosis of the knee. Sagittal (A) T1-weighted (800/20) and

(*continued*)

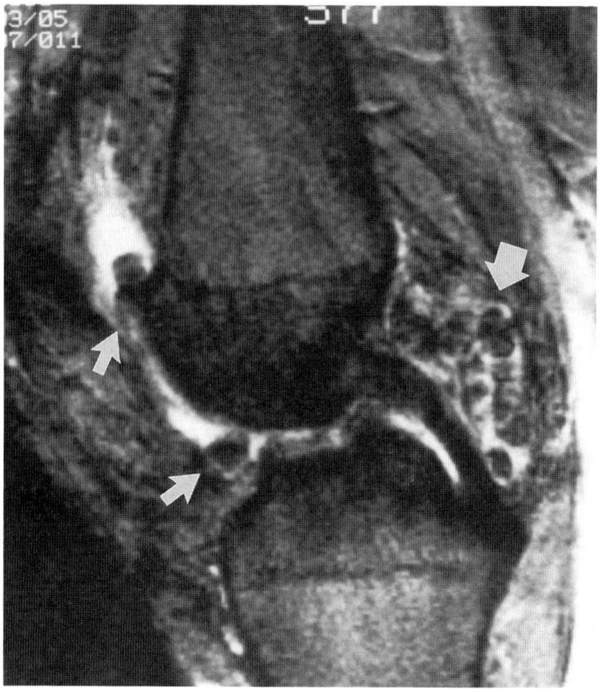

B

Figure 17.4 (continued) (B) MPGR (500/28, 20 degrees) images reveal numerous calcified/ossified intra-articular bodies of low signal intensity (arrows). The lesions are fairly uniform in size. A joint effusion is present.

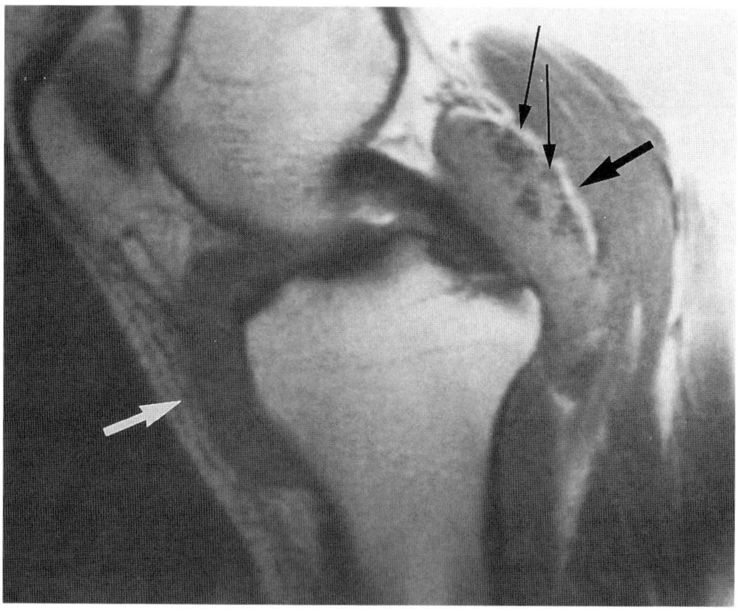

A

Figure 17.5 Synovial osteochondromatosis of the knee in a 27-year-old woman. Sagittal (A) T1-weighted (1000/20) and (B) T2-weighted (1500/70) images reveal synovial osteochondromatosis appearing as conglomerate masses at the periphery of the joint space anteriorly and posteriorly (arrows). The purely cartilaginous portions of the process exhibit intermediate signal intensity with T1-weighting and intermediate to high signal with T2-weighting. The posterior component extends into a popliteal cyst (gastrocnemiosemimembranosus bursa). Note the hypointense foci reflecting calcification/ossification (thin arrows). (C) Lateral radiograph demonstrates the calcified/ossified component posteriorly (wide arrows).

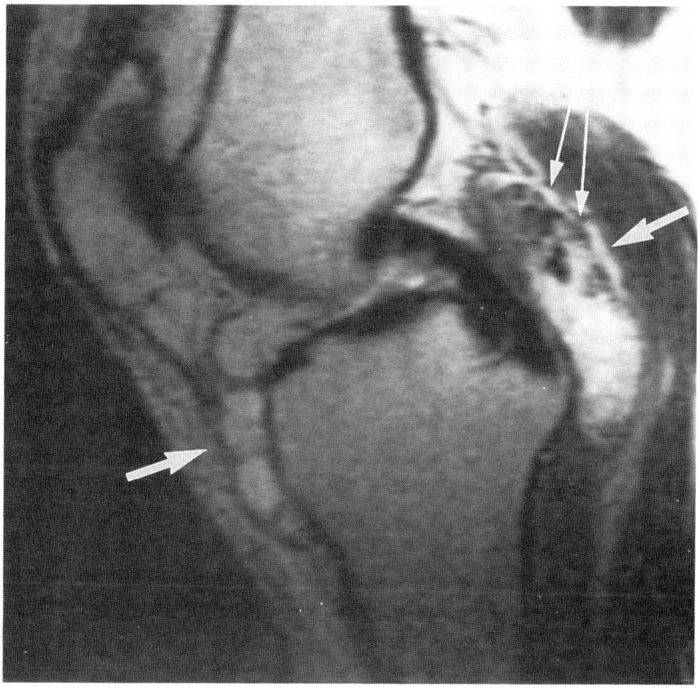

B

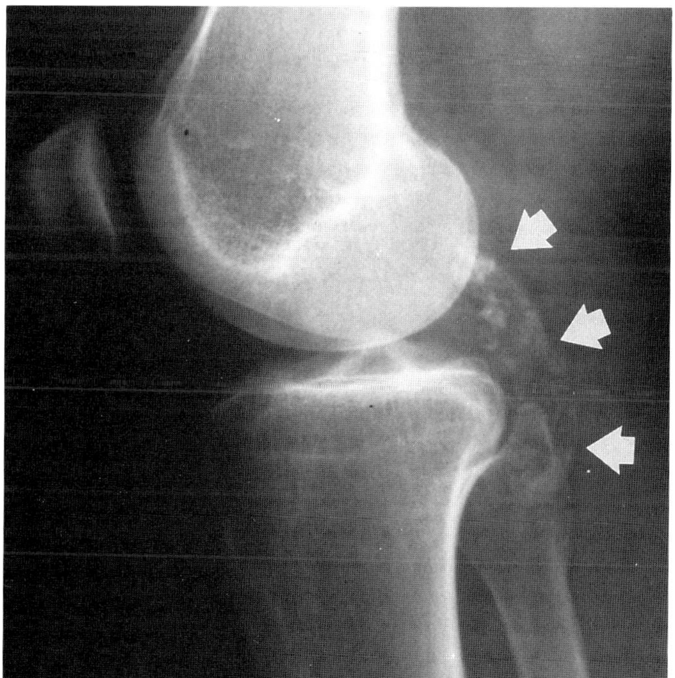

C

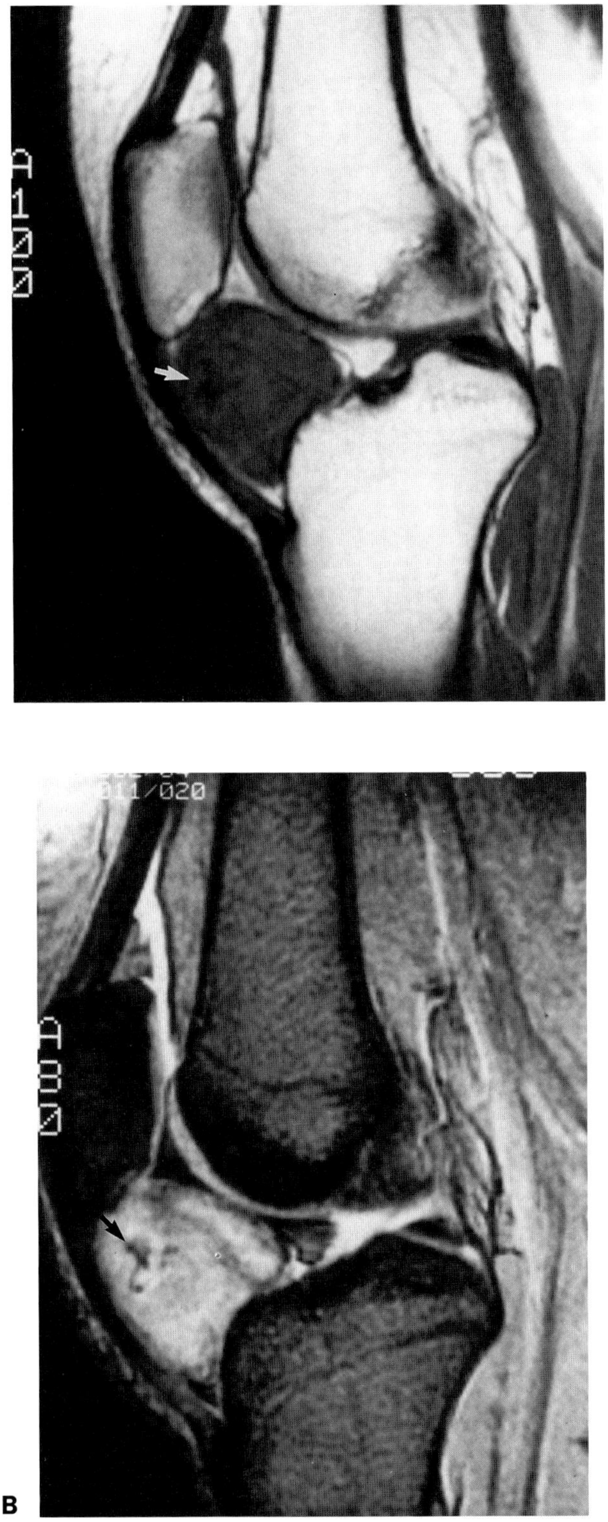

A B

FIGURE 17.6 A 39-year-old woman with focal synovial osteochondromatosis of the knee. Sagittal (A) T1-weighted (500/15) and (B) MPGR (500/15, 20 degrees) images reveal an isolated mass within Hoffa's fat pad. This lesion results in anterior bowing of the patellar tendon. The predominant signal intensity is approximately isointense to muscle with T1-weighting and hyperintense on the gradient-recalled echo sequence. Note the hypointense focus corresponding to calcification or ossification (arrows). A small joint effusion is present. Biopsy confirmed the diagnosis.

Lipoma Arborescens

Definition. Lipoma arborescens is a benign, hyperplastic condition in which mature adipose cells infiltrate the subsynovial tissue, resulting in proliferative villous projections. This intra-articular lesion is of unknown etiology with most cases arising apparently de novo, although there are associations with osteoarthritis, rheumatoid arthritis, and trauma.

Clinical Features. This rare condition typically presents with gradual joint swelling of many years duration and joint effusion. Pain and restricted range of motion may be present. Aspirated joint fluid is usually clear and yellow. This condition may be seen in nearly all ages with a reported age range of 9 to 90 years old. Males are more commonly affected.

Location. Lipoma arborescens usually affects the knee, particularly the suprapatellar recess. Cases involving the hip, wrist, and shoulder have also been reported.

Implications. MRI is useful in excluding other synovial processes that may present in a similar fashion clinically such as pigmented villonodular synovitis, synovial chondromatosis, rheumatoid arthritis, and synovial hemangioma. Treatment of this lesion consists of total synovectomy, which is considered curative. There has been only one reported case of recurrence after synovial resection and this patient was treated successfully by repeat synovectomy.

MRI Findings. The pathognomonic MR findings include a frond-like synovial mass with signal intensity which parallels fat on all pulse sequences and an associated joint effusion. In addition, chemical-shift artifact may be seen at the mass-fluid interface, confirming the fatty nature of this lesion.

Differential Diagnosis. The MRI findings are considered diagnostic. However, other synovial masses which contain fat include synovial lipoma and synovial hemangioma. While a simple synovial lipoma demonstrates identical signal characteristics to lipoma arborescens, it may be distinguished by the presence of a solitary, round or oval intra-articular mass. A synovial hemangioma may contain considerable fat, but the signal intensity would not be homogeneously fatty due to the presence of vascular channels and possibly calcifications.

References

Feller J, Rishi M, Hughes E. Lipoma arborescens of the knee: MR demonstration. *AJR* 163:162–164, 1994.

Laorr A, Peterfy C, Tirman P, et al. Lipoma arborescens of the shoulder: Magnetic resonance imaging findings. *Can Assoc Radiol J* 46:311–313, 1995.

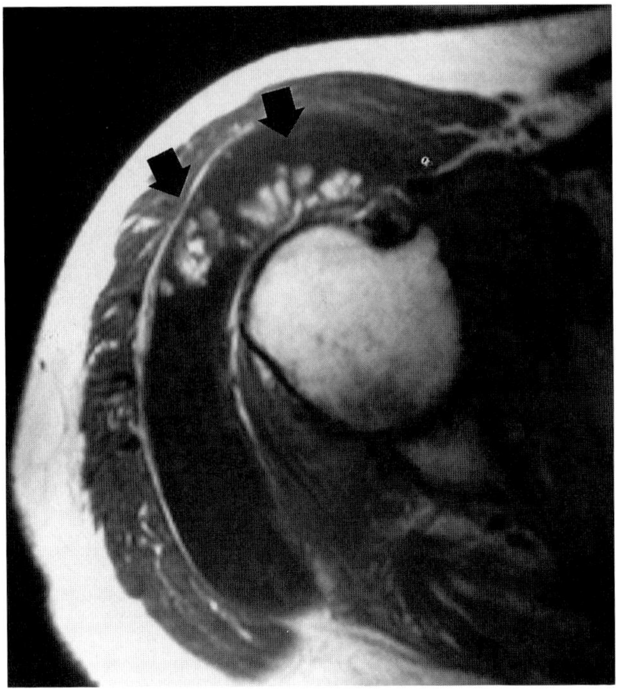

A

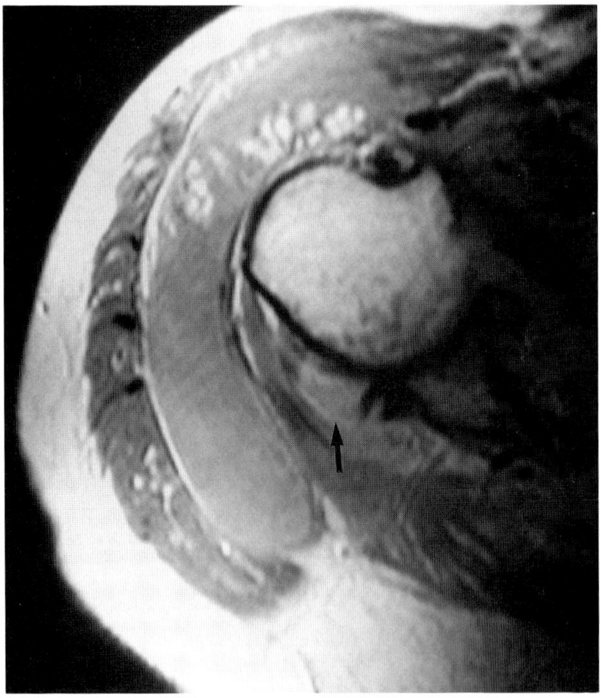

B

FIGURE 17.7 A 90-year-old woman with a history of chronic right shoulder pain and swelling. (A) Axial T1-weighted image demonstrates frond-like projections of high signal intensity (arrows) within a fluid-filled subacromial-subdeltoid bursa. (B), (C) Axial dual-echo T2-weighted images reveal that the lesion remains isointense to subcutaneous fat. A heterogeneous joint effusion is seen (thin arrows). (D) Coronal proton density image demonstrates chemical-shift artifact (long thin arrow) which confirms the fatty nature of this proliferative process. These findings are diagnostic of lipoma arborescens. A large full-thickness supraspinatus tendon tear is also present. (Courtesy of Antonio Rabassa, MD). (Reprinted from *CARJ* 46:311–313, 1995, with permission of the publisher.)

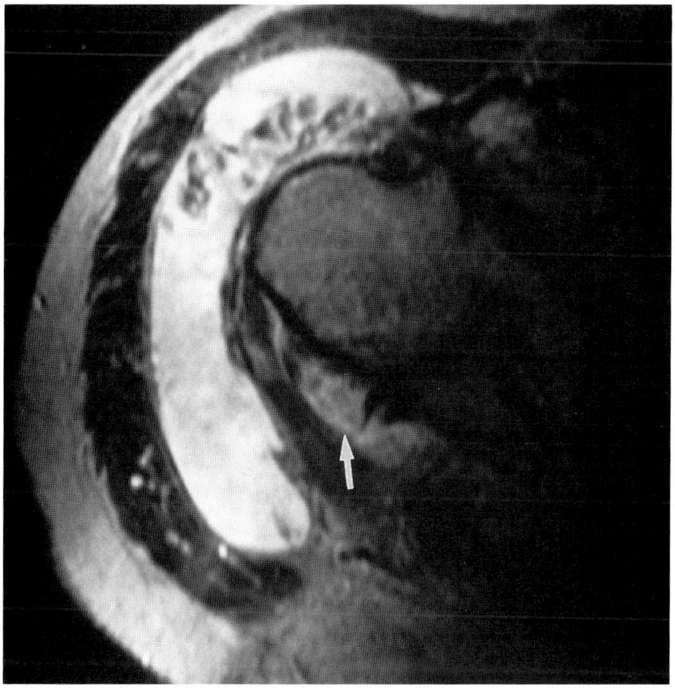

C

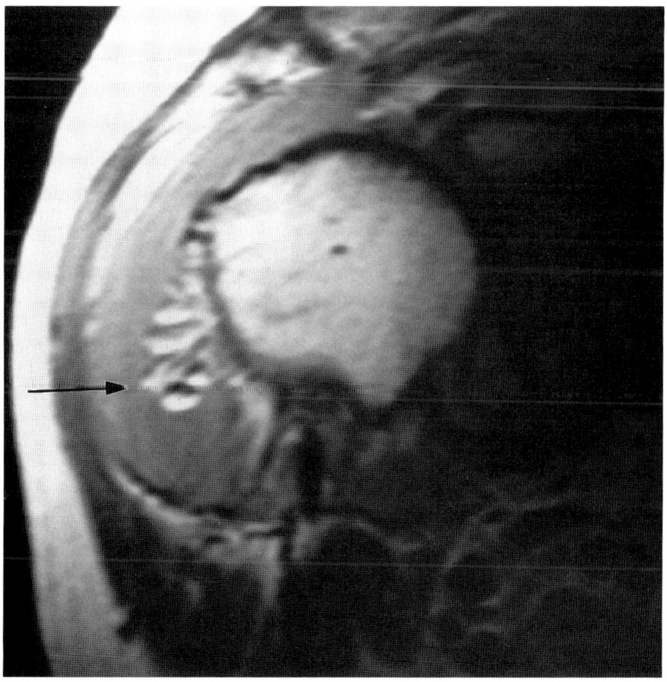

D

Synovial Hemangioma

Definition. Synovial hemangiomas are benign vascular neoplasms composed of vascular channels that may be cavernous, capillary, or venous in nature. They may be pedunculated or diffuse. Histologic examination reveals endothelial-lined vascular channels separated by fibrous and/or fatty linear strands. There are variable amounts of adipose and fibrous tissue. These lesions are histopathologically identical to soft tissue and osseous hemangiomas.

Clinical Features. Synovial hemangiomas are uncommon lesions usually affecting children, adolescents, or young adults, with a predilection for females. They are frequently misdiagnosed clinically, often delaying the correct diagnosis for many years. Nearly all patients are symptomatic and there is typically a history of recurrent joint pain and swelling. These lesions may also be associated with limited range of motion, limping, leg length discrepancy, a soft palpable mass, and adjacent cutaneous/soft tissue hemangiomas.

Location. The knee is the most frequently involved joint (97% of cases), although other sites may be affected including the elbow, ankle, wrist, temporomandibular joint, and various tendon sheaths.

Implications. Premature physeal closure, limb length discrepancy, and arthropathy may occur. The arthropathy probably results from recurrent episodes of hemarthrosis. The radiographic changes can mimic hemophilia. These lesions may spread to involve the entire synovium and even infiltrate surrounding muscle and fat. Diffuse lesions are best treated by surgical excision with partial or total synovectomy. Pedunculated masses can be excised arthroscopically.

MRI Findings. These lesions typically appear as poorly-marginated synovial masses without significant mass effect. They may be lobulated. On T2-weighted sequences, there is a heterogeneous appearance with bright vascular channels due to stagnant blood and intervening linear or rounded areas of lower signal intensity corresponding to fibrofatty septa and thrombosed vascular channels. On T1-weighted images, the vascular channels typically exhibit low or intermediate signal intensity and any predominantly fatty septa will appear hyperintense. Fluid-fluid levels can be seen. There may be invasion into Hoffa's fat pad or adjacent soft tissues. Erosions and osseous involvement may be identified. Phleboliths are characteristic of synovial hemangioma, appearing as areas of signal void, but are rarely present in the absence of surrounding soft tissue involvement.

Differential Diagnosis. If the characteristic MRI features are present, these lesions should be able to be differentiated from other synovial masses. The identification of phleboliths is essentially diagnostic.

References

Cotten A, Flipo R. Herbaux B, et al. Synovial haemangioma of the knee: A frequently misdiagnosed lesion. *Skeletal Radiol* 24:257–261, 1995.

Greenspan A, Azouz E, Matthews J, et al. Synovial hemangioma: Imaging features in eight histologically proven cases, review of the literature, and differential diagnosis. *Skeletal Radiol* 24:583–590, 1995.

Llauger J, Monill J, Palmer J, et al. Synovial hemangioma of the knee: MRI findings in two cases. *Skeletal Radiol* 24:579–581, 1995.

Suh J, Hwang G, Hahn S. Soft tissue hemangiomas: MR manifestations in 23 patients. *Skeletal Radiol* 23:621–625, 1994.

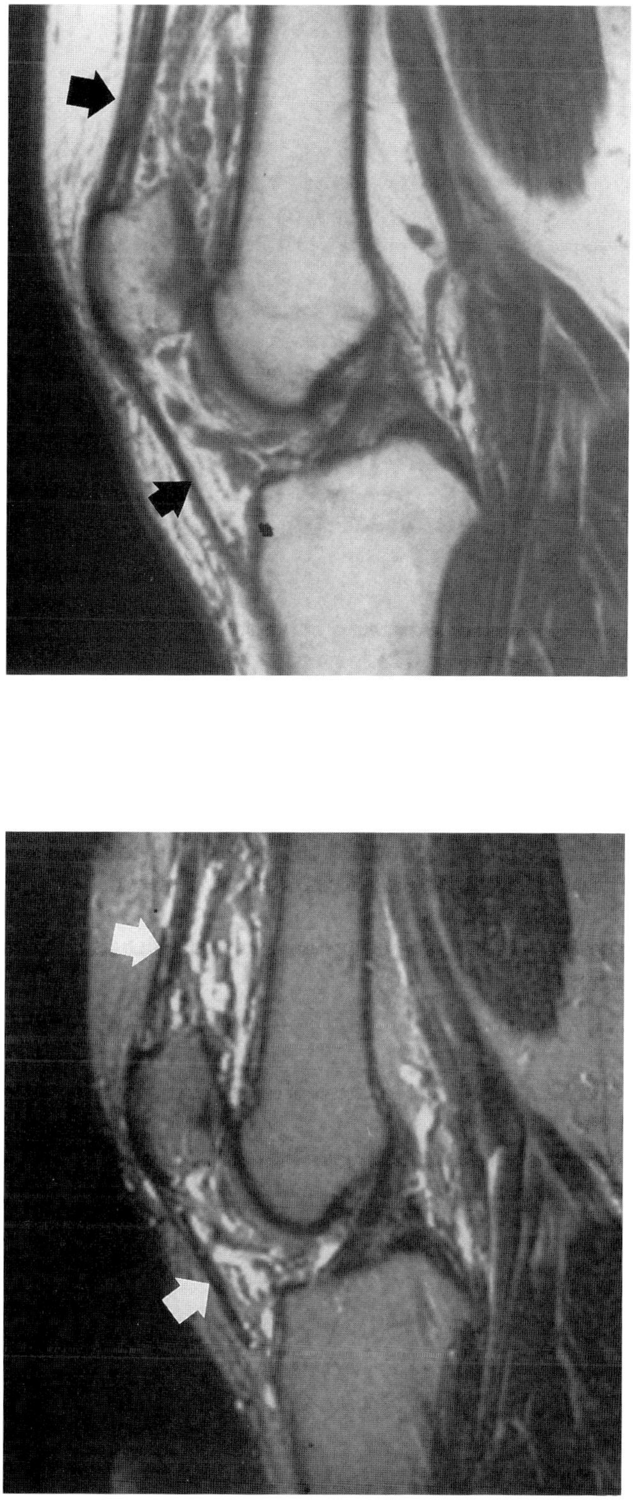

A

B

FIGURE 17.8 Synovial hemangioma of the knee in a 29-year-old woman. Sagittal (A) T1-weighted (600/16) and (B) T2-weighted (2200/80) images reveal a poorly-marginated synovial mass within the suprapatellar pouch and Hoffa's fat pad (arrows). The vascular channels exhibit intermediate signal intensity with T1-weighting and hyperintense signal with T2-weighting.

Intra-articular Ganglion Cyst (Cruciate Ligament Cyst)

Definition. Intra-articular ganglion cysts are also known as cruciate ganglia and cruciate ligament cysts. These lesions are ganglion cysts which arise from the cruciate ligaments. They are similar to ganglion cysts located elsewhere and are filled with clear, mucinous fluid. These cysts are lined with cells that are not true synovial cells. The exact pathogenesis of these lesions is unknown.

Clinical Features. Intra-articular ganglion cysts are uncommon lesions with an incidence of approximately 1% of knee MRI examinations. These lesions occur most commonly from early adulthood to middle age. They are most often asymptomatic but may present with pain and limited range of motion.

Location. Intra-articular ganglion cysts occur in the knee, arising from either the anterior or posterior cruciate ligament.

Implications. Most lesions are asymptomatic and do not require treatment. Symptomatic lesions should be treated surgically.

MRI Findings. The MR appearance of cruciate ganglia is distinctive, but dependent on whether the cyst arises from the anterior or posterior cruciate ligament. Cysts arising from the anterior cruciate ligament usually have a fusiform appearance extending along the course and interspersed within the fibers of the ligament. Ganglion cysts associated with the posterior cruciate ligament typically appear as well-marginated multilocular cysts which are located dorsal to the ligament. There may be a component ventral to the ligament as well. Occasionally, posterior cruciate ligament cysts may have an intraosseous component. These ganglia typically appear homogeneously hypointense with T1-weighting (approximately isointense to muscle) and homogeneously hyperintense on T2-weighted sequences. Occasionally, these cysts may contain hemorrhagic debris resulting in heterogeneous signal intensity.

Differential Diagnosis. In general, the MR appearance of these lesions is distinctive, with no significant differential diagnosis.

References

Recht M, Applegate G, Kaplan P, et al. The MR appearance of cruciate ganglion cysts: A report of 16 cases. *Skeletal Radiol* 23:597–600, 1994.

Steiner E, Helms C, Peterfy C, et al. Cruciate ligament cysts: MRI findings. (In Press.)

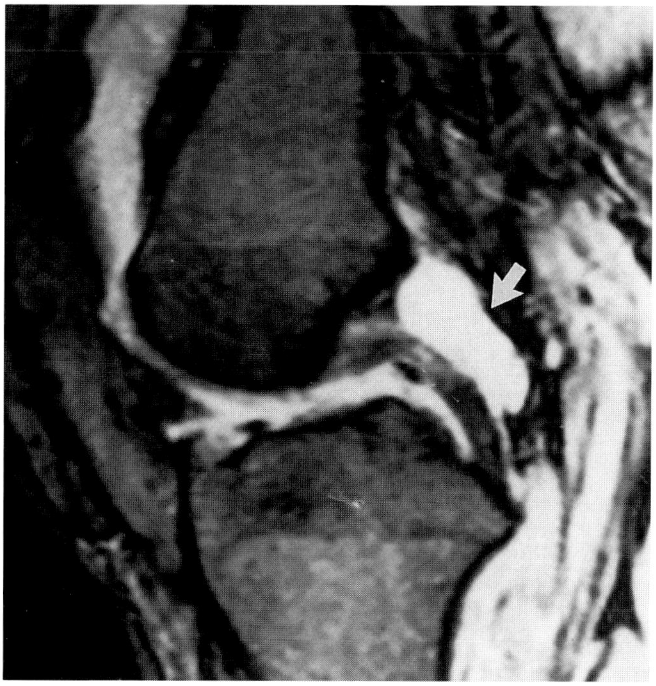

A

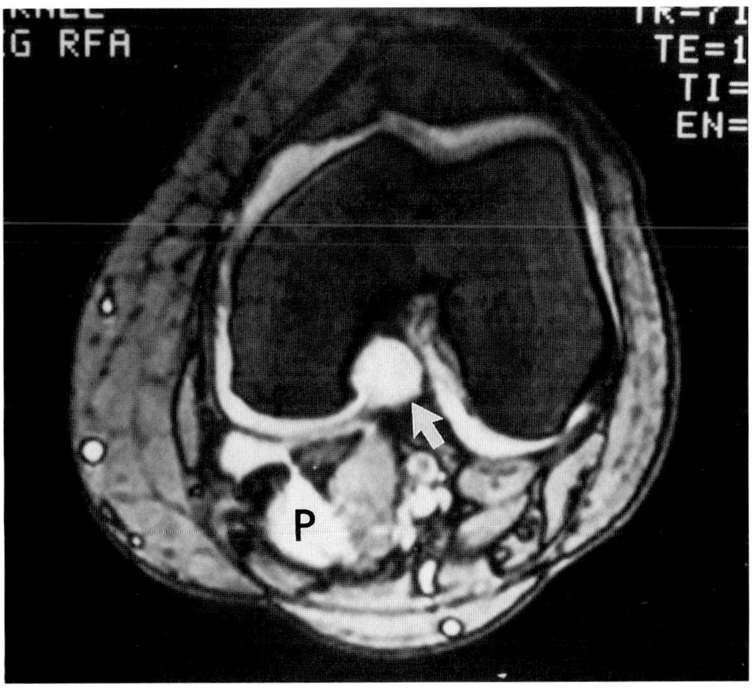

B

FIGURE 17.9 Posterior cruciate ligament cyst. MPGR (714/18, 20 degrees) (A) sagittal and (B) axial images reveal an elongated cyst (arrows) dorsal to the posterior cruciate ligament. The appearance and location are characteristic for an intra-articular ganglion cyst associated with the PCL. A joint effusion and popliteal cyst (P) are also present.

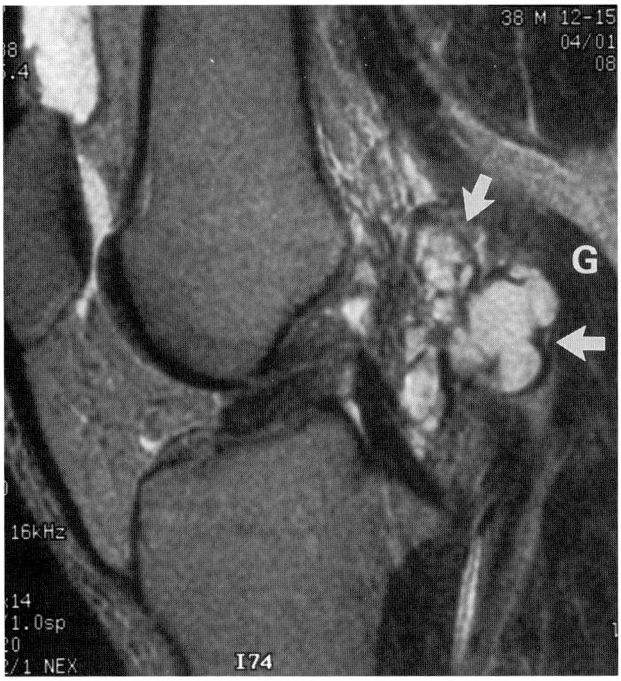

FIGURE 17.10 Intra-articular ganglion cyst in a 38-year-old male. Sagittal T2-weighted image (2000/80) demonstrates a large multiloculated lesion with bright signal intensity (arrows) located posterior to the PCL. The appearance is most consistent with a posterior cruciate ligament cyst. Note the mass effect on the gastrocnemius muscle (G). A joint effusion is also seen.

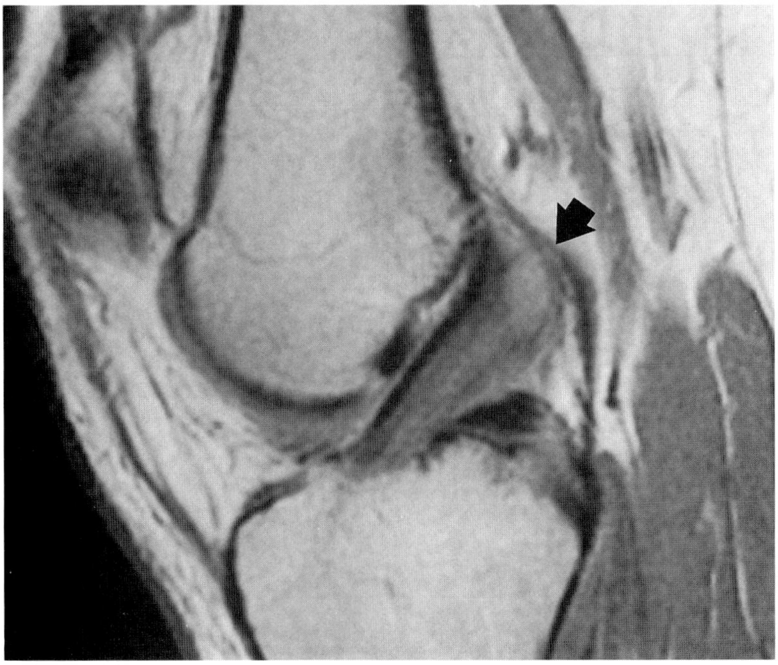

A

FIGURE 17.11 Anterior cruciate ligament cyst in a 17-year-old female who presented with knee stiffness and pain. (A), (B) Sagittal dual-echo T2-weighted images (2400/16,70) demonstrate a fusiform mass (arrows) extending along and interspersed within fibers of the ACL.

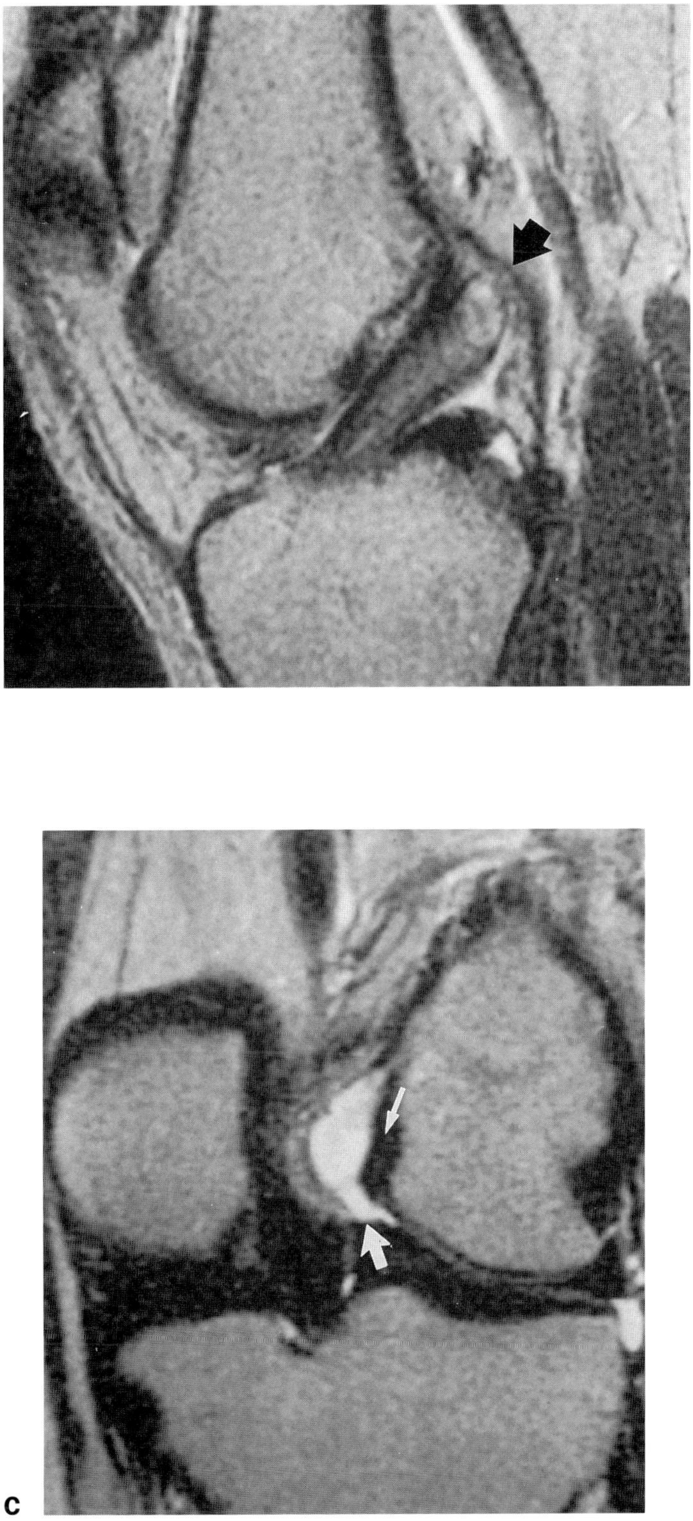

B

C

Figure 17.11 (continued) The signal intensity is approximately isointense to fat with conventional T2-weighting, but is very bright on (C) coronal FSE T2-weighted (4500/100) and

(continued)

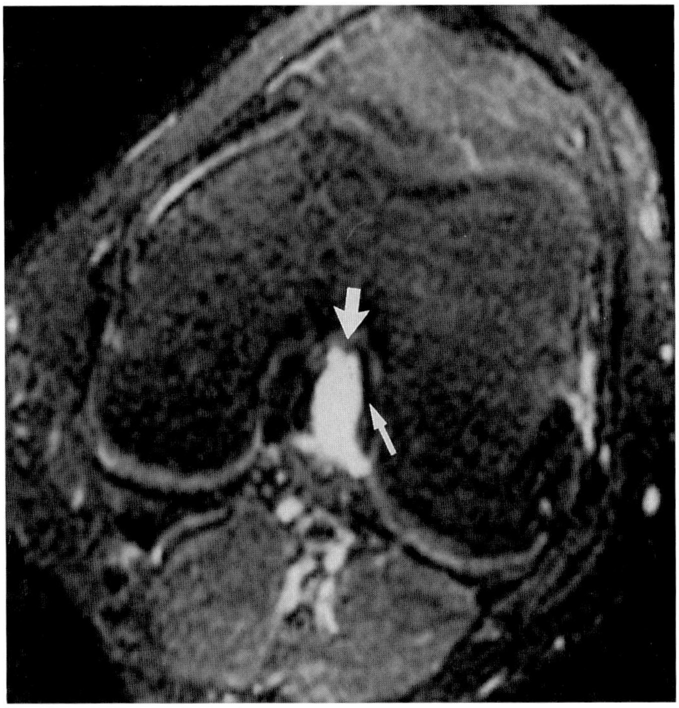

D

Figure 17.11 (continued) (D) axial FSE T2-weighted fat suppression (4000/68) images (white arrows). The cystic mass is intimately associated with the ACL (thin arrows).

Cyclops Lesion

Definition. A cyclops lesion is a fibrous or fibrocartilaginous mass which has been described in association with anterior cruciate ligament (ACL) reconstruction. It is a localized form of arthrofibrosis which may result in soft tissue impingement syndrome. It was named because of its bulbous appearance and characteristic focal areas of reddish-blue discoloration (due to venous channels), resembling an eye at arthroscopy. The precise etiology of a cyclops lesion is unclear. One proposed theory is that during the drilling of the tibial tunnel during ACL reconstruction, there is uplifting of fibrocartilaginous tissue from the tibia which serves as a nidus for the fibroproliferative process. An alternative mechanism is that the cyclops lesion arises from exposed ACL graft fibers which have been injured by impingement on the intercondylar notch. Pathologically, this lesion consists of dense fibrous or fibrocartilaginous tissue on the articular surface with some central granulation tissue. Although reported cases of cyclops lesions occur in the presence of ACL reconstruction, similar lesions can be seen in association with a chronic ACL tear or even with an intact ACL.

Clinical Features. The cyclops lesion occurs with an estimated frequency of 1–9.8% following ACL reconstruction. This proliferative soft tissue lesion may result in loss of full extension. Crepitation during terminal knee extension and pain are commonly present. The clinical differential diagnosis for loss of full extension also includes a loose body and displaced meniscal fragment.

Location. When associated with ACL reconstruction, a cyclops lesion occurs in the intercondylar notch, anterior or anterolateral to the tibial insertion of the reconstructed ligament.

Implications. A cyclops lesion is an important cause of soft tissue impingement following ACL reconstruction. MRI allows identification of this lesion and offers the potential to distinguish between different causes of extension block following ACL reconstruction, thereby assisting in treatment planning. Surgical debridement of this lesion results in restoration of full knee extension. A cyclops lesion can also cause articular cartilage damage through impingement and abnormal pressure during weight bearing. Debridement minimizes this damage and lessens the risk of subsequent osteoarthritis.

MRI Findings. On MRI, a soft tissue mass is seen anteriorly or anterolaterally in the intercondylar notch. Due to the fibrous content, a cyclops lesion typically appears intermediate in signal intensity on T1-weighted sequences and heterogeneously hypointense on T2-weighted images. Occasionally, there may be increased signal in the distal two-thirds of the graft due to graft impingement.

Differential Diagnosis. The differential diagnosis on MRI includes localized pigmented villonodular synovitis (PVNS), loose body, and displaced meniscal fragment. All of these lesions may demonstrate similar signal characteristics to a cyclops lesion. Since PVNS contains hemosiderin, its hypointense signal typically becomes more prominent on gradient-echo images due to magnetic susceptibility, which should differentiate this entity from a cyclops lesion. A displaced meniscal fragment can be ruled out by evaluating the menisci and excluding a bucket handle (or bucket handle-type) tear. A loose body may be difficult to distinguish, but the diagnosis of a cyclops lesion would be favored by the characteristic location in the anterior or anterolateral portion of the intercondylar notch.

References

Recht M, Piraino D, Cohen M, et al. Localized anterior arthrofibrosis (cyclops lesion) after reconstruction of the anterior cruciate ligament: MR imaging findings. *AJR* 165:383–385, 1995.

Campbell R, Tirman P, Stauffer A, et al. The cyclops lesion: MRI findings. (in press).

Cannon WD, Vittori J. The Role of arthroscopic debridement after anterior cruciate ligament reconstruction. *Arthroscopy* 7:344–349, 1991.

Jackson D, Schaefer R. Cyclops syndrome: Loss of extension following intraarticular anterior cruciate ligament reconstruction. *Arthroscopy* 6:171–178, 1990.

Fisher S, Shelbourne K. Arthroscopic treatment of symptomatic extension block complicating anterior cruciate ligament reconstruction. *Am J Sports Med* 21:558–564, 1993.

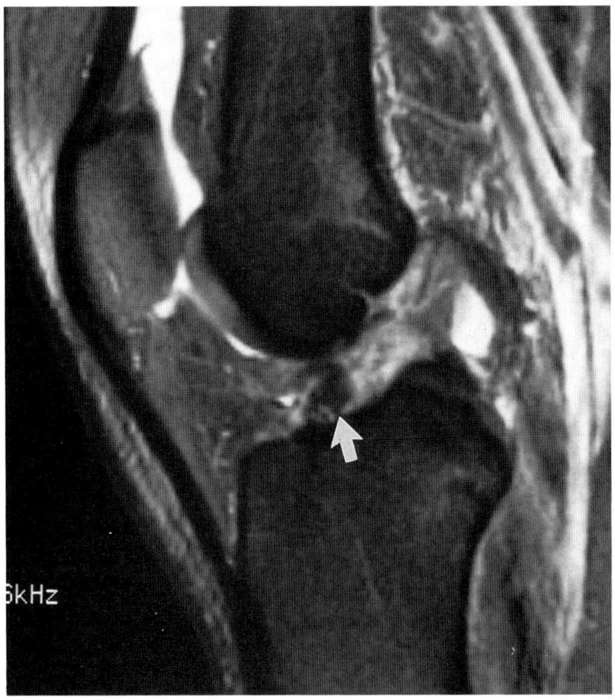

FIGURE 17.12 A 23-year-old woman with a chronic ACL tear and symptoms of mechanical impingement. No previous knee surgery. Sagittal FSE T2-weighted fat suppression image (4250/38) reveals an oval-shaped lesion of low signal intensity (arrow) within the intercondylar notch anteriorly near the tibial insertion of the ACL. A typical cyclops lesion was found at arthroscopy. A joint effusion is also present.

Loose Body

Definition. Intra-articular osteocartilaginous bodies ("joint mice") may arise from disintegration of the articular surface in osteoarthritis or from osteonecrosis. Fragments may be chondral or osteochondral. Osteocartilaginous bodies may remain on the joint surface, become dislodged or loose within the joint cavity, or become embedded at a distant synovial site. These lesions may increase or decrease in size, remain unchanged or disappear.

Clinical Features. These lesions may be asymptomatic or present with pain, locking, or limited range of motion.

Location. Loose bodies may occur in any joint. They tend to locate within joint recesses including the acetabular fossa of the hip, olecranon fossa of the elbow, proximal tibiofibular region of the knee, and subscapular recess of the shoulder. They may migrate into an adjacent synovial cyst, bursa, or tendon sheath.

Implications. Symptomatic lesions should be removed. In younger individuals, loose fragments should be removed to prevent the development of secondary osteoarthritis.

MRI Findings. Loose bodies are notoriously difficult to diagnose on MRI, especially in the absence of a joint effusion. Plain film correlation is recommended if there is concern for the presence of a loose body. Intra-articular injection of saline or dilute gadolinium may help identify these bodies. The signal intensity of a loose body depends on whether the fragment is chondral (noncalcified) or osteochondral (calcified or ossified). This distinction is usually possible with plain film correlation. Loose bodies tend to appear well-circumscribed with a predilection for joint recesses. Cartilaginous bodies (without calcification or ossification) appear as intermediate to high signal intensity lesions on T2-weighted sequences. Due to calcification, osteochondral bodies demonstrate hypointense signal on all pulse sequences. On gradient-echo images, due to magnetic susceptibility, calcified lesions become more conspicuous. For this reason, a gradient-echo sequence would be recommended if there is concern for the presence of a loose body.

Differential Diagnosis. An osteochondral body may resemble localized pigmented villonodular synovitis on MRI. Plain radiographs should enable this differentiation. Additionally, a loose body tends to be a more well-defined and discrete mass than does localized PVNS.

References

Resnick D. *Bone and Joint Imaging*. Philadelphia, PA: W.B. Saunders Company; 1989, p 390.

Munk P, Helms C. *MRI of the Knee*. Gaithersburg, MD: Aspen Publishers; 1992, p 174.

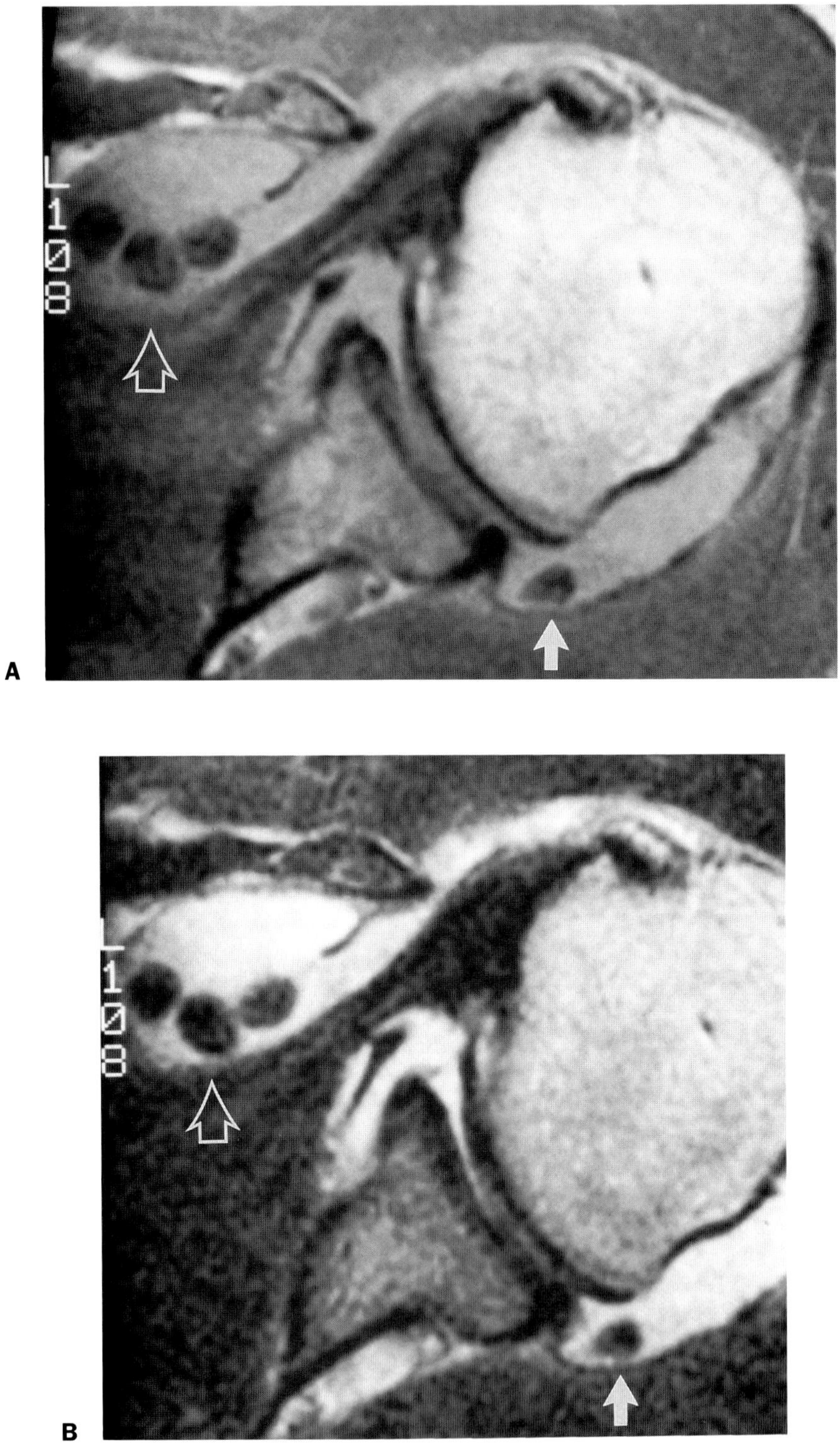

FIGURE 17.13 A 33-year-old male with chronic left shoulder pain. (A), (B) Axial dual-echo T2-weighted images (2000/30, 70) reveal four intra-articular loose bodies, which appear as round to oval-shaped, well-marginated, hypointense lesions. The associated joint effusion improves detection of these fragments. Three of the lesions are located within the subscapular recess (open arrows) and the other is seen posteriorly (arrows).

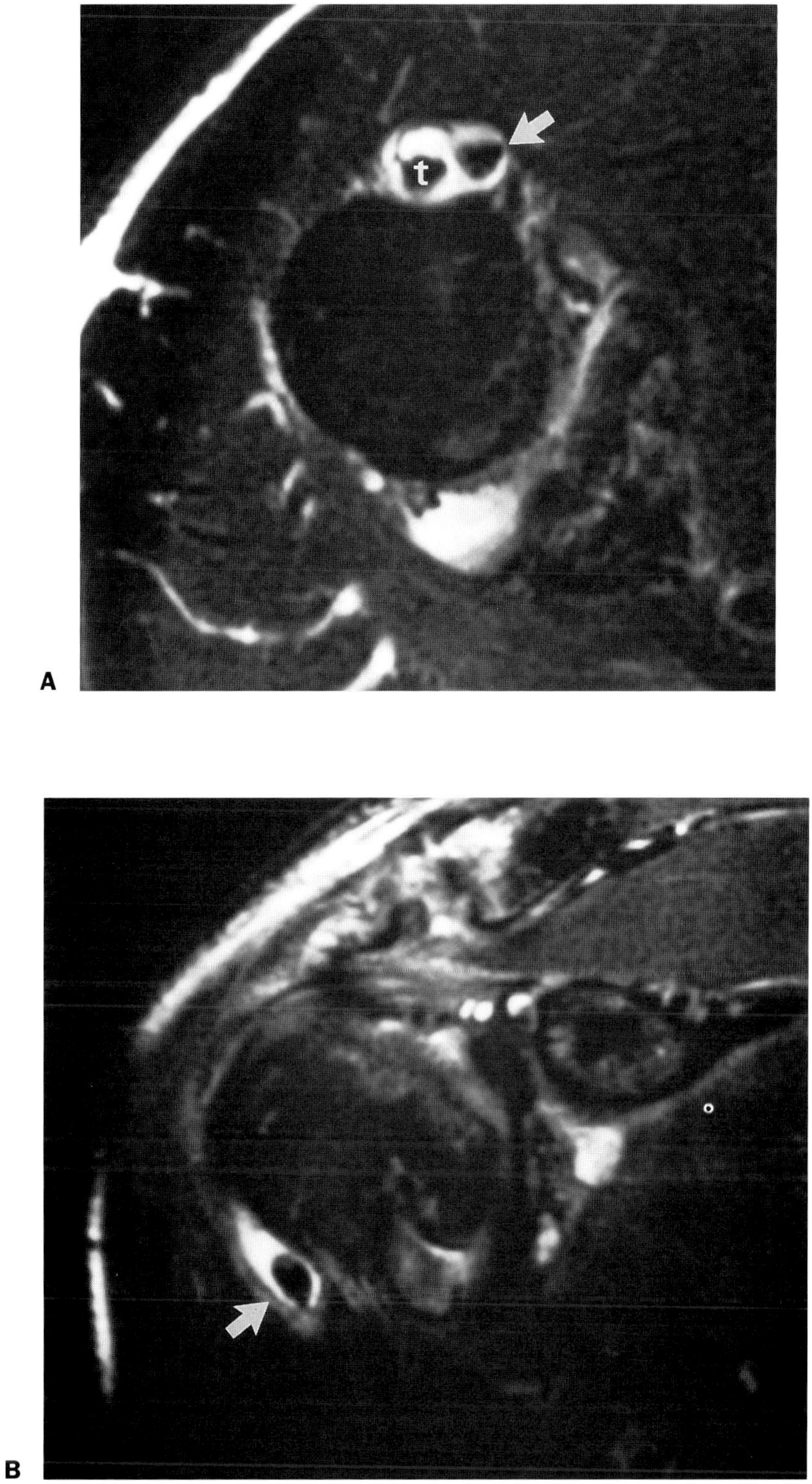

FIGURE 17.14 A 56-year-old male weightlifter with right shoulder pain. FSE T2-weighted fat suppression (A) axial and (B) coronal images reveal a loose body within the biceps tendon sheath (arrows), medial to the biceps tendon (t). Increased fluid within the tendon sheath is consistent with tenosynovitis. These findings were confirmed surgically.

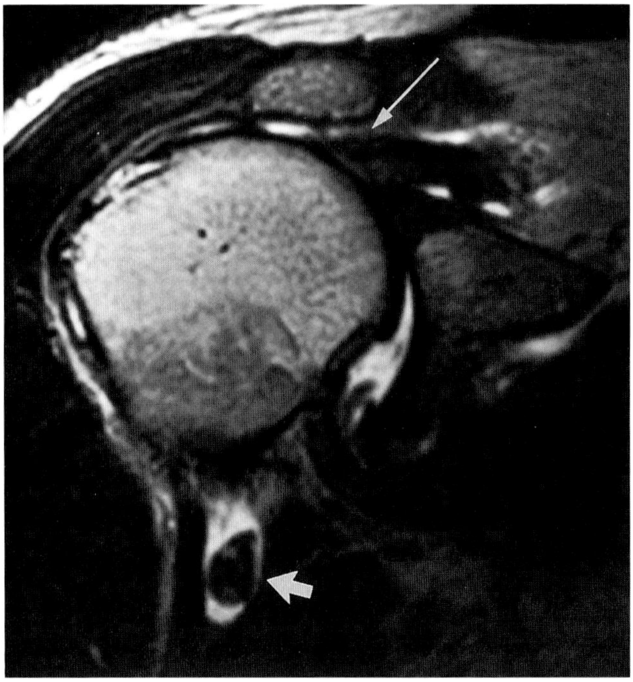

Figure 17.15 A 52-year-old male with right shoulder pain. Coronal FSE T2-weighted image (4000/140) demonstrates a loose body within the biceps tendon sheath (arrow). In addition, note the large full-thickness tear with retraction of the supraspinatus tendon (thin arrow). There were also tears involving the subscapularis and infraspinatus tendons.

Intra-articular Hemorrhage

Definition. Hemorrhage within a joint space acutely usually consists of a bloody joint effusion, possibly in different layers (fluid-fluid levels). Infrequently, one or more discrete intra-articular hematomas are present. Chronic repetitive hemorrhage into a joint may result in hypertrophied synovium which contains hemosiderin.

Clinical Features. Patients of all ages may be affected. Hemarthrosis is most commonly associated with trauma or bleeding diathesis. Following acute trauma, patients typically present with pain and swelling and may have limited range of motion. Patients with chronic repetitive bleeding into a joint, such as hemophiliacs, tend to have intermittent swelling and chronic progressive pain.

Location. The large joints are most commonly affected, especially the knee.

Implications. An acute traumatic hemarthrosis is often associated with internal derangement of the joint, such as ligamentous or capsular injury, cartilaginous (hyaline or fibrocartilage) injury, or intra-articular fracture. Therefore, identification of intra-articular hemorrhage should prompt careful evaluation for additional abnormalities. Chronic repetitive intra-articular bleeding (such as in hemophilia) leads to progressive joint degeneration.

MRI Findings. Intra-articular hemorrhage most commonly appears as a heterogeneous joint effusion or an effusion containing fluid-fluid levels. Infrequently, one or more focal hematomas is present with variable signal intensity depending on the age and blood product composition. In hemophilia, hyperplastic hemosiderin-laden synovium appears hypointense (hypointense or isointense to muscle) on both T1- and T2-weighted images. On gradient-echo images, due to magnetic susceptibility, the hypointense signal of the hemosiderin becomes more prominent. With hemophilia, associated cartilage loss and subchondral cystic lesions are often present.

Differential Diagnosis. The diagnosis of hemarthrosis is usually straightforward when the MR exam is correlated with the clinical history. However, intra-articular hematomas could have similar signal characteristics to loose bodies or meniscal fragments and a detailed evaluation of the hyaline articular cartilage and menisci should be performed for potential donor sites. Chronic intra-articular hemorrhage from hemophilia or repetitive trauma may resemble pigmented villonodular synovitis due to the presence of hyperplastic, hemosiderin-laden synovium, but the distinction should be apparent on clinical grounds.

Reference

Hermann G, Gilbert M, Abdelwahab I. Hemophilia: Evaluation of musculoskeletal involvement with CT, sonography, and MR imaging. *AJR* 158:119–123, 1992.

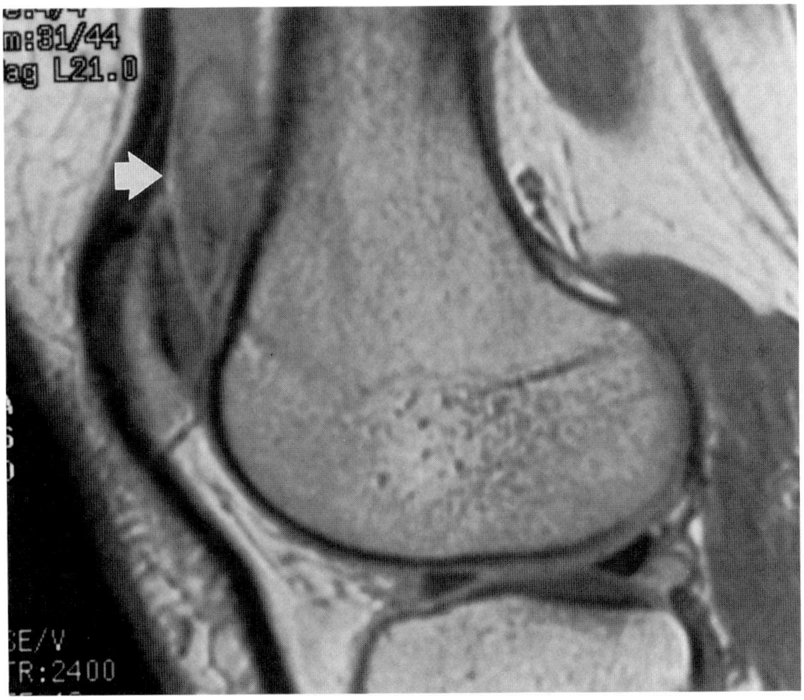

A

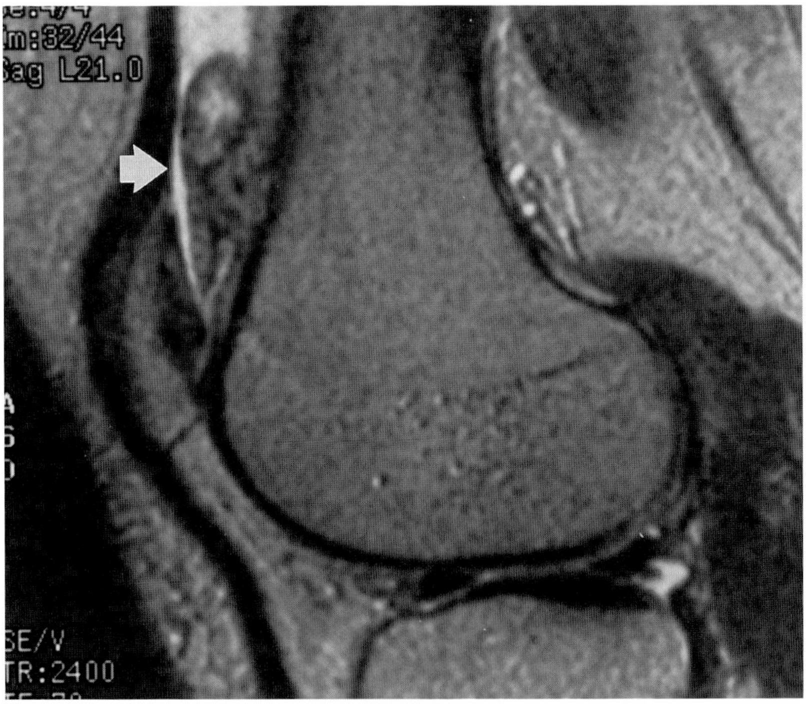

B

FIGURE 17.16 Intra-articular hematoma in a 49-year-old woman who sustained a knee injury one week prior to the examination. (A), (B) Sagittal dual-echo T2-weighted images (2400/16,70) reveal a joint effusion outlining a mass within the suprapatellar pouch (arrows). There are areas of low, intermediate, and bright signal intensity within the lesion. (C) Axial FSE T2-weighted fat suppression image (4000/51) shows the heterogeneous, well-marginated, elongated mass surrounded by joint fluid.

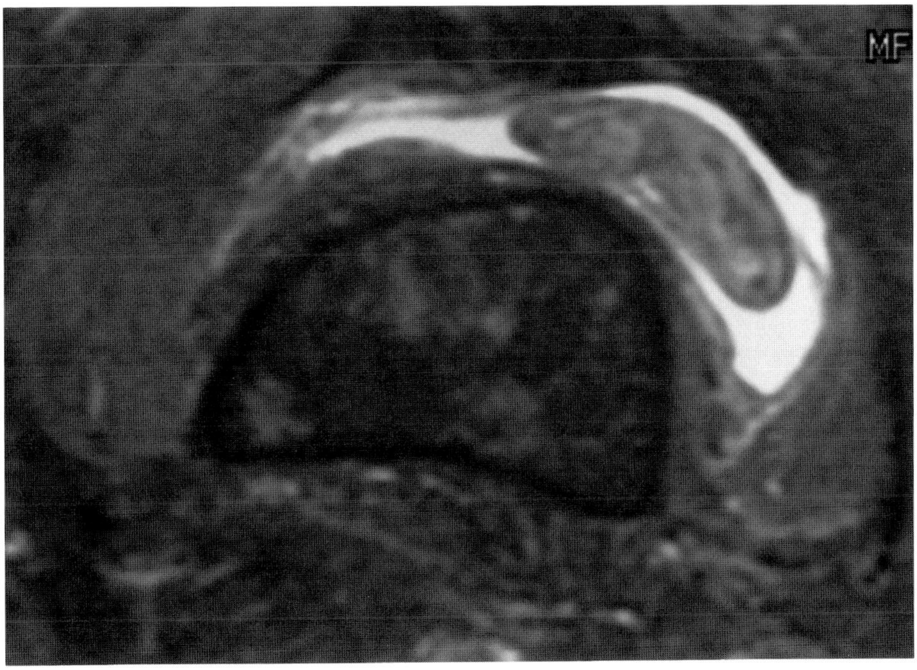

C

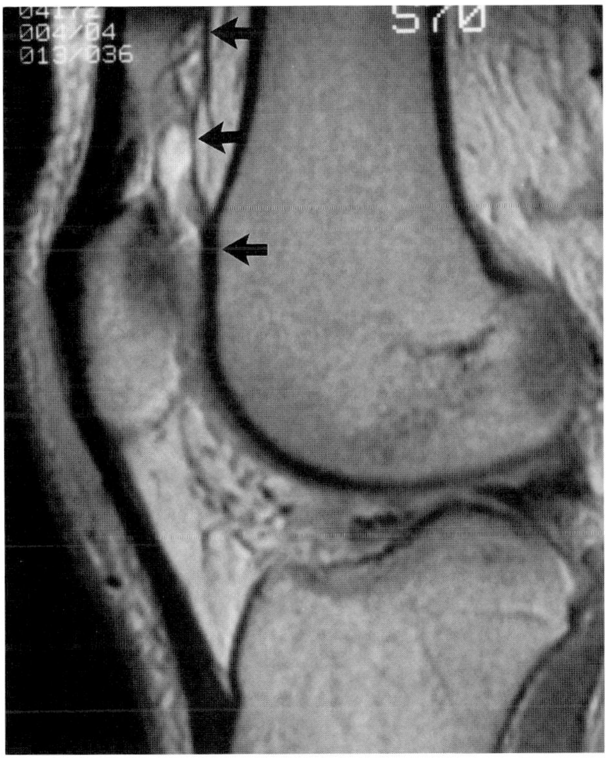

A

Figure 17.17 Intra-articular hematoma in a 19-year-old woman following a recent motorcycle accident. (A), (B) Sagittal dual-echo T2-weighted images (2000/19, 70) demonstrate an elongated

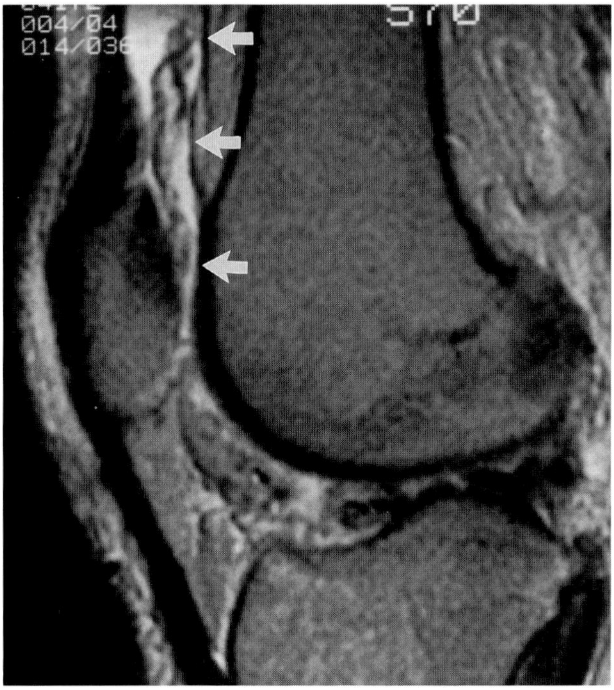

B

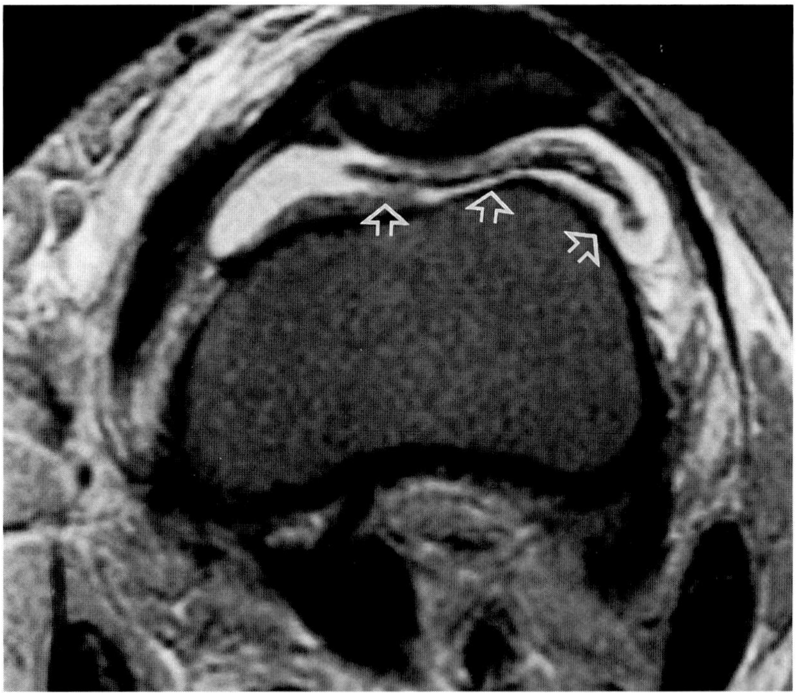

C

FIGURE 17.17 (continued) lesion within the suprapatellar pouch which exhibits heterogeneous signal intensity (arrows). This mass is surrounded by joint fluid which is of uniform signal intensity. (C) Axial T2-weighted image (2000/70) again reveals areas of low, intermediate, and high signal intensity within the lesion (open arrows). These findings are consistent with an intra-articular hematoma. Surrounding soft tissue edema is also noted.

Isolated Suprapatellar Bursa

Definition. During early embryologic development, the knee is partitioned into three compartments by septa of embryonic synovium. The suprapatellar plica represents a remnant of the embryonic septum which previously separated the suprapatellar cavity from the medial and lateral compartments. With failure of involution, the suprapatellar plica may persist as an intact septum which completely divides the suprapatellar bursa from the remainder of the knee joint cavity. An isolated suprapatellar bursa may also be acquired and occur following inflammation or trauma in this region.

Clinical Features. An isolated suprapatellar bursa is present in 4–16% of individuals. Synovitis, hemorrhage, trauma, or infection may cause accumulation of fluid in this bursa, which may present clinically as a suprapatellar mass that is firm, cystic, or rubbery on palpation.

Location. The location of an isolated suprapatellar bursa coincides with the expected position of the normal suprapatellar pouch.

Implications. Identification of this entity may have considerable importance to the orthopedist when planning an optimal surgical approach.

MRI Findings. MRI demonstrates fluid distending the suprapatellar bursa, which is separated from the remainder of the knee joint by a thin, imperforate suprapatellar plica. This plica may be flat or bowed inferiorly. The fluid collection usually appears homogeneous and isointense with knee joint fluid, which is hypointense on T1-weighted images and markedly hyperintense with T2-weighting. However, internal debris, hemorrhage, or osteochondral loose bodies may also be identified within the isolated bursa.

Differential Diagnosis. An isolated suprapatellar bursa may be distinguished from a large joint effusion by the identification of an imperforate suprapatellar plica. A ganglion cyst may have a similar appearance, however, it would be seen in the presence of a normal suprapatellar pouch.

References

Deutsch A, Resnick D, Dalinka M, et al. Synovial plicae of the knee. *Radiology* 141:627–634, 1981.

Janzen D, Peterfy C, Forbes J, et al. Cystic lesions around the knee joint: MR imaging findings. *AJR* 163:155–161, 1994.

Zidorn T, Schafer H. Morphologic variants of the proximal knee-joint cavity. An anatomical and radiological study. *Surg Radiol Anat* 14:141–146, 1992.

Zidorn T. Classification of the suprapatellar septum considering ontogenetic development. *Arthroscopy* 8:459–464, 1991.

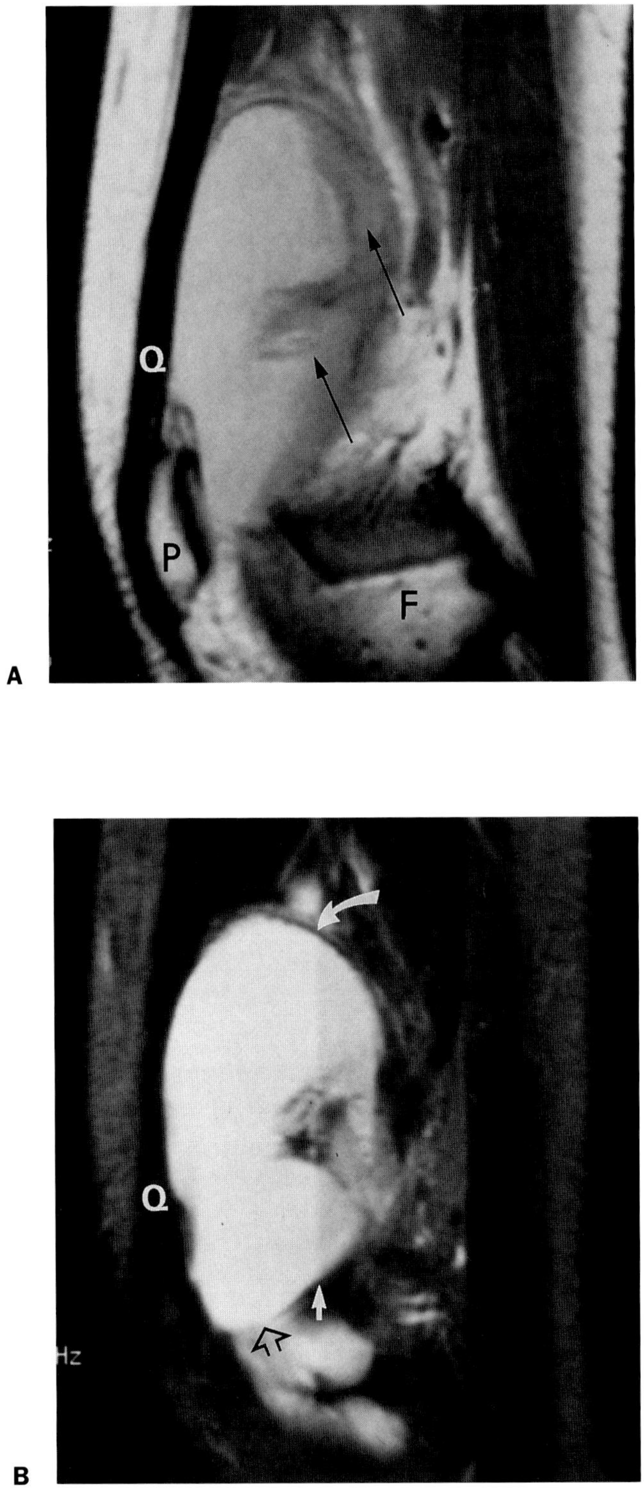

Figure 17.18 A 12-year-old female athlete presented with complaints of right knee swelling. Physical examination revealed soft tissue swelling superolateral to the patella. (A) Sagittal proton density image (2200/20) reveals marked distension of the suprapatellar pouch which contains fluid with heterogeneous signal intensity (arrows). (B) Sagittal T2-weighted image (2200/80) depicts a fluid-fluid level (white arrows) within the suprapatellar pouch as well as an internal area of predominantly low signal intensity. These findings suggest hemorrhage in this region. Note that there appears to be a very thin suprapatellar plica which is slightly bowed inferiorly (open arrow).

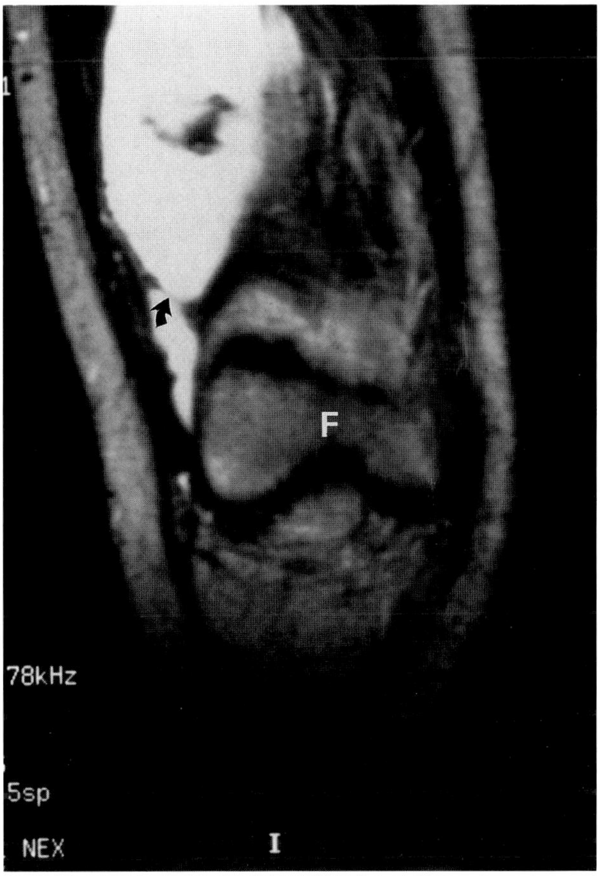

C

FIGURE 17.18 (continued) (C) Coronal T2-weighted image (2500/80) further delineates an apparent thin, imperforate suprapatellar plica (small curved arrow). These findings are highly suggestive of an isolated suprapatellar bursa. In this patient, the distended bursa is lateral in position. Patella (P), quadriceps tendon (Q), distal femur (F).

INDEX

Italicized numbers refer to figures.

G

H

S